Robotics in Neurosurgery

Jorge Alvaro González Martínez
Francesco Cardinale
Editors

Robotics in Neurosurgery

Principles and Practice

Springer

Editors
Jorge Alvaro González Martínez
Department of Neurological Surgery
and Epilepsy Center
University of Pittsburgh Medical Center
Pittsburgh, PA, USA

Francesco Cardinale
"Claudio Munari" Center
for Epilepsy Surgery
Azienda Socio-Sanitaria Territoriale Grande
Ospedale Metropolitano Niguarda
Milano, Italy

Department of Medicine and Surgery
Unit of Neuroscience
Università degli Studi di Parma
Parma, Italy

ISBN 978-3-031-08379-2 ISBN 978-3-031-08380-8 (eBook)
https://doi.org/10.1007/978-3-031-08380-8

This Springer imprint is published by the registered company Springer Nature Switzerland AG
The registered company address is: Gewerbestrasse 11, 6330 Cham, Switzerland

Our work is dedicated:
to our patients
to our wives, Andrea and Marina
to our sons, Sophia, Alessandro and Chiara
to our long-standing friendship

Jorge and Cico

Foreword

"Hopefully we won't have to use the Robot, today. It's true, Pr Benabid wants us to use it. We need to understand how it works and give him and the engineers directions for its fine-tuning, but what a pain! It means making the procedure much longer. For giving the coordinates, we only have X-rays in the two projections face and profile, and we practically have to input everything by hand. Then it doesn't always go smoothly, because the 'petits déplacements itératifs' are at order of the day. Each trajectory must practically always be adjusted to the final position by means of small shifts. With just few approaches, ok it is still feasible. But when up to twenty trajectories are required as for Stereoelectroencephalography, there is the risk of never leaving the room. Of course, we can say that we used the robot, but what a struggle! Fortunately, the most difficult approaches, i.e. those in double obliquity, are also the most successful, practically always on the first shot.

For the classic orthogonal trajectories of the Talairach frame, on the other hand, the simplicity and precision of the original approach remain unsurpassed, with the only limitation that the holes of the double grid allow only a limited and fixed number of trajectories. We will arrive at the usual compromise in order not to waste too much time, most of the approaches, the orthogonal ones with the double grid and the oblique ones with the robot …."

It was 1990, and I had just arrived in Grenoble with my Master Claudio Munari and had the good fortune to work in the neurosurgery department of Prof. Alim Louis Benabid. With Dominique Hoffman we shared the commitments of the stereotactic room, and we were at the same time fascinated and terrified by the use of the first robot I had ever seen in a neurosurgical room.

The robot is accurate, not that. The robot acts in the surgeon's place, taking work away from him, and I can assure you that that took up all our energy. The robot does not get tired, that is true; of course it does not, but we were exhausted.

But after only a short time, the results of constant work and fine-tuning were beginning to show the reliability and advantages of the surgical robot.

How much time has passed since then and how the world of surgical robotics has been transformed by the people who invented the robots and made them!

Now they do this and that, they align with sub-millimetric precision, they allow almost immediate and automatic registration of the patient's head position, and they are driven by a very sophisticated planning software that allows planning using models that are increasingly close to the actual anatomy of the individual patient.

The workflow has to be progressively implemented, but the advantages of using the robot are soon evident and there are also significant time savings. We, at the Claudio Munari Centre, also delayed until 2009 to switch completely to the use of the robot for SEEG, since then we can no longer do without it and the average time per implant has been reduced by several hours.

Of course, in other surgeries, the robot is also the arm of the surgeon who can, for example, operate in master-slave mode and, in some cases, has greater autonomy even though it is supervised by the surgeon. This is not yet the case in neurosurgery where the time does not seem to be ripe.

But even in our specialty, the robot in its various presentations has become part of the routine and its evolution seems unstoppable. The possibility of controlling the surgical act and the reliability seem to be the main goals to be achieved, and imagining a working robot is no longer confined to science fiction films. There is still a long way to go, but the continuous technological evolution allows us to glimpse at possible solutions and goals that are no longer unreachable.

This book by my dear friends JGM and F(C)C represents the current state of the art and an undoubted reference for the developments we are aiming at.

I wish them all the success I am sure they deserve.

"Claudio Munari" Center for Epilepsy Surgery
Azienda Socio-Sanitaria Territoriale Grande Ospedale
Metropolitano Niguarda
Milano, Italy

Giorgio Lo Russo

Introduction

The application of surgical robots in neurosurgery has been significant in the last decade, and it will likely continue to expand at an unparalleled rate. The development of computational engineering and adaptations to surgical methods related to the so-called minimally invasive surgical techniques have been the driving forces in recent years. The utilization of robotics in many surgical fields is becoming the new standard of care. Neurosurgery is not an exception.

Robots have been applied to the manufacturing industry as earlier as the 1960s where they performed tasks like welding, assembly, shipping, handling of raw materials, and product packing. Only recently have they been applied to medicine. Interestingly, the inception of robotic technology in the field of medicine was in neurosurgery. Authors often differ in their definition of the first robotic procedure of the modern era, but arguably, Kwoh and colleagues were the first to use the PUMA 560 robotic system in stereotactic brain biopsies with great accuracy. Since then, the application of robots in neurosurgery has taken a slow but continuous progression, until the very last two decades, when it acquired a fast and diverse pace, involving several subfields in neurosurgery.

Although the practical applications of robots are relatively recent, the concept is more than 100 years old. The word robot derives from the Czech word *robota*, which describes a forced labor or activity, in other words, a "slave machine." The term rapidly became corrupted to reflect a machine-oriented repetitive task with no associated artificial intelligence. The Czech writer Karel Capek introduced the concept in his play "Rossum's Universal Robots" in 1920, defining the term robot for the first time. In the play, the robots attempted to take control of their own destinies and taking independent decision. Although the science fiction nature of his play is evident, we can start realizing that it is closer in realization than we could possibly predict. The upcoming new technologies and the most recent human interactions with robots are triggering new adaptative behaviors in our societies, whether related to scientific, social, or legal spheres. To guide us into this journey and preserve the essence of our mission of improving the medical care and the quality of life of our societies, we could perhaps recall some initial concepts in robotics, resting at the nebulous interface between fiction and reality.

Many writers of robot stories, without actually quoting the three laws, take them for granted, and expect the readers to do the same.
Isaac Asimov

Isaac Asimov (1920–1992) was a prolific and provocative American writer. Many of his writings were related to science fiction, especially robots and their interaction with humans. In 1941, he wrote *Runaround*, the latest in a series of stories on robotic machines with positronic, humanlike brains in the era of space discoveries. In *Runaround*, three astronauts (two humans, *Powell and Donovan*, and a robot SPD-13—*Speedy*) are sent to an abandoned mining station on the apocalyptic planet of Mercury. While there, a compound necessary to power the station's life-giving photocells, selenium, alters SPD-13 and causes him to become dysfunctional and confused, unable to operate under the three laws of robots. According to Asimov's imagination, these laws are the following: (1) a robot must not injure a human being or allow a human to come to harm; (2) a robot must obey orders given by humans, except if the order conflicts with the first law; and (3) a robot must protect its own existence as long as it does not conflict with the first and second laws. In the end, Powell was able to fix the photocells and Speedy went back to a normal function, and the mission was saved. Over the course of his prolific career, Asimov's view on the sacredness of the three laws varied, from seeing them as simple rules and guidelines through to wholly uncompromising subroutines imprinted into the robot's operational system. What is interesting is the fact that the "three laws" lifted robots from the mindless cadre of Frankenstein-like machines and creatures with no guiding principles that had characterized horror and science fiction for decades and gave them the capacity of dealing with moral dilemmas, as humans. In 1985, Asimov added a fourth law, known as the "zeroth law," to precede the first law: a robot may not harm humanity or, by inaction, allow humanity to come to harm. Asimov's laws were so highly regarded that it was as though his three laws would, in the real ages of robotics to come, be a foundational stone in a positronic Brave New World (in reference to the famous Aldous Huxley book). In the current age of automation, artificial intelligence, and social distancing, our interactions with machines and "intelligent" operating systems have acquired a new importance and the 100-year-old robot concept has suddenly acquired a new interest. The reality is that no computer or robot has so far had the three laws built into its network. They were, and remain, little more than imaginary literacy concepts, designed to further the plot of the finest science fiction models ever written, but maybe applicable in the near future.

As opposed to science fiction, the collection of manuscripts present in this book attempts to describe the current state-of-the-art applications of robotic devices in neurosurgery. Our goal is to inform the readers regarding the new robotic technologies currently applied in neurosurgical interventions and research and perhaps guide them to new developments and applications for the next decade.

Department of Neurological Surgery and Epilepsy Center
University of Pittsburgh Medical Center
Pittsburgh, PA, USA
e-mail: gonzalezjo@upmc.edu

Jorge González Martínez

"Claudio Munari" Center for Epilepsy Surgery
Azienda Socio-Sanitaria Territoriale Grande
Ospedale Metropolitano Niguarda,
Milano, Italy

Department of Medicine and Surgery,
Unit of Neuroscience, Università degli Studi di Parma
Parma, Italy
e-mail: francesco.cardinale@ospedaleniguarda.it

Francesco Cardinale

Contents

Contributors

Hussam Abou-Al-Shaar Department of Neurological Surgery and Epilepsy Center, University of Pittsburgh Medical Center, Pittsburgh, PA, USA

Nitin Agarwal Department of Neurological Surgery and Epilepsy Center, University of Pittsburgh Medical Center, Pittsburgh, PA, USA

Khalid Al Orabi "Claudio Munari" Center for Epilepsy Surgery, Azienda Socio-Sanitaria Territoriale Grande Ospedale Metropolitano Niguarda, Milano, Italy

Department of Neurosurgery, King Abdullah Medical City, Al Mashair, Saudi Arabia

Ryan J. Austerman Department of Neurological Surgery, Houston Methodist Hospital, Houston, TX, USA

Michael Y. Bai Department of Neurological Surgery and Epilepsy Center, University of Pittsburgh Medical Center, Pittsburgh, PA, USA

Gene H. Barnett Rose Ella Burkhardt Brain Tumor and Neuro-Oncology Center, Department of Neurological Surgery, Neurological Institute, Cleveland Clinic, Cleveland, OH, USA

Cleveland Clinic Lerner College of Medicine of Case Western Reserve University, Cleveland, OH, USA

Neil Barua Department of Neurosurgery, Southmead Hospital, Bristol, UK

Luca Berta Department of Medical Physics, Azienda Socio-Sanitaria Territoriale Grande Ospedale Metropolitano Niguarda, Milano, Italy

Lorenzo Maria Giuseppe Bianchi Postgraduate School in Radiodiagnostics, Università degli Studi di Milano, Milano, Italy

Alison Bienemann Functional Neurosurgery Research Group, Learning and Research, University of Bristol, Bristol, UK

Guido Caccianiga Department of Electronics, Information and Bioengineering—DEIB, Politecnico di Milano, Milano, Italy

Haptics Intelligence Department, Max Planck Institute for Intelligent Systems, Stuttgart, Germany

Andrea Carai Neurosurgery Unit, Department of Neurosciences, Bambino Gesù Children's Hospital, IRCCS, Rome, Italy

Francesco Cardinale "Claudio Munari" Center for Epilepsy Surgery, Azienda Socio-Sanitaria Territoriale Grande Ospedale Metropolitano Niguarda, Milano, Italy

Department of Medicine and Surgery, Unit of Neuroscience, Università degli Studi di Parma, Parma, Italy

Laura Castana "Claudio Munari" Center for Epilepsy Surgery, Azienda Socio-Sanitaria Territoriale Grande Ospedale Metropolitano Niguarda, Milano, Italy

Aswin Chari Department of Neurosurgery, Great Ormond Street Hospital, London, UK

Developmental Neurosciences, Great Ormond Street Institute of Child Health, University College London, London, UK

Danielle Corson Department of Neurological Surgery and Epilepsy Center, University of Pittsburgh Medical Center, Pittsburgh, PA, USA

Massimo Cossu "Claudio Munari" Center for Epilepsy Surgery, Azienda Socio-Sanitaria Territoriale Grande Ospedale Metropolitano Niguarda, Milano, Italy

Alessandro De Benedictis Neurosurgery Unit, Department of Neurosciences, Bambino Gesù Children's Hospital, IRCCS, Rome, Italy

Elena De Momi Department of Electronics, Information and Bioengineering—DEIB, Politecnico di Milano, Milano, Italy

Piergiorgio d'Orio "Claudio Munari" Center for Epilepsy Surgery, Azienda Socio-Sanitaria Territoriale Grande Ospedale Metropolitano Niguarda, Milano, Italy

Department of Medicine and Surgery, Unit of Neuroscience, Università degli Studi di Parma, Parma, Italy

Amir H. Faraji Department of Neurological Surgery, Houston Methodist Hospital, Houston, TX, USA

Giancarlo Ferrigno Department of Electronics, Information and Bioengineering—DEIB, Politecnico di Milano, Milano, Italy

NeuroEngineering and Medical Robotics Lab – NearLab (POLIMI Leonardo Robotics Labs), Milano, Italy

Daryl P. Fields Department of Neurological Surgery and Epilepsy Center, University of Pittsburgh Medical Center, Pittsburgh, PA, USA

Zachary C. Gersey Department of Neurological Surgery and Epilepsy Center, University of Pittsburgh Medical Center, Pittsburgh, PA, USA

Jorge Alvaro González Martínez Department of Neurological Surgery and Epilepsy Center, University of Pittsburgh Medical Center, Pittsburgh, PA, USA

Marc Guénot Department of Functional Neurosurgery, P. Wertheimer Hospital, Hospices Civils de Lyon, University of Lyon, Lyon, France

Marc Harislur Service de Neurochirurgie, GHU Paris—Psychiatrie et Neurosciences—Hôpital Sainte-Anne, Paris, France

Université de Paris, Sorbonne Paris Cité, Paris, France

Yusuke S. Hori Rose Ella Burkhardt Brain Tumor and Neuro-Oncology Center, Department of Neurological Surgery, Neurological Institute, Cleveland Clinic, Cleveland, OH, USA

Sogha Khawari Victor Horsley Department of Neurosurgery, National Hospital for Neurology and Neurosurgery, London, UK

Department of Clinical and Experimental Epilepsy, Queen Square Institute of Neurology, University College London, London, UK

L. Dade Lunsford Department of Neurological Surgery, University of Pittsburgh Medical Center, Pittsburgh, USA

Arka N. Mallela Department of Neurological Surgery and Epilepsy Center, University of Pittsburgh Medical Center, Pittsburgh, PA, USA

Gordon Mao Department of Neurosurgery, Indiana University, Indianapolis, IN, USA

Department of Neurosurgery, The Johns Hopkins School of Medicine, Baltimore, MD, USA

Hani J. Marcus Victor Horsley Department of Neurosurgery, National Hospital for Neurology and Neurosurgery, London, UK

Wellcome EPSRC Centre for Interventional and Surgical Sciences, University College London, London, UK

Carlo Efisio Marras Neurosurgery Unit, Department of Neurosciences, Bambino Gesù Children's Hospital, IRCCS, Rome, Italy

Silvestro Micera Center for Neuroprosthetics and Institute of Bioengineering, School of Engineering, Ecole Polytechnique Federale de Lausanne, Lausanne, Switzerland

The Biorobotics Institute and Department of Excellence in Robotics and AI, Scuola Superiore Sant'Anna, Pisa, Italy

Ajay Niranjan Department of Neurological Surgery, University of Pittsburgh Medical Center, Pittsburgh, USA

Carlotta Ginevra Nucci Neurosurgery Unit, Department of Neurosciences, Bambino Gesù Children's Hospital, IRCCS, Rome, Italy

Cihat Ozhasoglu Department of Radiation Oncology, University of Pittsburgh Medical Center, Pittsburgh, PA, USA

Johan Pallud Service de Neurochirurgie, GHU Paris—Psychiatrie et Neurosciences—Hôpital Sainte-Anne, Paris, France

Université de Paris, Sorbonne Paris Cité, Paris, France

Inserm, UMR1266, IMA-Brain, Institut de Psychiatrie et Neurosciences de Paris, Paris, France

Angelo Pichierri Department of Neurosurgery, Southmead Hospital, Bristol, UK

Camilla Pierella Department of Neurosciences, Rehabilitation, Ophthalmology, Genetics, and Maternal and Children's Sciences (DINOGMI), University of Genoa, Genoa, Italy

Department of Informatics, Bioengineering, Robotics and Systems Engineering (DIBRIS), University of Genoa, Genoa, Italy

Sibi Rajendran Department of Neurological Surgery, Houston Methodist Hospital, Houston, TX, USA

Sergio Raspante Department of Neuroradiology, Azienda Socio-Sanitaria Territoriale Grande Ospedale Metropolitano Niguarda, Milano, Italy

Martina Revay "Claudio Munari" Center for Epilepsy Surgery, Azienda Socio-Sanitaria Territoriale Grande Ospedale Metropolitano Niguarda, Milano, Italy

Department of Biomedical and Clinical Sciences "L. Sacco", Università degli Studi di Milano, Milano, Italy

Karl Roessler Department of Neurosurgery, Medical University of Vienna, Vienna, Austria

Camilla Rossi-Espagnet Neuroradiology Unit, Imaging Department of Radiology, Bambino Gesù Children's Hospital, IRCCS, Rome, Italy

Neuroradiology Unit, NESMOS Department, Sapienza University, Rome, Italy

Giorgio Lo Russo "Claudio Munari" Center for Epilepsy Surgery, Azienda Socio-Sanitaria Territoriale Grande Ospedale Metropolitano Niguarda, Milano, Italy

Julia Shawarba Department of Neurosurgery, Medical University of Vienna, Vienna, Austria

Zaid A. Siddique Department of Radiation Oncology, University of Pittsburgh Medical Center, Pittsburgh, PA, USA

Giorgia Antonia Simboli Service de Neurochirurgie, GHU Paris—Psychiatrie et Neurosciences—Hôpital Sainte-Anne, Paris, France

Université de Paris, Sorbonne Paris Cité, Paris, France

James Sweat Department of Neurological Surgery and Epilepsy Center, University of Pittsburgh Medical Center, Pittsburgh, PA, USA

Nicholas Theodore Department of Neurosurgery, The Johns Hopkins School of Medicine, Baltimore, MD, USA

Martin M. Tisdall Department of Neurosurgery, Great Ormond Street Hospital, London, UK

Developmental Neurosciences, Great Ormond Street Institute of Child Health, University College London, London, UK

Vejay Vakharia Victor Horsley Department of Neurosurgery, National Hospital for Neurology and Neurosurgery, London, UK

Department of Clinical and Experimental Epilepsy, Queen Square Institute of Neurology, University College London, London, UK

Fabian Winter Department of Neurosurgery, Medical University of Vienna, Vienna, Austria

Marc Zanello Service de Neurochirurgie, GHU Paris—Psychiatrie et Neurosciences—Hôpital Sainte-Anne, Paris, France

Université de Paris, Sorbonne Paris Cité, Paris, France

Inserm, UMR1266, IMA-Brain, Institut de Psychiatrie et Neurosciences de Paris, Paris, France

Part I
General Principles

Chapter 1
Robotics in Neurosurgery: Overture

Francesco Cardinale, Piergiorgio d'Orio, Martina Revay, and Laura Castana

Introduction

Since the first robot-assisted CT-guided brain biopsy was stereotactically performed in 1985 by Kwoh and coworkers with an industrial PUMA robot [1], the adoption of robotic assistance in neurosurgical practice has progressively gained popularity. The above-mentioned system was quickly abandoned for safety issues, and the early years were signed mainly by the pioneering work of Alim Louis Benabid at Grenoble University, the father of the NeuroMate robotic assistant (Renishaw, Wotton-under-Edge, United Kingdom). Out of the several systems developed in the first two decades of neurosurgical robotics, only NeuroMate is still available in the market. It was the first neurosurgical robot certified by the US Food and Drug Administration at the beginning of the 2000s [2] and it is still one of the most

F. Cardinale (✉) · P. d'Orio
"Claudio Munari" Center for Epilepsy Surgery, Azienda Socio-Sanitaria Territoriale Grande Ospedale Metropolitano Niguarda, Milano, Italy

Department of Medicine and Surgery, Unit of Neuroscience, Università degli Studi di Parma, Parma, Italy
e-mail: francesco.cardinale@ospedaleniguarda.it; piergiorgio.dorio@ospedaleniguarda.it

M. Revay
"Claudio Munari" Center for Epilepsy Surgery, Azienda Socio-Sanitaria Territoriale Grande Ospedale Metropolitano Niguarda, Milano, Italy

Department of Biomedical and Clinical Sciences "L. Sacco", Università degli Studi di Milano, Milano, Italy
e-mail: martina.revay@ospedaleniguarda.it

L. Castana
"Claudio Munari" Center for Epilepsy Surgery, Azienda Socio-Sanitaria Territoriale Grande Ospedale Metropolitano Niguarda, Milano, Italy
e-mail: laura.castana@ospedaleniguarda.it

J. A. González Martínez, F. Cardinale (eds.), *Robotics in Neurosurgery*,
https://doi.org/10.1007/978-3-031-08380-8_1

accurate systems for stereotactic implantation of intracerebral devices, as suggested by recent papers reporting smallest errors in the implantation of stereoelectroencephalography (SEEG) electrodes for both children and adults [3–5].

For some decades, the neurosurgical use of robotic assistance has been limited to intracranial procedures. Subsequently, the range of available procedures has been widened, now including also spine surgery. Differently from the field of body surgery, robotic assistants are not commonly used for surgeon's motion replication aimed at performing tele-controlled micro-neurosurgical operations. Instead, most popular clinically available systems are passive robots able to hold a surgical tool along the vector of a pre-planned direction, exploiting the well-established technologies that have been developed in the field of image-guided surgery.

Besides surgical assistance, robotic systems can be used also in the fields of rehabilitation and prosthetics.

Clinical Applications

As already mentioned, most popular systems can passively assist the neurosurgeon holding a tool (e.g., a twist drill to prepare the intracranial path to implant recording or stimulating electrodes, laser fibers, or biopsy needles) along the direction of one or multiple pre-planned trajectories. In 1992, more than 20 years ago, Benabid and coworkers had already described the use of Neuromate robot in a number of stereotactic intracranial needle biopsies, intracerebral electrode implantations for SEEG or deep brain stimulation (DBS), and brachytherapy procedures [6]. In the same year, the same Grenoble group pioneered the use of the robot also in neuroendoscopy [7].

SEEG

SEEG gained popularity worldwide in the recent years, pushing the adoption of robotic assistance. We can also interpret this tendency in a "circular" view because a wider availability of robotic assistants made easier the birth of many SEEG programs even outside the countries where this method was traditionally adopted in the last decades, France and Italy [8, 9]. Since the number of SEEG trajectories is commonly high [10], this is the field in which robots can give their best because they do not suffer fatigue and cannot be affected by tremor. Moreover, most modern systems are characterized by high mechanical accuracy and therefore guarantee safe implantations when planning is based on high resolution images providing comprehensive multimodal information. In fact, numerous recent papers have reported a high safety profile for robot-assisted SEEG implantations [3, 11–15]. Non-inferior or superior accuracy and safety profiles against other types of framed or frame-less equipment have been also reported [5, 16, 17].

Neuromate and ROSA (Zimmer Biomet, Warsaw, Indiana) are the two most popular robots used for SEEG implantation. Both of them have been originally developed in France. Another similarly large robot, Sino Robot (Sinovation Medical Technology—Beijing—China), has been recently developed in China [18, 19]. A small form-factor robotic device, originally developed in Austria, has been also developed and reported: the Stealth Autoguide (Medtronic; Minneapolis, Minnesota, USA—formerly known as iSYS1) [20]. In particular, it has been compared against a manual arm-based technique in a single-blinded controlled randomized trial, showing shorter median operative time but lower stereotactic accuracy [21].

Besides the surgical aspects of electrode implantation, it remains dramatically important to understand that a rigorous technique can guarantee the necessary safety profile, but also that without an appropriate method for the selection of patients, the definition of topographical strategy and the interpretation of long-term monitoring findings, SEEG cannot give the expected results in terms of post-operative seizure-freedom [22], whatever the used stereotactic tools.

Radio-Frequency Thermocoagulation and Laser Interstitial Thermal Therapy

Strictly related to SEEG investigation, there is the possibility of ablating multiple small volumes of brain tissue surrounding the recording probes if an adequate power of electrical current is administered between two adjacent contacts. Radio-Frequency Thermocoagulation (RF-THC) was first published by Guénot and coworkers in 2004 [23] and has gained popularity particularly in the most recent years, as testified by a number of articles on larger and larger case series [24–28]. Robotic assistance provides the necessary accuracy, and the main advantage is the possibility of performing the ablation before removing the SEEG electrodes, thus coagulating the brain tissue surrounding the contacts best seated in the ictal onset zone. Thanks to RF-THC, SEEG is no longer only a diagnostic method but offers also a treatment option for malformations of cortical development [29–32]. Of particular interest is the reborn interest for SEEG-guided RF-THC of mesial temporal structures, reproposed with local high-density implantation and also with the opportunity of ablating between contacts lying on different probes thanks to special equipment [33–35]. Finally, robotic SEEG-guided RF-THC has been reported even in the field of pediatrics [36].

Tissue ablation performed by means of robot-implanted devices can be performed also independently from SEEG, following it as a second-stage procedure or performed without any prior intracranial recording. Mullatti et al. recently published their experience on the successful use of a larger electro-catheter implanted into an epileptogenic insular lobe to perform ablations in a variety of epileptogenic clinical conditions (tumor, focal cortical dysplasia (FCD), or unknown pathological substrate) [37]. Robotic RF-THC of hypothalamic hamartoma has been also described [38].

Robot-assisted Laser Interstitial Thermal Therapy (LiTT) is an emerging technique in the treatment of drug-resistant epilepsy. The first case, following SEEG in a patient presenting with a periventricular nodular heterotopy, was described by Gonzalez-Martinez et al. in 2014 [39]. LiTT is now used for ablating brain tissue also in other epileptogenic conditions, such as FCD [40, 41], hypothalamic hamartoma, [42] and mesial temporal lobe epilepsy (MTLE) [43, 44].

Out of epilepsy surgery, LiTT is largely used also for the treatment of many other brain lesions such as primary or metastatic malignant tumors and radiation necrosis [45–48]. Robotic assistance guarantees the necessary accuracy also in these cases, of course.

Deep Brain Stimulation

Chronic high-frequency DBS mimics the effect of surgical ablation of functional targets. Therefore, it is used to treat movement disorders and, more recently, also drug-resistant epilepsy (commonly targeting the anterior nucleus of thalamus or the hippocampus). Parkinson disease is certainly the most common indication for such treatment in adults. Thalamic nucleus ventralis intermedius (VIM) was the first reported target of robot-assisted DBS [6]. In early 90s, it was quickly replaced by the subthalamic nucleus (STN) because DBS of this structure improves not only tremor, but also rigidity and bradykinesia [49]. DBS with robot-assisted bilateral implantation of the stimulating electrodes in the STN is therefore the most common procedure for treating Parkinson disease in adults [50], while the globus pallidus internus is the target of choice for dystonia, often treated during pediatric age [51, 52].

All the subcortical structures that are targeted for DBS treatment in the field of movement disorders are small and characterized by a somatotopic arrangement that must be carefully considered in order to obtain the best balance between benefit and side effects. Thus, high accuracy at the target is critical. A recent meta-analysis, following a systematic review of the literature, suggested that robotic assistance significantly and independently provides better accuracy of implantation not only in the field of SEEG, but also in the DBS one [17].

Biopsy

As above mentioned, the history of robotic assistance in neurosurgery started with a brain biopsy surgery [1]. It is not surprising that at the present time, given the renewed enthusiasm likely due to the worldwide spread of SEEG, also stereotactic biopsies are often performed with the aid of robotic equipment. Even if the number of trajectories is usually very limited (only one in most cases), robots still guarantee the necessary accuracy and mechanical stability in such critical procedures. For multi-bite biopsy of the lesion, the arm of large robots not only aligns the tool holder with the vector of the planned trajectory. It also gives the possibility of advancing by small steps to sample different zones of the abnormal tissue, from the periphery to the core, as described by Zanello and coworkers in the largest study reporting on a robotic biopsy series [53]. The histopathological diagnosis has been obtained in 98.7% of 377 patients, with a favorable safety profile guaranteed by Neuromate robot. The use of ROSA system has been also reported [54], as long as the utilization of the Stealth Autoguide [55, 56].

Neuroendoscopy

The disconnection of hypothalamic hamartoma is one of the most common surgical techniques that takes advantage from robotic assistance. It was popularized by Delalande and coworkers in the early 90s for treating patients suffering from gelastic seizures, especially when the insertion of the hamartoma is pedunculate and the stalk is accessible [57]. Expanding from the original indication, robotic neuroendoscopy is used mostly in pediatric neurosurgery for ventriculostomies or septostomies aimed at treating obstructive hydrocephalus, for fenestration of intraventricular or extraventricular cysts, or for biopsies of intraventricular or midline tumors [58]. More recently, robotic endoscopy has been utilized also to perform hemispherotomy in patients suffering from catastrophic hemispheric epilepsy [59].

Spine Surgery

SpineAssist was the first robot to obtain Food and Drug Administration (FDA) clearance for spine surgery in 2004 [60]. Since then, the number of indications and procedures in this field of interest are progressively increasing. In fact, robotic equipment can guide the neurosurgeon to deep anatomical structures along a narrow path, making the avoidance of vessels and nerves easier. Moreover, robotic assistance offers intraoperative navigation, decrease of incision size, elimination of hand tremors, and reduction of neurosurgeon fatigue [61]. Throughout the years, the initial level of mistrust against the use of robotics in spine surgeries is decreasing, and the two most popular procedures are the pedicle-screw placement and the anterior lumbar interbody fusion. Likely, image-guided navigation is the most important advantage of robotics for pedicle-screw placement, as suggested by a large meta-analysis aimed at comparing conventional free-hand against navigated surgery [62]. While pedicle-screw placement is typically performed by means of supervisory-control robots [63–67], robotic anterior lumbar interbody fusion is done using Da Vinci Surgical System (Intuitive Surgical - Sunnyvale - California), a tele-controlled assistant for surgeon's motion replication very popular for abdominal and urological surgery [68].

Other Procedures

Robotic assistance has been described also in some other types of procedures, such as drug delivery [69], radiosurgery [70], laser osteotomy [71].

Moreover, neurosurgical robots not only can assist neurosurgeons during surgical procedures but can also support patients with impaired motor or sensory functions during rehabilitation or assist them in their daily life. The more complex implementation of such robots is the brain–machine interface-controlled exoskeleton for tetraplegic patients recently developed by Benabid and coworkers [72].

Final Remarks

Robots for cranial surgery are accurate and can assist the neurosurgeon in performing safe operations, reducing sources of inaccuracy and the probability of procedural errors. Most of them are passive supervisory-control robots able to align a tool holder along the vector of a pre-planned trajectory, as in the cases of stereotactic intracerebral electrode implantation or of a biopsy needle advancement into the cranial space. They are used also to constrain the movements of an endoscope in order to limit healthy brain injury. The accuracy of such robots is not the only component affecting the final accuracy of the procedure: it is also mandatory to plan the surgery on high-definition and undistorted images and to register correctly the image and the robotic spaces.

Compared to cranial surgery, robotics is still at an earlier stage in the field of spine surgery. Nonetheless, the use of supervisory-control robots is progressively gaining popularity, especially for pedicle-screw placement. Differently, anterior lumbar interbody fusion is performed with the assistance of a tele-controlled manipulation system.

Compared to the existing non-robotic standard of care, the main tradeoffs of robotics are the need for additional special training and the considerable start-up costs [9]. Especially for spine surgery, the cost-benefit balance is not yet well estimated and further studies are needed [73].

References

1. Kwoh Y, Hou J, Jonckheere G, Hayah S. A robot with improved absolute positioning accuracy got CT-guided stereotactic brain surgery. IEEE Trans Biomed Eng. 1988;55:153–60.
2. Li QH, Zamorano L, Pandya A, Perez R, Gong J, Diaz FG. The application accuracy of the NeuroMate robot—a quantitative comparison with frameless and frame-based surgical localization systems. Comput Aided Surg. 2002;7(2):90–8.
3. Mullin JP, Shriver M, Alomar S, et al. Is SEEG safe? A systematic review and meta-analysis of stereo-electroencephalography-related complications. Epilepsia. 2016;57(3):386–401.

4. Cardinale F, Rizzi M, D'Orio P, et al. A new tool for touch-free patient registration for robot-assisted intracranial surgery: application accuracy from a phantom study and a retrospective surgical series. Neurosurg Focus. 2017;42(5):E8.
5. Sharma JD, Seunarine KK, Tahir MZ, Tisdall MM. Accuracy of robot-assisted versus optical frameless navigated stereoelectroencephalography electrode placement in children. J Neurosurg Pediatr. 2019;23:297–302.
6. Benabid AL, Lavallée S, Hoffmann D, Cinquin P, Demongeot J, Danel F. Computer-driven robot for stereotactic neurosurgery. In: Kelly PJ, Kall BA, editors. Computers in stereotactic neurosurgery. Cambridge, MA: Blackwell Publishers, Inc.; 1992. p. 330–42.
7. Benabid AL, Lavallée S, Hoffmann D, Cinquin P, Demongeot J, Danel F. Potential use of robots in endoscopic neurosurgery. Acta Neurochir. 1992;54:93–7.
8. Joswig H, Steven DA, Parrent AG, et al. Intracranial electroencephalographic monitoring: from subdural to depth electrodes. Can J Neurol Sci. 2018;45(3):336–8.
9. Ball T, González-Martínez JA, Zemmar A, et al. Robotic applications in cranial neurosurgery: current and future. Oper Neurosurg. 2021;21:371–9.
10. Cardinale F, Casaceli G, Raneri F, Miller JP, Lo RG. Implantation of StereoElectroEncephaloGraphy (SEEG) electrodes: a systematic review. J Clin Neurophysiol. 2016;33(6):490–502.
11. Gonzalez-Martinez JA, Bulacio JC, Thompson S, et al. Technique, results, and complications related to robot-assisted Stereoelectroencephalography. Neurosurgery. 2016;78(2):169–80.
12. Ollivier I, Behr C, Cebula H, et al. Efficacy and safety in frameless robot-assisted stereo-electroencephalography (SEEG) for drug-resistant epilepsy. Neurochirurgie. 2017;63(4):286–90.
13. Cardinale F, Rizzi M, Vignati E, et al. Stereoelectroencephalography: retrospective analysis of 742 procedures in a single Centre. Brain. 2019;142:2688–704.
14. Tandon N, Tong BA, Friedman ER, et al. Analysis of morbidity and outcomes associated with use of subdural grids vs Stereoelectroencephalography in patients with intractable epilepsy. JAMA Neurol. 2019;76(6):672–81.
15. Spyrantis A, Cattani A, Woebbecke T, et al. Electrode placement accuracy in robot-assisted epilepsy surgery: a comparison of different referencing techniques including frame-based CT versus facial laser scan based on CT or MRI. Epilepsy Behav. 2019;2019(91):38–47.
16. Bourdillon P, Chatillon CÉ, Moles A, et al. Effective accuracy of StereoElectroEncephaloGraphy (SEEG): robotic tridimensional vs Talairach orthogonal approaches. J Neurosurg. 2019;131:1938–46.
17. Philipp LR, Matias CM, Thalheimer S, Mehta SH, Sharan AD, Wu C. Robot-assisted Stereotaxy reduces target error: a meta-analysis and meta-regression of 6056 trajectories. Neurosurgery. 2021;88(2):222–33.
18. Zheng J, Liu YL, Zhang D, et al. Robot-assisted versus stereotactic frame-based stereoelectroencephalography in medically refractory epilepsy. Neurophysiol Clin. 2021;51:111–9.
19. Zhang D, Cui X, Zheng J, et al. Neurosurgical robot-assistant stereoelectroencephalography system: operability and accuracy. Brain Behav. 2021;11(10):e2347.
20. Dorfer C, Minchev G, Czech T, et al. A novel miniature robotic device for frameless implantation of depth electrodes in refractory epilepsy. J Neurosurg. 2017;126:1622–8.
21. Vakharia VN, Rodionov R, Miserocchi A, et al. Comparison of robotic and manual implantation of intracerebral electrodes: a single-Centre, single-blinded, randomised controlled trial. Sci Rep. 2021;11:17,127.
22. Chabardès S, Abel TJ, Cardinale F, Kahane P. Commentary: understanding Stereoelectroencephalography: what's next? Neurosurgery. 2017;82(1):E15–6.
23. Guénot M, Isnard J, Ryvlin P, Fischer C, Mauguière F, Sindou M. SEEG-guided RF thermocoagulation of epileptic foci: feasibility, safety, and preliminary results. Epilepsia. 2004;45(11):1368–74.
24. Bourdillon P, Isnard J, Catenoix H, et al. Stereo electroencephalography–guided radiofrequency focal epilepsy: results from a 10-year experience. Epilepsia. 2017;58(1):85–93.

25. Cossu M, Cardinale F, Casaceli G, et al. Stereo-EEG-guided radiofrequency thermocoagulations. Epilepsia. 2017;58(Suppl 1):S66–72.
26. Dimova P, de Palma L, Job A-S, Minotti L, Hoffmann D, Kahane P. Radiofrequency thermocoagulation of the seizure-onset zone during stereoelectroencephalography. Epilepsia. 2017;58(3):381–92.
27. Catenoix H, Bourdillon P, Guénot M, Isnard J. The combination of stereo-EEG and radiofrequency ablation. Epilepsy Res. 2018;142:117–20.
28. Mirza FA, Hall JA. Radiofrequency thermocoagulation in refractory focal epilepsy: the MNI experience. Can J Neurol Sci/J Can des Sci Neurol. 2021;48(5):626–39.
29. Wellmer J, Kopitzki K, Voges J. Lesion focused stereotactic thermo-coagulation of focal cortical dysplasia IIB: a new approach to epilepsy surgery? Seizure. 2014;23(6):475–8.
30. Catenoix H, Mauguière F, Montavont A, Ryvlin P, Guénot M, Isnard J. Seizures outcome after stereoelectroencephalography-guided thermocoagulations in malformations of cortical development poorly accessible to surgical resection. Neurosurgery. 2015;77:9–15.
31. Cossu M, Fuschillo D, Cardinale F, et al. Stereo-EEG-guided radio-frequency thermocoagulations of epileptogenic grey-matter nodular heterotopy. J Neurol Neurosurg Psychiatry. 2014;85:611–7.
32. Cossu M, Fuschillo D, Casaceli G, et al. Stereoelectroencephalography-guided radiofrequency thermocoagulation in the epileptogenic zone: a retrospective study on 89 cases. J Neurosurg. 2015;123:1358–67.
33. Fan X, Shan Y-Z, Lu C, et al. Optimized SEEG-guided radiofrequency thermocoagulation for mesial temporal lobe epilepsy with hippocampal sclerosis. Seizure. 2019;71:304–11.
34. Wang Y-H, Chen S-C, Wei P-H, et al. Stereotactic EEG-guided radiofrequency thermocoagulation versus anterior temporal lobectomy for mesial temporal lobe epilepsy with hippocampal sclerosis: study protocol for a randomised controlled trial. Trials. 2021;22:425.
35. Losarcos NG, Miller J, Fastenau P, et al. Stereotactic-EEG-guided radiofrequency multiple hippocampal transection (SEEG-guided-RF-MHT) for the treatment of mesial temporal lobe epilepsy: a minimally invasive method for diagnosis and treatment. Epileptic Disord. 2021;23(5):682–94.
36. Chipaux M, Taussig D, Dorfmüller G, et al. SEEG-guided radiofrequency thermocoagulation of epileptic foci in the paediatric population: feasibility, safety and efficacy. Seizure. 2019;70(July):63–70.
37. Mullatti N, Landré E, Mellerio C, et al. Stereotactic thermocoagulation for insular epilepsy: lessons from successes and failures. Epilepsia. 2019;60(8):1565–79.
38. Tandon V, Chandra PS, Doddamani RS, et al. Stereotactic radiofrequency thermocoagulation of hypothalamic hamartoma using robotic guidance (ROSA) coregistered with O-arm guidance—preliminary technical note. World Neurosurg. 2018;112:267–74.
39. Gonzalez-Martinez JA, Vadera S, Mullin JP, et al. Robot-assisted stereotactic laser ablation in medically intractable epilepsy: operative technique. Oper Neurosurg. 2014;10(2):167–72.
40. Ellis JA, Mejia Munne JC, Wang SH, et al. Staged laser interstitial thermal therapy and topectomy for complete obliteration of complex focal cortical dysplasias. J Clin Neurosci. 2016;2016(31):224–8.
41. Jain P, Ochi A, Mcinnis C, et al. Surgical outcomes in children with bottom-of-sulcus dysplasia and drug-resistant epilepsy: a retrospective cohort study. J Neurosurg Pediatr. 2021;28(3):295–305.
42. Bourdillon P, Ferrand-Sorbets S, Apra C, et al. Surgical treatment of hypothalamic hamartomas. Neurosurg Rev. 2021;44(2):753–62.
43. Youngerman BE, Oh JY, Anbarasan D, et al. Laser ablation is effective for temporal lobe epilepsy with and without mesial temporal sclerosis if hippocampal seizure onsets are localized by stereoelectroencephalography. Epilepsia. 2018;59:595–606.
44. Gross RE, Stern MA, Willie JT, et al. Stereotactic laser amygdalohippocampotomy for mesial temporal lobe epilepsy. Ann Neurol. 2018;83(3):575–87.
45. Patel NV, Jethwa PR, Shetty A, Danish SF. Does the real-time thermal damage estimate allow for estimation of tumor control after MRI-guided laser-induced thermal therapy? Initial experience with recurrent intracranial ependymomas. J Neurosurg Pediatr. 2015;15:363–71.

46. Ivan ME, Mohammadi AM, De Deugd N, et al. Laser ablation of newly diagnosed malignant gliomas. Neurosurgery. 2016;79(Suppl 1):S17–23.
47. Lee I, Kalkanis S, Hadjipanayis CG. Stereotactic laser interstitial thermal therapy for recurrent high-grade gliomas. Neurosurgery. 2016;79(Suppl 1):S24–34.
48. Smith CJ, Myers CS, Chapple KM, Smith KA. Long-term follow-up of 25 cases of biopsy-proven radiation necrosis or post-radiation treatment effect treated with magnetic resonance-guided laser interstitial thermal therapy. Neurosurgery. 2016;79(Suppl 1):S59–72.
49. Krack P, Batir A, Van Blercom N, et al. Five-year follow-up of bilateral stimulation of the subthalamic nucleus in advanced Parkinson's disease. N Engl J Med. 2003;349:1925–34.
50. Benabid AL, Chabardès S, Mitrofanis J, Pollak P. Deep brain stimulation of the subthalamic nucleus for the treatment of Parkinson's disease. Lancet Neurol. 2009;8(1):67–81.
51. Alteman RL, Shils JL. Pallidal stimulation for dystonia. In: Starr PA, Barbaro NM, Larson PS, editors. Neurosurgical operative atlas. Functional neurosurgery. New York: Thieme Medical Publishers; 2011. p. 195–203.
52. Furlanetti LL, Ellenbogen J, Gimeno H, et al. Targeting accuracy of robot-assisted deep brain stimulation surgery in childhood-onset dystonia: a single-center prospective cohort analysis of 45 consecutive cases. J Neurosurg Pediatr. 2021;27(6):677–87.
53. Zanello M, Roux A, Senova S, et al. Robot-assisted stereotactic biopsies in 377 consecutive adult patients with supratentorial diffuse gliomas: diagnostic yield, safety and postoperative outcomes. World Neurosurg. 2021;148:e301–13.
54. Lefranc M, Capel C, Pruvot-Occean A-S, et al. Frameless robotic stereotactic biopsies: a consecutive series of 100 cases. J Neurosurg. 2015;122(February):342–52.
55. Legnani FG, Franzini A, Mattei L, et al. Image-guided biopsy of intracranial lesions with a small robotic device (iSYS1): a prospective, exploratory pilot study. Oper Neurosurg. 2019;17(4):403–12.
56. Minchev G, Kronreif G, Ptacek W, et al. Frameless stereotactic brain biopsies: comparison of minimally invasive robot-guided and manual arm-based technique. Oper Neurosurg. 2020;19(3):292–301.
57. Procaccini E, Dorfmüller G, Fohlen M, Bulteau C, Delalande O. Surgical management of hypothalamic hamartomas with epilepsy: the stereoendoscopic approach. Neurosurgery. 2006;59(4 Suppl 2):ONS336-344.
58. De Benedictis A, Trezza A, Carai A, et al. Robot-assisted procedures in pediatric neurosurgery. Neurosurg Focus. 2017;42(5):E7.
59. Chandra PS, Subianto H, Bajaj J, et al. Endoscope-assisted (with robotic guidance and using a hybrid technique) interhemispheric transcallosal hemispherotomy: a comparative study with open hemispherotomy to evaluate efficacy, complications, and outcome. J Neurosurg Pediatr. 2019;23(2):187–97.
60. Theodore N, Ahmed AK. The history of robotics in spine surgery. Spine (Phila Pa 1976). 2018;43(7S):S23.
61. D'Souza M, Gendreau J, Feng A, Kim LH, Ho AL, Veeravagu A. Robotic-assisted spine surgery: history, efficacy, cost, and future trends. Robot Surg Res Rev. 2019;6:9–23.
62. Verma R, Krishan S, Haendlmayer K, Mohsen A. Functional outcome of computer-assisted spinal pedicle screw placement: a systematic review and meta-analysis of 23 studies including 5,992 pedicle screws. Eur Spine J. 2010;19(3):370–5.
63. Ringel F, Stüer C, Reinke A, et al. Accuracy of robot-assisted placement of lumbar and sacral pedicle screws: a prospective randomized comparison to conventional freehand screw implantation. Spine (Phila Pa 1976). 2012;37(8):E496–501.
64. Molliqaj G, Schatlo B, Alaid A, et al. Accuracy of robot-guided versus freehand fluoroscopy-assisted pedicle screw insertion in thoracolumbar spinal surgery. Neurosurg Focus. 2017;42(5):E14.
65. Solomiichuk V, Fleischhammer J, Molliqaj G, et al. Robotic versus fluoroscopy-guided pedicle screw insertion for metastatic spinal disease: a matched-cohort comparison. Neurosurg Focus. 2017;42(5):E13.

66. Schatlo B, Molliqaj G, Cuvinciuc V, Kotowski M, Schaller K, Tessitore E. Safety and accuracy of robot-assisted versus fluoroscopy-guided pedicle screw insertion for degenerative diseases of the lumbar spine: a matched cohort comparison—clinical article. J Neurosurg Spine. 2014;20(6):636–43.
67. Lieberman IH, Kisinde S, Hesselbacher S. Robotic-assisted pedicle screw placement during spine surgery. JBJS Essent Surg Tech. 2020;10(2):1–15.
68. Lee Z, Lee J, Welch WC, Eun D. Technique and surgical outcomes of robot-assisted anterior lumbar interbody fusion. J Robot Surg. 2013;7(2):177–85.
69. Lewis O, Woolley M, Johnson DE, et al. Maximising coverage of brain structures using controlled reflux, convection-enhanced delivery and the recessed step catheter. J Neurosci Methods. 2018;308(June):337–45.
70. Adler JR, Chang SD, Murphy MJ, Doty J, Geis P, Hancock SL. The Cyberknife: a frameless robotic system for radiosurgery. Stereotact Funct Neurosurg. 1997;69:124–8.
71. Roessler K, Winter F, Wilken T, Pataraia E, Mueller-Gerbl M, Dorfer C. Robotic navigated laser craniotomy for depth electrode implantation in epilepsy surgery: a cadaver lab study. J Neurol Surg Part A Cent Eur Neurosurg. 2021;82:125–9.
72. Benabid AL, Costecalde T, Eliseyev A, et al. An exoskeleton controlled by an epidural wireless brain-machine interface in a tetraplegic patient: a proof-of-concept demonstration. Lancet Neurol. 2019;18:1112–22.
73. Fiani B, Quadri SA, Farooqui M, et al. Impact of robot-assisted spine surgery on health care quality and neurosurgical economics: a systemic review. Neurosurg Rev. 2020;43(1):17–25.

Chapter 2
Historical Perspectives

Elena De Momi

History of Robotic Surgery

A robot is "a reprogrammable multifunctional manipulator, designed to move material, parts, tools or specialized devices through variable programmed motions for the performance of a variety of tasks" (Robot Institute of America) [1]. First industrial robots started to be developed in the early 60s in order to replace labor-intensive tasks previously carried out by humans.

The definition of "surgical robot" given in [2], is "a powered computer-controlled manipulator with artificial sensing that can be reprogrammed to move and position tools to carry out a range of surgical tasks." Robots do not replace surgeons, rather they assist during surgical task execution, under his/her supervision, allowing increasing accuracy and safety, while alleviating surgeon fatigue. Given their intrinsic repeatability and maneuverability, their potential advantage in high-accuracy requiring procedures was first demonstrated in the 80s.

The first robot-assisted surgical procedure was reported by Kwoh et al. in 1988 [3]. This historical milestone is represented by a CT-guided stereotactic brain tumor biopsy performed in 1985 on a 52-year-old man with a suspicious brain lesion. The robotic system, i.e., an industrial Puma 560, Unimation Limited, with stated relative accuracy of 0.05 mm, autonomously reached the desired position, and the task execution was based on the CT-based preoperative plan. Once the robot reached the planned pose, the biopsy probe was manually inserted into the skull by the surgeon. Thus, the surgeon's actions were limited to straight-line insertions and axial rotations. The authors claim that the procedure resulted faster than the manually adjustable frame and they improved the targeting accuracy. Since manufacturing

E. De Momi (✉)
Department of Electronics, Information and Bioengineering – DEIB, Politecnico di Milano, Milano, Italy
e-mail: elena.demomi@polimi.it

J. A. González Martínez, F. Cardinale (eds.), *Robotics in Neurosurgery*,
https://doi.org/10.1007/978-3-031-08380-8_2

companies refused to allow the use of the robot outside protective barriers, due to the lack of safety measures, the project was dismissed.

Another industrial robot was used for hip surgery [4]: a SCARA robot autonomously reamed out the proximal femur to accommodate the femoral component of a hip prosthetic implant. The system, so-called ROBODOC, was then tried on a human being in 1991.

In the late 80s, the PROBOT system was used to assist in transurethral prostatectomies [5] and represented the first attempt to translate the surgical robotic activities to "soft-tissue." In essence, the PROBOT represented a framework to direct a rotating blade to autonomously resect the prostate. The system was clinically used on 40 patients by 1991. Key advantages to the PROBOT were its small size, cutting accuracy, and no-fatigue for the surgeon when performing the surgery.

After these first attempts, a new era of robotic tools and computer assisted procedures was revolutionizing surgery, creating the needs of experts in technology within the medical doctors, and the need of shortening learning curves to be proficient in benefitting from the clear advantages represented by such instruments.

Surgical Applications

Orthopedics

Orthopedic surgery is ideally performed using robotic systems: the robot can generate high cutting forces on hard tissue, based on the preoperative or the intraoperative plan. If the movement of the robot is constrained applying virtual walls/constraints, the robot is prevented from entering in contact with soft tissues.

The abovementioned ROBODOC system for hip surgery was then commercialized by Integrated Surgical Supplies Limited, Sacramento, USA [6]. While planning phase is performed on CT dataset, the intraoperative rigid registration is performed attaching "fiducial" markers into the bone in both the proximal head of the femur and the distal femoral condyles, so that, given their coordinates in the preoperative CT scans and in the intra-operative settings, the spatial transformation can be estimated. Long-term reported benefits for robotic procedures were good alignment of the implant stem in the femur and a very good contact area between bone and stem [2], which could offer improved bone growth. Short-term benefits, however, were more difficult to demonstrate as the time for the procedure was longer, resulting in increased anesthesia times and blood loss.

The "Caspar" system, developed by Orto-Maquet, used an anthropomorphic Stäubli-Automation industrial clean-room robot and was tested on 75 patients for hip replacement procedures. Other projects using robots for orthopedic surgery include Rizzoli Orthopaedic Institute, Bologna [7], which used a Puma 560 robot, and Helmholtz-Institute, Aachen, which started to develop a special-purpose parallel link robot for hip surgery in the early 2000s [8].

As far as the knee implant is concerned, the system developed by Imperial College in [9] allowed the surgeon to hold a force-controlled lever placed at the end-effector, together with a motorized cutter. The surgeon could use the lever to back-drive the robot motors within software-based virtual constraints so that an appropriate cutting shape is performed. The "Active constraint" robot (known as "Acrobot") allows the surgeon to feel directly the forces experienced by the cutter. Acrobot represented a new type of robotic system for surgery, known as a "synergistic" system, in which the surgeon's skills and judgment are combined with the controller-provided spatial constraint capabilities to enhance the performance of the robot/surgeon [2]. The concept has been now brought to the market by the Mako (Striker, USA) system, which has proven to offer better surgical results in terms of clinical outcome with respect to the manual approach.

Neurosurgery and Spine Surgery

Robots excel at handling spatial information, and are, thus, obvious candidates in the guidance of instrumentation along precisely planned trajectories. The above-mentioned milestone achieved in 1985 is in fact related to neurosurgery, where high positioning accuracy is demanded, and the robot can be seen as a replacement for the stereotactic frame. Faria et al. [10] reviewed robotic systems specifically developed for or capable of executing stereotactic neurosurgery, describing specific characteristics and workflows. As future perspective, the authors stated that the trend of technological progress is pointing toward the development of miniaturized cost-effective solutions with more intuitive interfaces.

Back in the late 80s, Benabid and colleagues [11, 12] in Grenoble, France, stereotactically reached several intracranial targets for biopsy, stereoelectroencephalography (SEEG), or brachytherapy procedures. An industrial robot was fitted with additional large-ratio gearboxes so that the robot could move slowly and safely. The addition of a preoperative planning facility based on CT imaging has made this a powerful system. The intraoperative registration was performed using X-ray projection and a so-called calibration cage held by the robot. By 1992, 140 cases were performed, including image guided robotic endoscopy. The special-purpose robot, later called "Neuromate," to be used "passively," was later distributed commercially by IMMI Limited, Lyon, and received FDA approval for cranial procedures in the early 2000s. The original French company was then acquired by Integrated Surgical Systems Inc. (USA), by Mayfield (USA) and finally by Renishaw (UK). The robot can be used for stereotactic procedures, such as deep brain stimulation, and has been extensively used for SEEG [11–16]. Median application accuracy (and Inter-Quartile Range—IQR) at the cortical entry point in frame-based or frame-less modality was reported to be 0.78 mm (IQR 0.49–1.08) and 0.59 mm (IQR 0.25–0.88), respectively. Median application accuracy at the deepest target in frame-based or frame-less modality was reported to be 1.77 mm (IQR 1.25–2.51) and

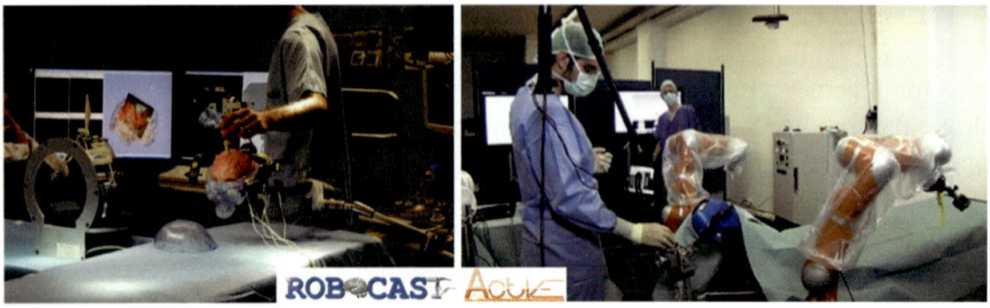

Fig. 2.1 Research activities performed at Politecnico di Milano in the framework of robotic surgery. On the left, the platform developed within the ROBOCAST project and, on the right, the ACTIVE system

1.49 mm (IQR 1.06–2.4), respectively. Of note, accuracy at the deepest point of trajectories is affected not only by image and robotic properties, but also by possible intracerebral deviations of the semi-rigid SEEG electrodes.

A further example of an active robot was the "Minerva" project, which was clinically applied for stereotactic neurosurgery [17]. This was a special-purpose system developed by the precision mechanisms group at the University of Lausanne. A powered robot, operating in a dedicated CT imaging system, was used in 8 neurosurgery clinical experiments. The operation is entirely performed by the robot, i.e., skin incision, bone drilling, dura perforation, and probe manipulation. This single axis then linearly advances the tool into the region of the patient's head which is fixed in a stereotactic frame.

The ROSA system (Zimmer Biomet, USA)[1] is a 6-degrees-of-freedom (DoF) system which can be directly manipulated by the surgeon in any desired direction. It received FDA approval in 2010. The system can be used for a wide range of clinical applications, including endoscopy and SEEG.

Among the systems which remained at a research phase with experimental studies completed in lab environments (reaching TRL[2] 6), the ROBOCAST EU[3] project is worth being mentioned (Fig. 2.1, on the left) since it introduced novel insight in robotic neurosurgery, namely the possibilities of (1) adopting an intelligent and automatic preoperative plan to compute the best trajectory for the surgical probe [18–20], (2) providing haptic perception during the active advancement of the surgical probe within the brain soft tissue [21, 22], and (3) performing curvilinear paths within the brain, using a steerable catheter, in order to reach the target with a greater number of possible paths. This last concept was then explored and translated into preclinical trials within the EDEN2020 EU project[4] [23].

[1] https://www.zimmerbiomet.com/medical-professionals/cmf/rosa-brain.html

[2] https://ec.europa.eu/research/participants/data/ref/h2020/wp/2014_2015/annexes/h2020-wp1415-annex-g-trl_en.pdf

[3] https://cordis.europa.eu/project/id/215190

[4] https://www.eden2020.eu/

With the aim of introducing the possibility of increasing the spectrum of possible operations on brain tissue, with respect to stereotactic procedures, the ACTIVE EU project (Fig. 2.1, on the right) was aimed at performing delicate tissue manipulation being able of actively compensating the small movements of the brain and of the skull, which might occur during awake neurosurgery [24].

Recent developments in neurosurgery have been dedicated to spine surgery. The first-ever spine robot, the SpineAssist (Mazor Robotics Ltd., Caesarea, Israel), gained FDA approval in 2004. With its ability to provide real-time intraoperative navigation and rigid stereotactic guidance, robotic-assisted spinal surgery has the potential to increase accuracy while decreasing radiation exposure, complication rates, operative time, and recovery time. Currently, robotic assistance is mainly dedicated to spinal fusion and instrumentation procedures, but, recently, complex procedures such as spinal tumor resections and ablations, vertebroplasties, and deformity correction have been performed. D'Souza et al. reviewed and discussed the history of spinal robots along as well as currently available systems [25].

From Cardiac Surgery to General Surgery/Urology/Gynecology

The advent of laparoscopy (or "minimally invasive surgery") at the beginning of the XXI century has seen several benefits over open surgery but also several drawbacks: a steep learning curve, a bidimensional view, and rigid instrumentation with a fulcrum effect and 4 degrees of freedom. The solution to the problems of laparoscopy was to be found with the rise of robotic surgery [26].

None of the systems mentioned in previous sections, however, was specifically designed for laparoscopic procedures. Initially, this technology was created by NASA in order to ensure surgical assistance to astronauts in space, thanks to the telepresence, avoiding the physical presence of a surgeon, which was allowed by immersive viewers. Consequently, NASA's Ames Research Centre, which was then joined by the Stanford Research Institute in 1990s which had developed a robotic telemanipulation system, designed the first phase robotic prototype based on telesurgery, which served as the starting platform for the future systems.

The US military recognized the potential significance of performing remote surgery (distant from the battlefield) to patients via a robotic platform, thus reducing the mortality and morbidity from service personnel serving in fields of conflict. Further support was offered by the Defense Advanced Research Project Agency (DARPA) for developing a system aimed at performing vascular surgery from remote [27]. Another project funded by DARPA gave birth to the voice-controlled robotic laparoscopic camera system, named AESOP® (Automated Endoscopic System for Optimal Positioning) (Computer Motion, Inc., Goleta, CA) and received FDA approval in 1994.

To improve surgeon dexterity during minimally invasive procedures, the same company developed an integrated robotic system composed of a control console connected to three robotic arms attached to the operating table, forming a tele-manipulator system. The endoscope holder arm was voice-controlled and the two other arms, with 4 DoFs each, hold a variety of instruments manipulated with joysticks from the surgeon console. The main clinical application was cardiovascular surgery, two aortocoronary bypasses were performed in 1999 [28].

In 1995, F. Moll and R. Young founded Intuitive Surgical in California and developed a new robotic surgical system, which they called MONA. In 1997, the first cholecystectomy was performed on a 72-year-old patient. The system was able to reproduce the surgeon's hand movements within the patient, giving the surgeon the impression of being immersed in the operative field. The first version of the da Vinci® surgical system with three arms became available in Europe in January 1999 and obtained FDA approval in July 2000.

Cardio-Thoracic

Despite first robotic devices were specifically designed for cardiovascular procedures, as already described, that surgical segment was not greatly pervaded by such technologies. Recently, robotic endovascular catheters for minimally invasive procedures have been proposed, but the spectrum of possible applications is being increased, as well as the possibility of reflecting the haptic feeling to the remote cardiologists (such as the Magellan system from Hansen Medical[5]).

F. Moll also founded Auris Health, aimed at developing micro-instrumentation (so-called Monarch) for diagnostic and therapeutic bronchoscopic procedures.

At the same time, Intuitive Surgical (CA, USA) is releasing the ion system, for a similar surgical application.

The Future of Robotic Surgery

The rise in robots used to assist surgical operations in the last 20 years is undoubted. Global surgical robots market size stood at USD 1463 million in 2018 and is projected to reach USD 6875 million by 2026, exhibiting a CAGR of 21.4% between 2018 and 2026.[6] Surgeons are recognizing that robots can increase the surgical outcome and decrease the possibility of errors. Patients are less and less skeptical of being operated by surgeons assisted by robots and the general tendency is to trust technology in exchange for increased results, reduced invasiveness and hospital stay.

[5] Hansen Medical was bought in 2016 by Auris Health, which was then bought in 2019 by Johnson & Johnson.

[6] fortunebusinessinsights.com/industry-reports/surgical-robots-market-100948

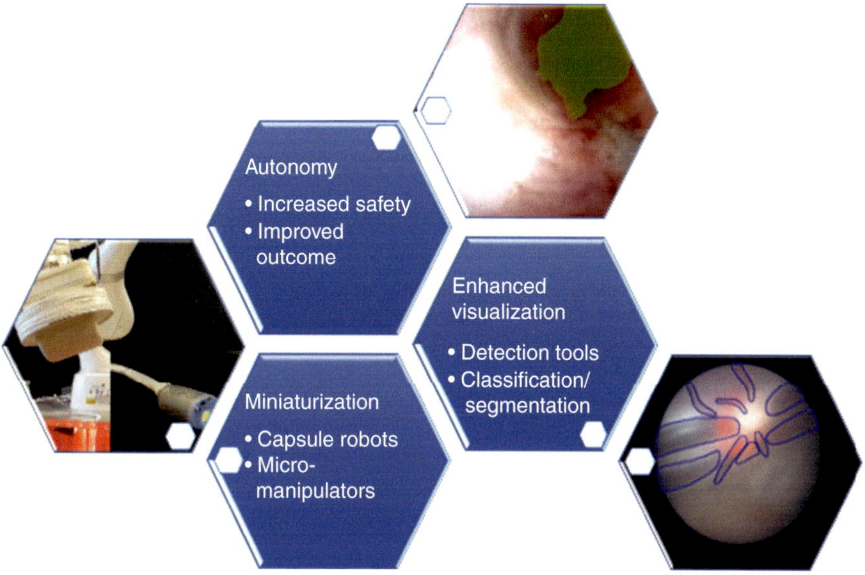

Fig. 2.2 Research directions for new robotic systems used in surgery

The three main directions towards which worldwide research and development are pointing at can be summarized in: (1) increased tools miniaturization, allowing reaching narrow spaces further reducing the size of the needed surgical access; (2) enhanced vision capabilities, and (3) greater autonomy (Fig. 2.2).

Miniaturization

Medical MicroInstruments (MMI) (Italy) is developing a robotic platform for reconstructive microsurgery for lymph vessel anastomosis and micro-neurosurgery. The platform has been preclinically validated.

Preceyes BV[7] is developing a system for vitreoretinal eye surgery, with stated precision of 10 microns. The system is currently tested in clinical trials.

From swallowed capsule robots for gastroscopy, we are now close to see magnetically actuated capsule robots, for colonoscopy. Human trials will start soon with the aim of proving that such approaches can be more efficient in detecting malignant tissue and less painful for the patients.

Smaller and smaller robotic devices are being designed, which could also be implanted, and which could be aimed at target personalized therapies.

[7] http://www.preceyes.nl/

Vision

The possibilities offered by artificial intelligence in image processing astonish (e.g., the reconstruction of a black hole achieved in April 2019). Filters on the endoscopic light and contrast media have allowed enhancing malignant tissue in the collected images in several surgical applications [29]. Artificial intelligence tools based on, e.g., deep learning allow for the automatic classification of tissues, detection of anatomical lesions, surgical tools and, in general, identification of the surgical step of the workflow [30]. This research line (called "surgical-data-science") will allow enhancing the surgeon awareness of the context and the possibility of preventing errors [31].

Autonomy

From the milestone paper describing the 5 levels of autonomy of robots in surgery [32] and the review paper listing all the attempts in literature towards the inclusion of autonomous control in surgical robotics [33], it is clear that increased autonomy means increased safety.

As reported, autonomy spans a broad range of possibilities. Several attempts have been performed and already translated into clinical practice for what concerns planning of safest paths in needle insertion, avoiding anatomical structures at risk. A review has been recently published by Scorza et al. [34].

Researchers have been also working on making some surgical gestures such as stapling, suturing, tissue retraction autonomously performed by the robotics arms, without the surgeon control, based on the processing of endoscopic images. Autonomous control will offer a further safety overlay, likewise autonomous control is offering to the automotive industry. The surgeon will always be in the loop, having the possibility to stop and change to manual surgery. Attention should be paid in training young surgeons, so that doctors are trained to go back to the manual approach in case of need.

Conclusion

In general, in the surgical robotics environment, the need for clinical evidence is recognized. Although the existing robotic platforms have an important role in other surgical interventions such as prostatectomies, clinical and economic benefit or at least equivalence must be demonstrated by properly conducted randomized controlled trials.

References

1. Hunt VD. Introduction to robotics. In: Hunt VD, editor. Industrial robotics handbook. New York: Industrial Press Inc; 1983. p. 3–21.
2. Davies B. A review of robotics in surgery. Proc Inst Mech Eng Part H J Eng Med. 2000;214(1):129–40.
3. Kwoh Y, Hou J, Jonckheere G, Hayah S. A robot with improved absolute positioning accuracy got CT-guided stereotactic brain surgery. IEEE Trans Biomed Eng. 1988;55:153–60.
4. Taylor RH, Paul HA, Mittelstadt BD, Glassman E, Musits BL, Bargar WL. Robotic total hip replacement surgery in dogs. Annu Int Conf IEEE Eng Med Biol Proc. 1989;11 pt 3(1):887–9.
5. Davies BL, Hibberd RD, Coptcoat MJ, Wickham JEA. A surgeon robot prostatectomy—a laboratory evaluation. J Med Eng Technol. 1989;13(6):273–7.
6. Mittelstadt BD, Kazanzides P, Zuhers J, Cain P and Williamson B. Robotic surgery: achieving predictable results in an unpredictable environment. In: Proceedings of 6th international conference on advanced robotics Tokyo, November 1993, pp. 367–372.
7. Martelli SM, Marcacci M, Nofrini L, et al. Computer- and robot-assisted total knee replacement: analysis of a new surgical procedure. Ann Biomed Eng. 2000;28(9):1146–53.
8. Brandt G, Radermacher K, Lavallée S, Staudte HW, Rau G. A compact robot for image guided orthopedic surgery: concept and preliminary results. In: Troccaz J, Grimson E, Mösges R, editors. CVRMed-MRCAS'97. CVRMed 1997, MRCAS 1997. Lecture Notes in Computer Science, vol. 1205. Berlin, Heidelberg: Springer.
9. Davies B, Fan K, Hibberd R, Jakopec M, Harris S. ACROBOT—using robots and surgeons synergistically in knee surgery. Int Conf Adv Robot Proceedings, ICAR. 1997:173–8.
10. Faria C, Erlhagen W, Rito M, De Momi E, Ferrigno G, Bicho E. Review of robotic technology for stereotactic neurosurgery. IEEE Rev Biomed Eng. 2015;3333:1–13.
11. Benabid AL, Cinquin P, Lavallée S, JF LB, Demongeot J, de Rougemont J. Computer-driven robot for stereotactic surgery connected to CT scan and magnetic resonance imaging. Technological design and preliminary results. Appl Neurophysiol. 1987;50:153–4.
12. Benabid AL, Hoffmann D, Lavallée S, et al. Is there any future for robots in neurosurgery? In: Symon L, Calliauw L, Cohadon F, et al., editors. Advances and technical standards in neurosurgery, vol. 18. Vienna: Springer; 1991. p. 3–45.
13. Cardinale F, Cossu M, Castana L, et al. Stereoelectroencephalography: surgical methodology, safety, and stereotactic application accuracy in 500 procedures. Neurosurgery. 2013;72(3):353–66.
14. Cardinale F, Rizzi M, D'Orio P, et al. A new tool for touch-free patient registration for robot-assisted intracranial surgery: application accuracy from a phantom study and a retrospective surgical series. Neurosurg Focus. 2017;42(5):E8.
15. Cardinale F, Rizzi M, Vignati E, et al. Stereoelectroencephalography: retrospective analysis of 742 procedures in a single Centre. Brain. 2019;142:2688–704.
16. Sharma JD, Seunarine KK, Tahir MZ, Tisdall MM. Accuracy of robot-assisted versus optical frameless navigated stereoelectroencephalography electrode placement in children. J Neurosurg Pediatr. 2019;23:297–302.
17. Glauser D, Fankhauser H, Epitaux M, Hefti J, Jaccottet A. Neurosurgical robot Minerva: first results and current developments. J Image Guid Surg. 1995;1:266–72.
18. De Momi E, Ferrigno G. Robotic and artificial intelligence for keyhole neurosurgery: the Robocast project, a multi-modal autonomous path planner. Proc Inst Mech Eng Part H J Eng Med. 2010;224(5):715–27.
19. De Momi E, Caborni C, Cardinale F, et al. Automatic trajectory planner for StereoElectroEncephaloGraphy procedures: a retrospective study. IEEE Trans Biomed Eng. 2013;60(4):986–93.

20. De Momi E, Caborni C, Cardinale F, et al. Multi-trajectories automatic planner for StereoElectroEncephaloGraphy (SEEG). Int J Comput Assist Radiol Surg. 2014;9:1087–97.
21. Vaccarella A, Comparetti MD, Enquobahrie A, Ferrigno G, De Momi E. Sensors management in robotic neurosurgery: the ROBOCAST project. Proc Annu Int Conf IEEE Eng Med Biol Soc EMBS.
22. Comparetti MD, Vaccarella A, Dyagilev I, Shoham M, Ferrigno G, De Momi E. Accurate multi-robot targeting for keyhole neurosurgery based on external sensor monitoring. Proc Inst Mech Eng Part H J Eng Med. 2012;226(5):347–59.
23. Favaro A, Cerri L, Galvan S, Rodriguez y Baena F, De Momi E. Automatic optimized 3D path planner for steerable catheters with heuristic search and uncertainty tolerance. Proc—IEEE Int Conf Robot Autom. 2018:9–16.
24. Beretta E, DeMomi E, Rodriguez Y, Baena F, Ferrigno G. Adaptive hands-on control for reaching and targeting tasks in surgery. Int J Adv Robot Syst. 2015;12:1–9.
25. D'Souza MD, Gendreau J, Feng A, Kim LH, Ho AL, Veeravagu A. Robotic-assisted spine surgery: history, efficacy, cost, and future trends. Robot Surg Res Rev. 2019;6:9–23.
26. Marino MV, Shabat G, Gulotta G, Komorowski AL. From illusion to reality: A brief history of robotic surgery. Surg Innov. 2018;25(3):291–6.
27. George EI, Brand TC, LaPorta A, Marescaux J, Satava RM. Origins of robotic surgery: from skepticism to standard of care. JSLS J Soc Laparoendosc Surg. 2018;22(4):e2018.00039.
28. Watanabe G, Takahashi M, Misaki T, Kotoh K, Doi Y. Beating-heart endoscopic coronary artery surgery. Lancet. 1999;354:2131–2.
29. Araújo T, Santos CP, De Momi E, Moccia S. Learned and handcrafted features for early-stage laryngeal SCC diagnosis. Med Biol Eng Comput. 2019;57(12):2683–92.
30. Nakawala H, Bianchi R, Pescatori LE, De Cobelli O, Ferrigno G, De Momi E. "Deep-onto" network for surgical workflow and context recognition. Int J Comput Assist Radiol Surg. 2019;14(4):685–96.
31. Maier-Hein L, Vedula SS, Speidel S, et al. Surgical data science for next-generation interventions. Nat. Biomed Eng. 2017;1(9):691–6.
32. Yang GZ, Cambias J, Cleary K, et al. Medical robotics—regulatory, ethical, and legal considerations for increasing levels of autonomy. Sci Robot. 2017;2(4):1–3.
33. Attanasio A, Scaglioni B, De Momi E, Fiorini P, Valdastri P. Autonomy in surgical robotics. Annu Rev Control Robot Auton Syst. 2021;4(1):651–79.
34. Scorza D, El Hadji S, Cortés C, et al. Surgical planning assistance in keyhole and percutaneous surgery: a systematic review. Med Image Anal. 2021;67:101820.

Chapter 3
General Principles of Robotics

Guido Caccianiga and Giancarlo Ferrigno

Abbreviations

AA	Anthropomorphic arm
AI	Artificial intelligence
AR	Anthropomorphic robot
AV	Autonomous vehicle
CAS	Computer-aided surgery
CBCT	Cone beam computer-aided tomography
CT	Computer aided tomography
DBS	Deep brain stimulation
DIH	Digital innovation hub
DIH-HERO	DIH for HEalthcare RObotics
DoF	Degree of freedom
EE	End effector
FB	Feedback

G. Caccianiga (✉)
Department of Electronics, Information and Bioengineering – DEIB, Politecnico di Milano, Milano, Italy

Haptics Intelligence Department, Max Planck Institute for Intelligent Systems, Stuttgart, Germany
e-mail: guido.caccianiga@mail.polimi.it

G. Ferrigno
Department of Electronics, Information and Bioengineering – DEIB, Politecnico di Milano, Milano, Italy

NeuroEngineering and Medical Robotics Lab – NearLab (POLIMI Leonardo Robotics Labs), Milano, Italy
e-mail: giancarlo.ferrigno@polimi.it

J. A. González Martínez, F. Cardinale (eds.), *Robotics in Neurosurgery*,
https://doi.org/10.1007/978-3-031-08380-8_3

FF	Feedforward
FK	Forward kinematics
FM	Fiducial marker
IEC	International electrotechnical committee
IK	Inverse kinematics
ISO	International standard organization
JWG	Joint working group
LoA	Level of autonomy
LVDT	Linear variable differential transformer
MRI	Magnetic resonance imaging
OR	Operating room
RASE	Robot-assisted surgical equipment
RASS	Robot-assisted surgical system
sEEG	Stereo electroencephalography

Introduction to Medical Robotics

Notwithstanding the wide number of already existing clinical applications matured in the last three decades, defining a medical robot is a hard challenge that still depends upon the medical application and the technology. A very recent analysis of robotic surgical systems for keyhole and endoscopic procedures, for example, has been published by Chen et al. in July 2020 [1]. A survey about this definition is important for properly framing the history and prospective uptake of robotics systems in neurosurgery, as well as in other fields.

A help in this sense comes from the work carried out since the beginning of 2010 by Joint working groups (JWG) of ISO (International Organization for Standardization) and IEC (International Electrotechnical Commission) committees, which have defined two main standards about medical robots (published in 2019).

The need of setting up JWGs for this purpose raised from the fact that ISO has been largely involved in industrial robot standards, while, on the other hand, IEC has been committed to medical electrical equipment standards (e.g., the IEC 60601 series), so a common effort was indeed needed.

Further definitions of medical robots have been brought about or fostered, recently, by European Commission (EC) funding schemes managed by unit A1 of the DG CONNECT (Directorate-General for Communications Networks, Content and Technology). Between 2018 and 2020, several ICT[1] calls have addressed the Robotics and Artificial Intelligence (AI) challenges including and promoting healthcare domain topics.

The interest of EC conjugates a better healthcare delivery for citizens at a reduced cost for the providers, with the concurrent development of new industrial markets

[1] ICT - Information and Communication Technology

and technologies in the framework of Industry 4.0. Among the projects started under that umbrella, the Digital Innovation hub in Healthcare Robotics (DIH-HERO) is relevant for medical robotics. DIH-HERO is an independent platform, funded by EC, which connects Digital Innovation Hubs across Europe to create a sustainable network for helping all those who are active in the healthcare robotics sector. The project consortium consists of 17 core partners spread across 11 pan-European countries.[2] This consortium has defined five paradigmatic application areas for robotics, which are helpful in the definition of medical robots (see "Fields of Application of Robotics in Health-Care" Section).

In order to define and classify a medical robot, a unique definition of Robot, though possibly changing in the years, is mandatory.

Robots at a Glance

Definition of Robot and Robotic Devices has been developed by ISO 8373:2012, "*Robots and Robotic Devices—Vocabulary*" in 2012. At that time, the vocabulary was managed by Subcommittee SC 2 (Robots and Robotic Devices) under the umbrella of the Technical Committee (TC) ISO/TC 184 (Automation Systems and Integration). Nowadays the increasing importance of robots in their wide range of applications, including professional robots for healthcare, has pushed to create a new Technical Committee ISO/TC 299 completely dedicated to Robotics.

Following ISO 8372 definition, a robot is an "*actuated mechanism programmable in two or more axes with a degree of autonomy, moving within its environment, to perform intended tasks.*" It "*includes the control system and its interface with the operator.*"

While also laypeople are quite familiar with the control system (basically perceived as a big box) and the interface (becoming more and more user friendly), the required autonomy needed to be classified as a robot is still a critical and nebulous point. Only recently this topic has been brought to a wide audience by discussing safety in Autonomous Vehicles (AV, e.g., Tesla autonomous cars).

On the one hand, autonomy is expected to speed up operation time and relieve cognitive load (for a surgeon or car driver), on the other, it raises ethical and legal problems related to the possibility of errors, possibly fatal, the responsible of which (human or machine error) is hard to define. An example is choosing, for a sentient car, between killing somebody crossing the street or killing the driver (who paid for the car!) crashing on a wall to dodge the undisciplined pedestrian. Extension to neurosurgery would be, as an example, the well-known trade-off between sparing eloquent areas and avoiding relapse.

---

[2] https://dih-hero.eu/; https://www.deib.polimi.it/eng/research-projects/details/339 (retrieved on 15/1/2021)

Standards for Medical Robots

As mentioned above, in 2019, two "particular"[3] standards for medical robotics have been published after an almost ten-year-long process, started in June 2011 in Torrance, CA, at "Toyota Motor Sales" premises, involving expert, mainly industrial and freelance, of standardization, medical electronic devices, and robots. Some medical experts participated from time to time as well.

These standards allow for a comprehensive definition of medical robots (see abstracts here below). They are available at ISO and IEC with the following identifiers:

- IEC 80601-2-77:2019[4]—Medical electrical equipment—Part 2-77: Particular requirements for the basic safety and essential performance of robotically assisted surgical equipment.
- IEC 80601-2-78:2019[5] Medical electrical equipment—Part 2-78: Particular requirements for basic safety and essential performance of medical robots for rehabilitation, assessment, compensation or alleviation.

The abstract of the "particular" 2-77 mentions

> "*IEC 80601-2-77:2019 applies to the* ***basic safety*** *and* ***essential performance*** *of* ***Robotically Assisted Surgical Equipment*** *(RASE) and* ***Robotically Assisted Surgical Systems*** *(RASS), referred to as* ***ME equipment*** *and* ***ME systems*** *together with their* ***interaction conditions*** *and* ***interface conditions****.*"

The abstract of the "particular" 2-78 states the following

> "*IEC 80601-2-78:2019 applies to the general requirements for* ***basic safety*** *and* ***essential performance*** *of* ***medical robots*** *that physically interact with a* ***patient*** *with an* ***impairment*** *to support or perform* ***rehabilitation, assessment, compensation*** *or* ***alleviation*** *related to the* ***patient's movement functions****, as intended by the* ***manufacturer****. IEC 80601-2-78:2019 does not apply to external limb prosthetic devices (covered in ISO 22523), electric wheelchairs (covered by ISO 7176 (all parts)), diagnostic imaging equipment (e.g. MRI, covered in IEC 60601-2-33), and personal care* ***robots*** *(covered in ISO 13482).*"

Although the "particular" which is better related to the robots in neurosurgery is the 80601-2-78, both abstracts highlight two important concepts in standardization: "Basic Safety" and "Essential Performance."

Basic Safety is related to the elimination or mitigation of all the possible risks for whom is defined in the vocabulary ISO 8373:2012 as Beneficiary (usually the patient, unless he or she falls in the User category as for in some home-based treatments) and for the User (usually the medical operator). Basic Safety thus accounts

---

[3] A particular standard is an add on to a family of standards, which includes provisions for a particular device. As an example a collection of requirements for the basic safety and essential performance of cardiac defibrillators is a particular of medical electrical equipment.

[4] https://www.iso.org/standard/68473.html (retrieved on 15/1/2021)

[5] https://www.iso.org/standard/68474.htm (retrieved on 15/1/2021)

for risk related to system malfunctioning, which can generate harm to the people involved (not only the patient).

Essential Performance is that way of functioning of the RASS or RASE, which, if not respected, may not cause direct immediate harm to the people involved, but does not ensure proper use of the system. This can potentially threaten the effectiveness of a therapy leading to morbidity or death instead of a healthy life.

As a general example, the loss of accuracy in surgical tool positioning is a lack of Essential Performance, which must be checked at each use with proper registration tools.

A force transmission cable breakage is a lack of Basic Safety, which must be prevented, for example, by defining the maximum number of uses of a surgical tool, which does not likely cause such a breakage. It is intended that the breakage not only stops the operation, but potentially may hurt the patient in his/her internal organs possibly leading not only to a failure of treatment, but to permanent damage or death. In the example, a maximum number of uses should be counted by the system hardware to avoid user misuse.

The impact of these adverse events strongly depends upon the field of application. As an example, the need for Basic Safety and Essential Performance is particularly important for neurosurgery, where the delicate and highly interconnected neural cells may, in a small area, control important functions, which, if lost, can affect dramatically the life of the patient. Indeed 5 mm of error in tool positioning may be in this case intolerable and the effect devastating. This example confirms the dependence of Basic Safety and Essential Performance upon the application. Indeed, in an orthopedic intervention, 5 mm error in hip joint center location creates an error lower than 1° of error in femur functional axis positioning, which is fully tolerable.

Robotic Autonomy

Robot autonomy, explicitly mentioned in ISO 8372 definition as a robot component, has recently been a hot topic for application domains such as AI and AV. Defining and regulating autonomy in surgery represent an even more delicate and challenging task. While introducing the automation of certain procedures and a more comfortable human–robot interaction should provide a remarkable step forward in terms of efficiency, safety, and usability of surgical robots, the actual deployment of autonomous systems remains, as of today, mostly limited to research applications.

Levels of Autonomy (LoA) have been widely discussed in the past decades. An example among the most cited is the paper of Sheridan and Verplank [2] that in 1978 proposed a ten LoA scale for describing the cooperation of generic operator and computer (the application to the case of surgical robots is straightforward, replacing "computer" with "robotic system control").

The ten LoA of the Sheridan paper are the following, starting with the lowest (1) and ending with the highest (10) LoA (where the word "computer" can be substituted with "Robot Control and Planning system"):

1. Computer offers no assistance; human does it all.
2. Computer offers a complete set of action alternatives.
3. Computer narrows the selection down to a few choices.
4. Computer suggests a single action.
5. Computer executes that action if human approves.
6. Computer allows the human limited time to veto before automatic execution.
7. Computer executes automatically, then necessarily informs the human.
8. Computer informs human after automatic execution only if human asks.
9. Computer informs human after automatic execution only if it decides to.
10. Computer decides everything and acts autonomously, ignoring the human.

More recently, AV, drones, and underwater robots development raised a similar problem including strong ethical and legal issues. The most popular LoA scale for AV is on 6 levels, from 0 meaning no autonomy, to 5 which means complete autonomy (level 10 in Sheridan's table). The intermediate levels are:

Level 1, driver assistance (already exists) including support functions as brake assistance and cruise control.

Level 2, partial automation, includes vehicles assisting with functions like steering, braking, and speed control, although drivers still need to have both hands on the wheel and be ready to take control if necessary. No other constraints must be applied.

Level 3, conditional automation, allows drivers to release hands and let the car do all the driving. Many Level 3 cars do not require any human intervention when driven at a moderate speed of less than 60 km/h.

Level 4, high automation, AV manage steering, accelerating, and braking. They're also able to monitor road conditions and respond to obstacles, determining when to turn and when to change lanes. Level 4 autonomous driving can only be activated when road conditions are ideal.

In 2017, Guang-Zhong Yang and other 12 authors published an editorial [3] discussing the "Regulatory, ethical, and legal considerations for increasing levels of autonomy" in Medical Robotics. They proposed, for the discussion, a paradigm of 6 LoA (starting from 0, the lowest as for AV) that will be only partially commented here recommending the reader to access the cited paper for further in-depth information (see Table 3.1).

Elaborating the similarities between medical robots and AV LoA, we can see that also for medical robots, the "road conditions" are important. So we can expect that LoA can increase only if the anatomy and physiology are well known and detectable (better intelligent imaging systems), the procedure is standardized and the expected adverse events are very rare and at some extent predictable, so that a risk/benefit ratio can be easily evaluated.

Table 3.1 The six levels of autonomy for medical robots, as defined by Yang et al. [3]. The lowest level is no autonomy, level 5 is complete autonomy. As can be seen, there are many resemblances with the AV scale reported in the text

Level of autonomy	Description	Specifications
0	No autonomy	This level includes tele-operated robots or prosthetic devices
1	Robot assistance	The robot provides some mechanical assistance during a task. Examples include surgical robots with virtual fixtures (also known as active constraints, electronic corridors, etc.)
2	Task autonomy	The robot is autonomous for specific tasks initiated by a human, for example, suturing
3	Conditional autonomy	A system generates task strategies but relies on the human to approve and/or select from among different strategies
4	High autonomy	The robot can make medical decisions but under the supervision of a qualified doctor, like it was a resident
5	Full autonomy	No human intervention is needed

Fields of Application of Robotics in Health-Care

As anticipated above, a very recent taxonomy of robotics application areas in healthcare has been brought about (although the last two are probably going to change the name for a better understanding of the meaning) by the EC-funded project DIH-HERO. In brackets some paradigmatic examples.

- DIAGNOSTIC ROBOTICS
  (Human function analysis, automated imaging, capsule endoscopy, blood sampling)
- INTERVENTIONAL ROBOTICS
  (Surgical robotics, image-guided robotics, dry or wet training robotics)
- REHABILITATION ROBOTICS
  (Wearable exoskeletons, mobile training devices)
- ROBOTICS SUPPORTING PATIENTS
  (Functional support, robot assistant, communication robots, social robots)
- ROBOTICS SUPPORTING HEALTHCARE PROFESSIONALS
  (Ergonomical robots, telepresence robots)

Although almost all the application areas can fit in neurosurgery, we will focus in this chapter on interventional robotics, while leaving a deep analysis of robotics exoskeletons in rehabilitation, training devices, BCI, and functional electrical stimulation in other dedicated chapters.

Robot-Assisted Surgery

Robot-assisted surgery has been introduced as a natural evolution of the "computer assisted surgery—CAS." The main difference is that in CAS the motion of the surgical instruments is controlled and generated by the surgeon, while, when the robot enters into play, it moves, with different modes, as we will see hereafter, the tool or at least controls the trajectory leaving to the surgeon the responsibility to move or not along the controlled path.

The first brain biopsy guided by images executed by a robot holding the surgical tool [4, 5] was performed in 1985. The robot base was registered with the reference system of the images of the patient, and the tool was directed toward the lesion by controlling the position of said tool. The evolution in time of the functions and approach are reported in the chapter "Historical Perspectives," but it is worth mentioning the RoboDoc® that in the same years was developed for total hip arthroplasty and was based on CT images [6].

Anyway, notwithstanding the very different requirements for the medical use of the robots (think of the difference between RoboDoc® and an endoscopic catheter insertion system), basic properties, control methods, Human–Robot Interface, etc. share some basic robotics fundamentals that will be introduced in the next section.

Fundamentals of Robotics

Basic Concepts

Starting from the robot definition given in "Robots at a Glance" Section, we see that a robot is a mechanical system supposed to have "Degrees of Freedom" (DoF), which allow it to move and carry tools in the Cartesian space (with a dimensionality up to six independent DoF, three translations, and three rotations).

A classical robot has a base, which is its global reference frame, and a kinematic chain of links, each one defined by a frame, which ends with an "end effector" (EE). This latter, in surgery, is itself, or brings, the surgical instrument to carry out the operation. The EE moves in the patient's centered space, easily registered by medical image space registration to robot base (Fig. 3.1).

A Robot is made of links connected among them by joints, the actuation of which moves the EE in space in a pose (Cartesian position x, y, and z and orientation angles such as the three Euler angles or Nautical Angles—roll, pitch, and yaw). In the three-dimensional space, the pose is specified by six independent values, three of which represent the Cartesian Position and the other three represent the Cartesian Orientation.

Joints can be rotational, i.e., the $link_{i+1}$ is moved with respect to $link_i$ thanks to a rotary actuator (e.g., an electrical motor with a gear-down box), or prismatic where

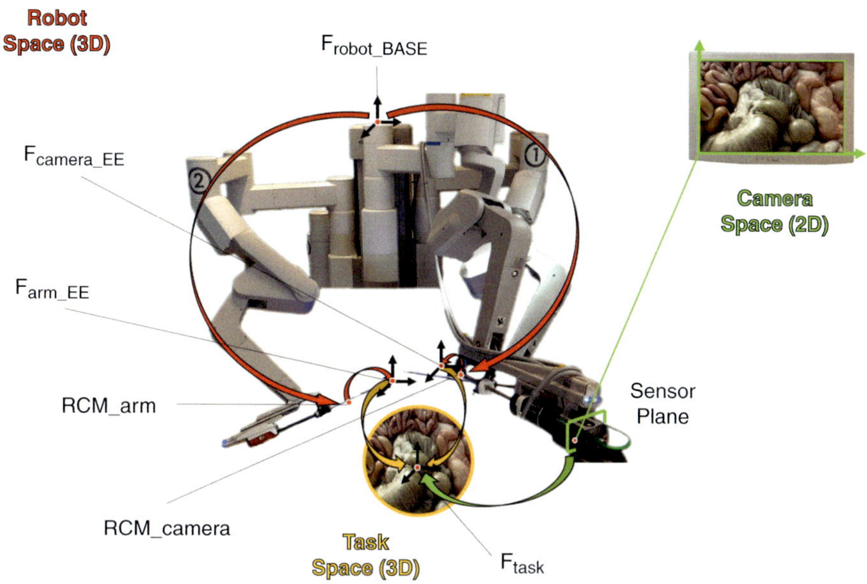

Fig. 3.1 Relationships among the OR reference frames in robotics-assisted surgery. Three spaces, opportunely registered, are highlighted: robot, task (i.e., patient), and camera reference frames. In general, the first two are three-dimensional, while camera space is a two-dimensional projection on an optical sensor. Anyway, being two projections available in the modern endoscope, surgeon's eyes let the brain perceive a stereoscopic view of the scene. The reference frames (denoted as F with subscript) of robot base, arm EE, task, and camera EE are denoted by black Cartesian axes while the relationship among them (transform) is denoted by curved, colored arrows. This information allows to easily shift from one frame to another. RCM (arm and camera) will be introduced later on in the chapter

$link_{i+1}$ slides with respect to $link_i$ thanks to a linear actuator (e.g., a slide screw or a hydraulic piston). Figure 3.2 represents the behavior for a rotational ($link_{i+1}$ is rotated with respect to $link_i$ of an angle α) and one prismatic ($link_{i+1}$ is translated of a distance d with respect to $link_i$).

Figure 3.3 presents two classic kinematic configurations that can be, in their wholeness, serial (the most used in the following examples) or parallel [7]. A well-known parallel robot for neurosurgery is the Renaissance MARS® [8], which is now under further development at Medtronic.

Links are generally supposed to be rigid rods (or other fancy shapes) and joints are supposed to be ideal mechanical hinges or prismatic coupling. There are anyway robots, also studied for surgery, which address tendons and flexible links [9].

Other robots for surgery do not present a well-defined link-joint structure, but rather a quasi-continuous deformation. An example is represented by concentric tubes [10], steerable needles [11], and snakes [12], which will not be dealt with here.

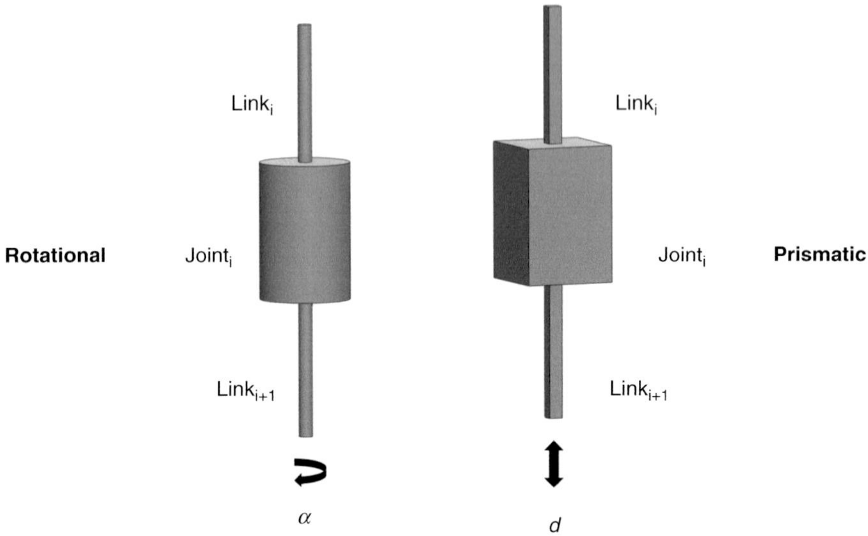

Fig. 3.2 A Robot is made of Links, which are connected among them by joints, the actuation of which moves the EE in space in a pose. In rigid robots (the one we are acquainted with) the displacement among two links is composed of rotary (rotating joint) or sliding movement (prismatic joint) relative to the previous position (link$_{i+1}$ with respect to link$_i$). Rotation is reported as α and sliding by d

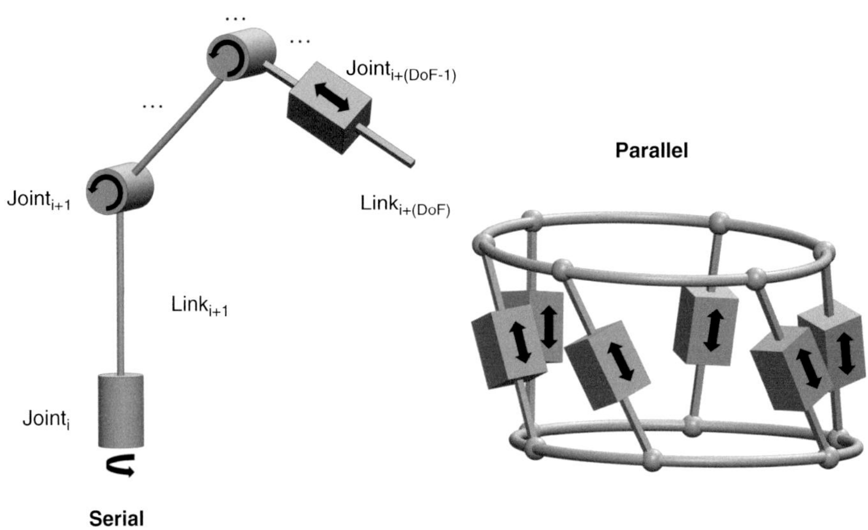

Fig. 3.3 Robots can have a serial or parallel kinematic chain. In the left part of the figure, an example of multiple link serial chain including rotary and prismatic joints is reported. Each link is connected to only one other link of the chain. In the right part, a six DoF fully parallel robot encompassing six prismatic joints is depicted

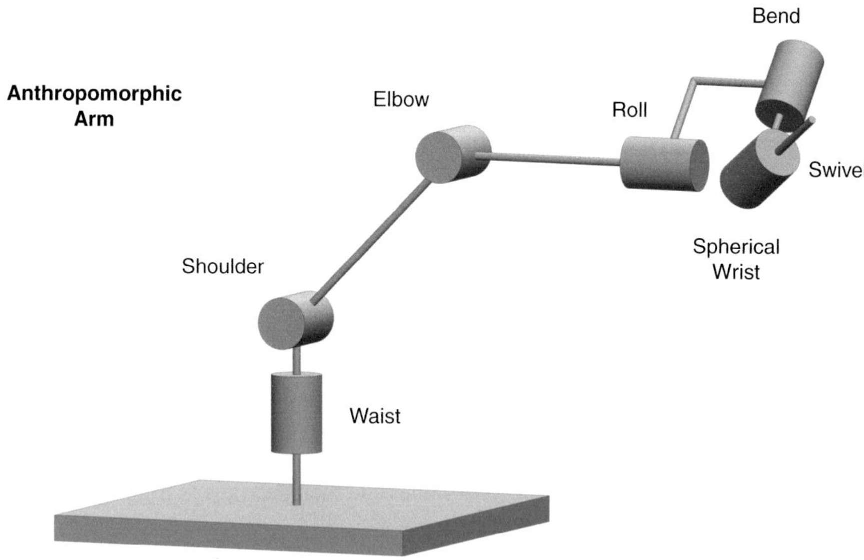

Fig. 3.4 CAD representation of a classical industrial anthropomorphic, 6 DoF, serial robot. It works by actuating 6 rotary motors. The intersection between adjacent joint axes lets us define a "waist," "shoulder," and "spherical wrist" (composed by roll, bend, and swivel). One can observe that with respect to the human arm, one DoF is missing at the shoulder (only two DoFs). Six DoFs are indeed enough to establish a pose of the EE (on the third link of the spherical wrist in the picture) in the so-called dexterity space

Robot Kinematics

One particular kind of serial robot is the "Anthropomorphic Arm" (AA). Anthropomorphism does not mean human-like in the aspect, a robot with such characteristic is rather called a humanoid.[6] Anthropomorphism is, instead, related to the similarity to the function of the human arm. A classic AA has, in fact, six rotational DoF (joints) and six links (plus a link 0, which supports the global reference frame in space). The first and second joints axes intersection define the center of the "shoulder" of the robot. The rotation axis of the first joint is called waist, while the rotation axis of the second is the shoulder. The following joint is the elbow, and the last three joints define the spherical wrist. They are defined as wrist roll, bend, and swivel (Fig. 3.4).

The full similarity with the human arm lacks one DoF at the shoulder. Seven DoF AA mimic better the human arm, but for many applications this is not required since six DoF are enough to reach any point in a sub-space (called dexterity space) with an arbitrary orientation of the EE, so apparently the seventh DoF is useless, but we will put it in the game later on.

[6] https://icub.iit.it/ (retrieved on 15/1/2021)

Simplifying the math behind the positioning of the EE in a desired position (let say an endoscope in the center of a burr hole) and orientation (pointing to a target within the body), we simply realize that we want to send the EE in a well-specified pose in the Cartesian Space, but the robot assembly can only receive angles (or sometimes translation) at the joints (Joint Space) as operational input.

Therefore, to perform the basic control of the robot, a precise Joint-to-Cartesian Space transformation (and vice versa) is needed, and this is achieved through specific kinematic formalisms.

Kinematic is the branch of mechanics that performs the rigid objects motion description without regard to the forces which cause it. Within the science of kinematics, position, velocity, and higher derivatives of motion are mathematically dealt with [13].

The Forward Kinematics (FK) represents the process of obtaining the Cartesian Space pose (position and orientation) and its derivatives from a given Joint Space configuration (angles).

The inverse process (computing joint values and their derivatives from a Cartesian Space pose) is called, instead, Inverse Kinematics (IK).

A full kinematic chain is built up by specifying the dimensional (by the links formalism) and mechanical (by the joints formalism) properties of each structural component of the robotic assembly (Denavit-Hartenberg, or D-H, parameters [14]).

Within the space of dexterity FK has always solutions, (they may be more than one depending on the so-called configuration like elbow up, elbow down, etc.), while IK, for example, in setting Cartesian velocity from joint space velocity, could fall in singularities, which make the computation impossible, basically requiring almost infinite velocity to reach a specific configuration. Singularities are often related to the collinearity of two or more links, in such configuration the robotic structure cannot guarantee the designed dexterity, and the number of actual DoFs is reduced. The potential presence of such singularities inside the workspace often leads to a modification in the design of the robot consisting of the introduction of one or more additional degrees of freedom (the structure is therefore defined as redundant) which improves the manipulability, versatility, and stability of the robot. Redundancy on a robotic arm allows, in fact, the possibility of reaching the same desired pose with different alternative values of the joints. This could, for example, be used to rearrange a robotic arm to avoid unwanted contacts potentially harmful to the OR personnel and instrumentation while keeping the EE steady [15].

Architecture

The functionality, geometry, potential field of application, and many other characteristics of a robotic system strongly impact its low-level mechanical design.

A robot can be defined as serial when its structure is composed of an end effector having multiple degrees of freedom and a fixed base linked together by a single kinematic chain where each link is connected only to the previous and the following link (Fig. 3.3).

A serial manipulator is, in fact, also defined as an open-loop manipulator since each link is never connected to more than one of the previous links in the kinematic chain.

A parallel manipulator can be defined, instead, as a closed-loop mechanism composed of an end effector having n degrees of freedom and a fixed base, linked together by at least two independent kinematic chains [16].

A widely adopted closed-loop architecture is the parallelogram; such a mechanical structure is composed of at least four links with equal pairwise dimensions interconnected by rotational joints.

The peculiarity of the parallelogram design is that of generating, when properly configured (Fig. 3.5), a mechanical Remote Center of Motion (RCM).

An RCM can be seen as a point inside the kinematic chain which is stationary in position but follows the orientation changes of the link in which it is located. Such an entity provides a kinematically constrained pivoting motion (also said fulcrum) at the point where the endoscope or tool enters the patient's body [17, 18].

The RCM turns out to be fundamental in most of the surgical keyhole and minimally invasive robotic applications where a surgical tool has to be inserted inside the body and no perpendicular forces with respect to the tool entrance direction want to be exerted on the tissue surrounding the entrance hole.

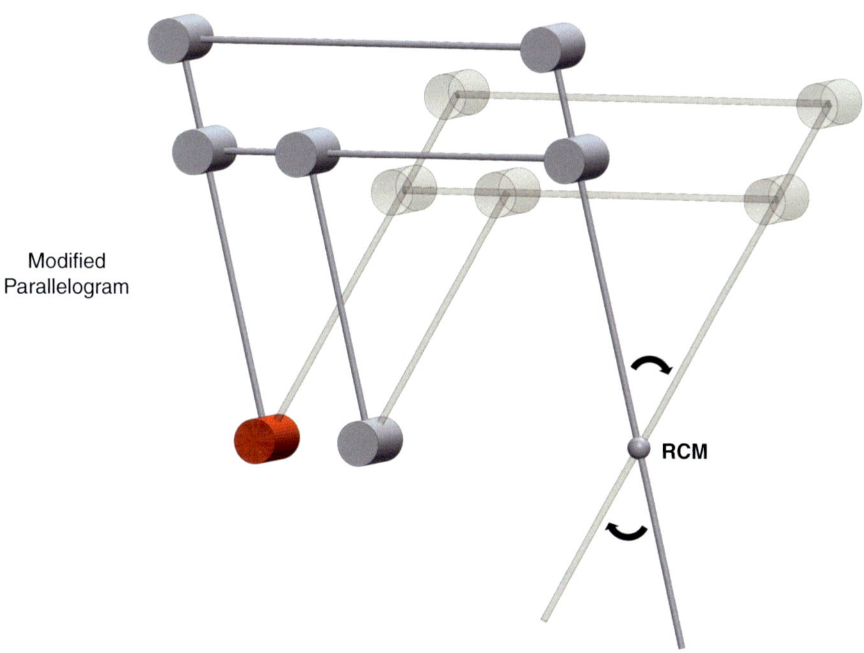

Fig. 3.5 A modified parallelogram structure allows the establishment of "physical" RCM. In the figure two different positions (solid and shaded) of a parallelogram, which preserve the position (not the pose) of RCM, are shown. The actuating joint is reported in red, while all the other joints are passive

Inserting a tool inside a body without aligning correctly, the RCM and the tool entrance site would lead to potential tissue damages or limits to the EE workspace.

Note that a virtual RCM (oppositely to mechanical) can be obtained through proper control of a serial manipulator [19].

Well-known commercial serial robots deployed for neurosurgery are the NeuroMate® and the Rosà® (Medtech S.A. Montpellier, France) while a parallel configuration is used in the spine robot MARS® (Mazor Robotics Ltd. Orlando, USA) and Surgiscope® (ISIS Robotics, Grenoble, France). They all have no mechanical RCM [20]. A widely adopted robot both serial and parallel with RCM is the daVinci Surgical System® (Intuitive Surgical Inc. Sunnyvale, USA).

Control and Interfacing

When considering a robot from the control perspective, we can see it as an input-output system where we model three fundamental components: a sensor, a controller, and an effector.

A sensor is an apparatus, electromechanical in most applications, deployed to the measurement and transduction of a specific physical variable (i.e., force, light, angular position, etc.) into an electrical signal.

Sensor outputs can be deployed as simple "watchdogs" to prevent system damage when a value goes over-threshold or can be used continuously by the controller to modulate a response or an action (perception-action paradigm).

The controller is, in fact, a computational unit where one or more codes are run to interpret the sensors signals following a specific control strategy to constantly obtain the desired operational outputs.

The effector, finally, is the component deployed to the transduction of the controller output signal into a behavioral effect of the robotic system (i.e., the activation of an electrical motor or a hydraulic or pneumatic piston).

This control scheme holds true both at the low level when considering the simple single joint angular positioning (Fig. 3.6), and at the high level when, for example, considering an autonomous car perceiving the environment through multiple advanced sensors and actuating hundreds of mechanical systems to keep the correct trajectory.

A robotic system is, in fact, composed of many elementary control loops with different control strategies and feedback modalities, and the complexity of the subsystems interconnection increases with the growing number of joints, arms, interfacing modalities, and, finally, degrees of autonomy featured by the system.

A controller can deploy mostly an infinite number of different control strategies, and each application finds its specific architecture, anyhow, the three main branches of control loops are FeedBack (FB) or error-based, FeedForward (FF) or model-based, and Adaptive or data-driven (or a combination of all of them) [21].

The first two modalities represent the classic architectures and most of the robotic control systems can be modeled through FB, FF, or combinations of those loops (Fig. 3.7).

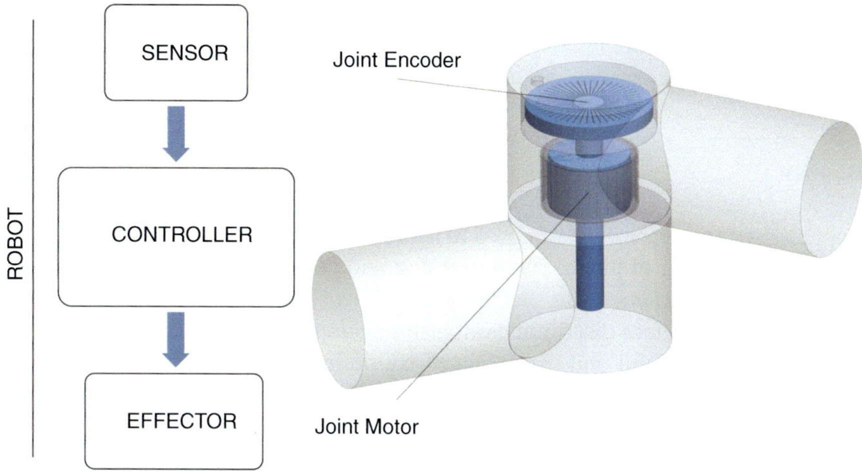

Fig. 3.6 The general control system (left block diagram) for robots encompasses sensor, controller, and effector. In the figure, an example including only one joint and two links is reported. At this very low level of control, the effector is the joint motor actuator, which should ideally send the link to the desired pose, while the actual position is read by the joint encoder. The controller reduces the possible errors in positioning, also avoiding any oscillations around the target position

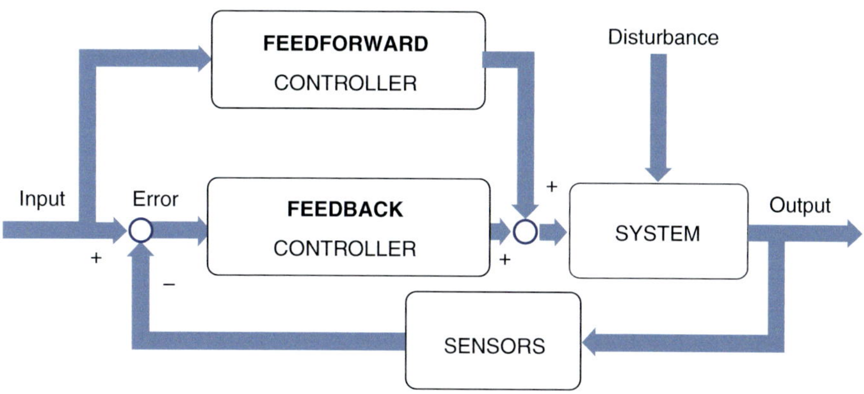

Fig. 3.7 Robot controller example. The controller is split into two parts, the feedback and feedforward blocks. Feedforward exploits the a priori knowledge, so the output is directly dependent on the input, while the feedback loop is driven by the residual error. This latter is built on the difference between input and actual output. The dynamics of the system could give rise to high errors or instability of the overall loop. This latter can be avoided by properly designing the "Feedback Controller" block

The third class refers to the most recently trending field of Machine Learning and Artificial Intelligence where the input-output transfer function is trained, tested, and constantly tuned according to a variety of internal and external variables and their temporal evolution [22].

Besides the aforementioned groupings, a further distinction can be made depending on the variables being controlled between the most widely used we can find motor current, force, gravity, position, and velocity.

Haptics

Haptics is a comprehensive term used to address the aspects of perception linked to the sensory domain of touch. Haptic sensing and perception are innate in humans and represent key elements to success in activities such as workspace exploration, consistency and pattern discrimination, manipulation, or force modulation.

The most successful and sophisticated haptic interface available is the human hand, where a high spatial resolution in the skin receptors coupled with the joint action of self-perceiving tendons and muscles generate a complex closed-loop, fully actuated, multi-joint/multi-DoF mechanical system.

In traditional (open) surgery, the surgeon's hand acts both as a sensor and actuator deploying an accurate and reliable action-perception loop. Minimally invasive approaches introduced a medium between the actor (the hand) and the object (the anatomical target) forcing the surgeon to re-learn the mapping of the different haptic cues.

In laparoscopy, for example, palpation and force modulation are biased by the fulcrum effect generated by the instrument and the tissue entry point (trocar); only some of the haptic cues can be transmitted by the instrument to the surgeon's hand [23].

The robotization of the surgical instruments increases the decoupling layers between the hand of the surgeon and the anatomical target; this is especially true for fully tele-operated systems where such interaction is totally decoupled. In robotic minimally invasive surgery, in fact, the action-perception loop relies only on vision: haptic cues (such as tissue properties, thread resistance, or exerted forces) need to be estimated indirectly through real-time images leading to a feedback mechanism called pseudo-haptic [24].

For what concerns neurosurgery, the use of haptics in robotics is mostly exploited to achieve stabilization of the end effector, weight reduction of the tool (i.e., gravity compensation of a drill assembly), guidance through a specific trajectory, and spatial constraint generation.

The two latter aforementioned haptic augmentations are most commonly referred to as virtual fixtures, or more specifically as haptic guidance and haptic constraints. Haptics is mainly deployed in neurosurgery in shared-control systems (see "Shared-Control Systems" Section).

Robots in the Operating Room

Medical robots have been adopted to assist in the most various types of surgery, ranging from, just to mention some, urogynecological, vascular, pulmonary, orthopedic, spinal, and cranial surgery, up to the most recent introduction in fields like ophthalmology or dental surgery [25].

Classifying medical robots, therefore, results in a non-trivial task especially considering that their structural complexity, technical features, and degree of applicational specificity are in constant growth. Nevertheless, a series of functional and morphological characteristics can always be highlighted and deployed to attempt a basic classification.

A first classification could be made depending on the size and the overall footprint of the robotic surgical system in the operating room. A distinction is worth mentioning in this context is between small robots directly attached to the patient (i.e., Mazor's MARS) or to the operating bed (i.e., Medtronic's Stealth Autoguide), or compactly transportable through wheels (i.e., Renishaw's NeuroMate), and robots that are large, heavy, and mostly grounded or not easily removable from the operating room (i.e., Intuitive's daVinci). For these two categories, we will refer to "small footprint" and "large footprint" (respectively).

While this chapter aims at delivering an as-broad-as-possible knowledge on medical robotics, a specific focus is also directed towards interventional neurosurgery robots, for which at least two other major distinctions can be made: considering (i) how the robotic manipulation is performed (passive/active), (ii) the level of autonomy in performing such manipulation (tele-surgical, shared-control, supervisory controlled) [26].

The motion strategy and the level of autonomy a robot deploys during surgery are, in fact, a direct result of both its architectural/technological features and the type of surgeon–robot interaction it was designed for. Other important aspects of the robot integration in the surgical workflow, such as the preoperative planning, the visualization methods, or the registration with the patient, are mostly dependent on the technological solutions deployed in each computer-integrated/robot-assisted operating room, as well as the specific surgical target.

For these reasons, the following subsections aim at delivering a general and hardware-oriented set of definitions and considerations, hoping to allow the reader to navigate the world of neurosurgical robots with the needed knowledge. The last one serves, specifically, as a general introduction to the concept of stereotaxis and the neurosurgical workflow. Further and more specific analyses from a functional/clinical perspective will be given in the next chapters.

Passive and Active Robots

A **passive robot** is an electromechanical system in which the intraoperative movement of the end effector is always a consequence of the end effector manipulation by the surgeon. Therefore, the robotic joints only modulate the level of backdrivability of the system (compliance to external manipulation) but do not perform "voluntary" movements directed towards the interaction with the human tissue [27].

Note that the end effector is moved in the Cartesian space by the user, while the actuation is in the joint space, so it is there that backdrivability is generated and controlled. Thus, the level of backdrivability of the robot mainly depends on fine control of actuators or application of the brakes. A good level of backdrivability is reached when the end effector applies no forces or torques to the hand, which is displacing it. It is straightforward that the gravity effect on the end effector should be canceled by the control system.

In the case of non-actuated passive robots, the level of backdrivability can be:

(i) Full backdrivability when no mechanical brakes are deployed. The structure serves only for metrology/localization purposes (e.g., using encoders or linear transducers).
(ii) Null backdrivability when brakes are deployed. The structure is mainly used to hold a guide or an instrument in a fixed configuration after manual positioning; metrology can be added through encoders and sensors [28].

In the case of actuated passive robots, it can be:

(i) Full backdrivability when joint actuators provide only the effort to keep the end effector stationary (gravity compensated), but no movement constraints are imposed (i.e., the surgeon-side manipulators of the daVinci).
(ii) Constrained backdrivability when joint actuators limit the operational workspace of the end effector resulting in haptic augmentation. Gravity compensation can be either performed or not but is present in most haptic applications to deliver more uniform and meaningful feedback.

An **active robot** is an electromechanical system in which the movement of the end effector is not exclusively a consequence of the manipulation of the surgeon when interacting with the anatomical target. Therefore, the robotic joints need to be actuated and can actively take part, intraoperatively, in the manipulation of the end effector.

The end effector of an active robot is usually backdrivable only during those applications that imply collaborative tasks between the robot and the surgeon (shared-control, "Shared-Control Systems" Section). Most frequently while an active robot is performing a task, it does not allow external perturbations (i.e., the hand of the surgeon) to modify the end effector planned trajectory.

It has to be noted that both active and passive robots, when redundant, can allow reconfiguration of the links without modifying the end effector pose (joint backdrivability).

Tele-surgical Systems

Tele-operation can simply be described as the act of controlling a moving system from a remote location [29]. This technique has been widely used through years in different contexts such as, just to mention some, robotic rescue and hazard handling, excavators and construction cranes, unmanned aerial and amphibious vehicles [30]. While its application outside the operating room is ubiquitous, the use of tele-operation in the medical field has been mostly directed towards minimally invasive robot-assisted surgery [31].

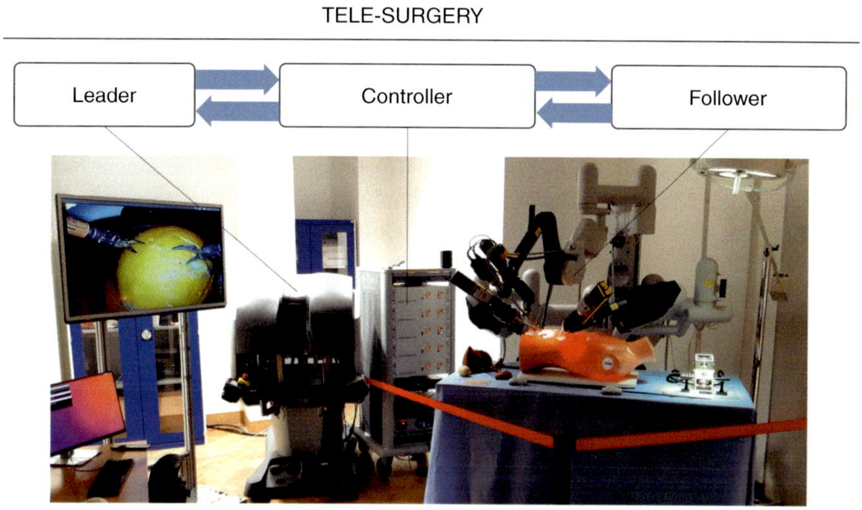

Fig. 3.8 Tele-surgical system. It usually encompasses a passive master leader unit where the surgeon inputs the motor controls, and an active patient follower unit where surgical instruments are driven by a mechanical system to reproduce the surgeon's hands motion. In the figure, the operation is simulated on the red phantom (laparoscopy). Note that the leader acts as a passive and transparent manipulandum, but in order to be really transparent, a gravity compensation is implemented. The image has been taken by authors in the dVRK room of the NeuroEngineering And medical Robotics Laboratory (NEARLab) of Politecnico di Milano

Intuitive integrated in the early 2000 the concept of tele-operation on an FDA-approved surgical system, the daVinci®. The system was submitted for approval as a sophisticated endoscopic device instead of a surgical robot. With the futuristic vision of physically decoupling, the patient and the surgeon allowing ideally for cross-oceanic tele-surgery, a Defense Advanced Research Project Agency spinoff project for surgical assistance in remote war field locations [32] has brought to the commercialization of a clinical robotic system with more than 5000 units installed in healthcare facilities all over the world.[7]

A tele-surgical system is usually composed of a passive leader unit where the surgeon inputs the motor controls, and an active follower unit where surgical instruments are driven by a mechanical system to reproduce the surgeon's hands motion (Fig. 3.8).

The original DaVinci® had, for example, two 8DoF passive, gravity compensated, fully backdrivable, redundant leaders on the surgeon side, and a multi-arm patient side (follower) composed of four passive backdrivable setup joints used for the positioning of four non-backdrivable active manipulators (three 7 DoF tool manipulators and a 4 DoF camera manipulator). Even though the most recent daVinci Xi® has reduced its overall size and introduced many technological

[7] https://isrg.gcs-web.com/ (retrieved on 15/1/2021)

advancements, the system still has a large footprint in the operating room and it lacks any form of haptic feedback.

NeuroArm is one of the most advanced tele-surgical systems ever developed for neurosurgery; it is the world's first MRI-compatible tele-operated robot and it was developed by the University of Calgary [33]. Its active patient side arms can both perform biopsy and microsurgery while performing real-time intraoperative MRI imaging guidance. The robot can perform haptic feedback through sensors applied to the patient side in the proximity of the neurosurgical tools attached to the end effector. This type of robot-imaging system fusion is a clear example of how technology is going towards a rapid integration in the operating theater. The project has been taken over by IMRIS in 2010 and up to now, the system has still to transition from research to the clinical market.

Shared-Control Systems

Following the initial tendency to deploy only passive robots, especially for keyhole neurosurgery, with the simple aim of trajectory alignment and instrument support, an intermediate step towards the integration of more advanced passive and sometimes even active systems has found its way through the operating room in what is defined as shared-control modality.

The trivial explanation of such a method is that the robot and the surgeon share either continuously or during specific steps of a procedure the control of the surgical tool.

The role of the surgical system in this collaborative context is anyhow limited to the delivery of haptic cues, as the robot is never allowed to perform the task on its own. The system can perform haptic augmentation of the surgeon's hand motion either in the form of stabilization/constraint (passive robots) or active guidance (active robots). Override should be always possible.

A well-known commercial shared-control surgical system is the ROSA® a 6DoF passive robot used in different contexts ranging from spine neurosurgery, stereotactic biopsy, Deep Brain Stimulation (DBS), to ventricular and trans-rectal endoscopy. Moreover, the system can perform haptic collaboration in the form of isocentric (through a virtual RCM), axial, and speed constraint (the latter also defined as "free-hand").

An example of mixed human-only and shared-control application is sEEG: while drill guide positioning is robot-assisted, the actual drilling and depth electrodes insertion are performed by the surgeon alone. Another example in a different field (orthopedics) is represented by Stryker's Mako SmartRobotics® with AccuStop® haptic technology, allowing the precise milling of bones in lower limb joint total or partial replacement surgery. The end effector of the robot, driven by the surgeon's hand, moves freely or gets stuck in space based on preoperative images of the bones.[8]

[8] https://www.stryker.com/us/en/portfolios/orthopaedics/joint-replacement/mako-robotic-arm-assisted-surgery.html (retrieved on 15/1/2021)

Supervisory Controlled Systems

A supervisory controlled framework is realized when one or more human operators are in charge of the decision-making process and setup of the initial conditions necessary for a procedure (e.g., the preoperative planning and the operating room setup) while supervising one or more computer-driven systems (e.g., a robot, an imaging device) performing low-level tasks. Supervisory control is also more generally defined as "…intermittently adjusting and receiving information from a computer that itself closes an inner control loop through electromechanical sensors, effectors, and the task environment." [34].

Under this definition, together with most of the human–computer–robot interaction activities investigated in the last decades, the majority of the actuated surgical robots can be classified as supervisory controlled. A crucial distinction is therefore to be made depending on the nature of the task that is left for the robot to perform.

Remaining in the neurosurgical context, sticking with the active/passive definitions of "Passive and Active Robots" Section, most of the diffused commercial systems limit their contribution to actuated, passive, tool positioning/alignment tasks (e.g., NeuroMate®, Stealth Autoguide®, Mazor X Stealth®, MARS®).

As the level of allowed autonomy grows, the surgeon moves step by step further aside from the manual control of the surgical tool. The surgical robot is no more just a sophisticated extension of the surgeon's hand (as in Tele-surgical systems), or a tool to support it (passive supervisory controlled) and to constrain/guide it (passive/active collaborative). Robots can finally start to actively and independently ("supervisedly"!) interact with the surgical target.

A classical method for supervision is the execution confirmed by the pressure on a pedal. Whenever the pedal is released, the system stops in a safety position, e.g., applying brakes. Further pressure starts the process again.

As of 2020, while high-level robotic decisional and operational autonomy are still far from realistic applications (both from technological and ethical perspectives), medical robotic research is moving towards demonstrating the feasibility of small autonomous surgical tasks such as tissue manipulation [35, 36], suturing [37, 38], or camera motion [39].

An early exception to this trend, showing already full autonomy in following the whole pre-planned and real-time re-planned treatment is the Cyberknife® (Accuray Incorporated, Sunnyvale, USA). Such a system is used to perform radiation therapy of lung tumors and it is capable of adjusting autonomously and in real-time the irradiation target accounting for both the respiratory cycle and the small movements of the patient. Cyberknife® couples a 6DoF robotic arm supporting the LINAC (linear accelerator—the source of the radiation), a localization system, and a 6DoF patient positioning system called RoboCouch®.

It has to be noted that Cyberknife® represents a unicum in 2020, as a fully autonomous interventional system on the market, and this is only possible because the risks connected to not performing such movement compensation, both in terms of missed irradiation of the target and unwanted irradiation of the surrounding healthy tissues, clearly exceed the potential risks deriving from inaccuracy of the autonomous system.

As in tele-surgery before, partially and fully autonomous systems may allow surgeons to control or supervise an increasing variety of procedures from a remote location. These far-from-the-patient modalities take even more relevance today, in the light of global pandemic outbursts, potentially removing or drastically reducing the risk of mutual infectious agents exchange in the operating room.

Stereotactic Workflow

The stereotactic technique has, since the beginning, been a fundamental methodological scaffolding for the development of keyhole neurosurgery and many other computer-assisted procedures [40]. Such a technique envisions the use of geometric-mathematical approaches to defining points in the three-dimensional space utilizing three orthogonal planes [41].

The main goal of stereotaxis is to allow for quantitative approaches to the spatial localization and reciprocal registration between the key elements in the operating room (i.e., imaging devices, anatomical targets, surgical instruments, etc.).

Nowadays, stereotaxis, together with advanced 3D imaging techniques and sophisticated robotic devices, allows surgeons to perform preoperative planning and registration, intraoperative navigation, multimodal imaging fusion, and postoperative assessment as a whole optimized computer-integrated surgical workflow [42–45] (Fig. 3.9).

Preoperative planning: Initially, a few weeks before the intervention, a radiologist performs manual or semi-automated segmentation of volumetric slices coming

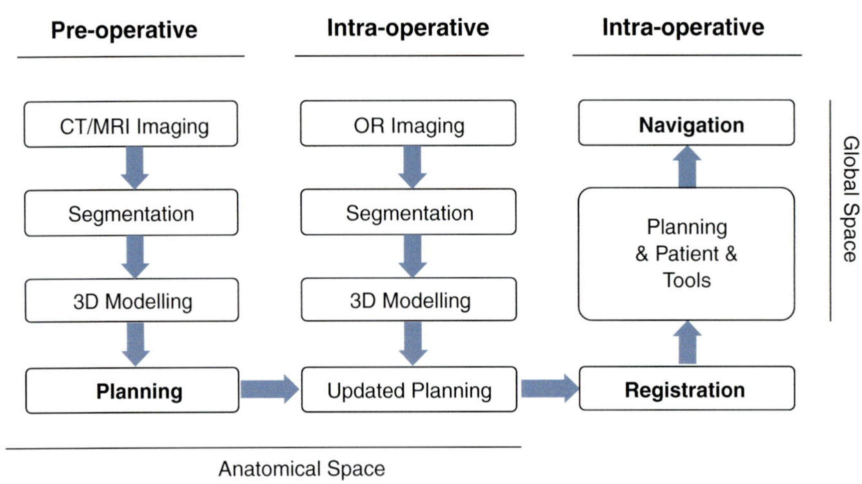

Fig. 3.9 The stereotactic workflow in the OR is reported. The two first columns refer to planning in the anatomical space. The first column happens before the intervention, while the second represents the update in the OR. The last column shows the operations carried out after in-OR registering of the updated planning to patient and tools (passive or robotized) deploying the in-OR navigation. "&" symbols highlight co-registration among planning, patient, and tools

from CT/MRI scanners with dedicated software. Subsequently, the resulting high-accuracy 3D model of the patient's pathology is evaluated by the surgical specialists and enriched with labels, annotations, and ad-hoc planned interventional strategies (i.e., trajectories, safety boundaries, targets, etc.).

Intraoperative model update: The preoperative model might vary significantly from the actual anatomy right before or during the intervention, due both from natural degeneration of the pathology and surgery-induced deformation (i.e., brain shift, insufflation, patient positioning, changes in morphology, etc.). For this reason, the model is always updated intraoperatively, ideally utilizing the same imaging technique used to build the planning. Such smooth intraoperative update (where pre- and intraoperative 3D volumes obtained with the same imaging device are compared) is difficult to obtain in most cases due to various technological incompatibilities, first of all, the complexity of integrating large CT/MRI systems into regular operating rooms. A different imaging method (i.e., 2D X-rays, ultrasound, CBCT, etc.) is therefore used to update the preoperative anatomical model. An exception to this trend is represented by modern hybrid operating rooms that are specifically built to accommodate both surgical technologies and imaging devices (i.e., CT/MRI) [46].

Intraoperative registration and navigation: The final step is to bring the planning, which is defined in the image coordinate system in the room coordinates system (also referred to as global space, tool space, frame space, or robotic space) to allow for correct alignment of the surgical tools and execution of the planned procedure.

The image space can be registered to the robotic space in frame-based or frameless modality.

In **frame-based** modality, the stereotactic frame serves not only as a rigid head holder, but it also provides its own coordinate system. It is usually secured to the anatomical region of interest (i.e., the head) through screws or conical pins. 2D or 3D localizers are fixed to the frame in order to be visualized in the planning images, thus guaranteeing a software-based procedure to transform the stereotactic coordinates from the image space to the robotic space. The most modern framed systems provide both 2D and 3D localizers for projective X-rays or MR/CT scans, respectively. Of note, the Talairach frame, the most popular stereotactic frame until the 90s, provides only 2D localizers. However, 2D and 3D image datasets can be "fused" in the planning software by means of a point-to-point rigid registration based on extrinsic or anatomical FM visible on both modalities [47].

Probably due to the lack of a 3D localizer, the Talairach frame is likely not used any longer at any neurosurgical center as a true stereotactic frame. It is rather still used only as a head-holder in some centers performing stereoelectroencephalography implantations in **frame-less** modality [48]. The patient's head is rigidly secured to the robotic assistant and different tools and methods can be adopted to register the image space to the robotic space. In the NeuroLocate® system, for example, the robotic system handles, as an end effector, a tridimensional support for multiple FM; the support is positioned close to the anatomical target and a 3D imaging method and software are used to directly register the anatomical and the robot coordinates spaces in the OR. The rest of the surgical workflow remains un-altered. Other methods for frame-less registration involve the use of a laser scanner (or other

3D reconstruction modalities) attached to the robot end effector to scan the anatomical target surface (i.e., the skull and face of the patient) allowing for single-step direct 3D/3D patient-robot-planning registration.

Intraoperative registration techniques are further detailed in the next chapter.

Conclusions

In conclusion, this chapter presented the robotics foundations, which represent the basic knowledge needed to understand the design and operation of medical robots. Starting from the definition, through the new standards and the future aspects of autonomy, the reader is supported with surgical robots taxonomy, based on different criteria and basic architectures. Basic control and human–robot interface issues are presented and discussed. This information allows medical professionals and technology providers to share a common language on surgical robots. The lack of such unified and accessible knowledge usually represents a barrier in medical robot's uptake and full exploitation.

References

1. Chen Y, Zhang S, Wu Z, Yang B, Luo Q, Xu K. Review of surgical robotic systems for keyhole and endoscopic procedures: state of the art and perspectives. Front Med. 2020;14:382–403.
2. Sheridan TB, Verplank WL. Human and computer control of undersea teleoperators. Massachusetts Inst of Tech Cambridge Man-Machine Systems Lab; 1978.
3. Yang GZ, Cambias J, Cleary K, et al. Medical robotics—regulatory, ethical, and legal considerations for increasing levels of autonomy. Sci Robot. 2017;2(4):1–3.
4. Kwoh YS. A new computerized tomographic aided robotic stereotactic system. Robot Age. 1985;7:17–21.
5. Kwoh YS, Hou J, Jonckheere EA, Hayati S. A robot with improved absolute positioning accuracy for CT guided stereotactic brain surgery. IEEE Trans Biomed Eng. 1988;35:153–60.
6. Bargar WL. Robots in orthopaedic surgery: past, present, and future. Clin Orthop. 2007;463:31–6.
7. Dasgupta B, Mruthyunjaya TS. The Stewart platform manipulator: a review. Mech Mach Theory. 2000;35:15–40.
8. D'Souza MD, Gendreau J, Feng A, Kim LH, Ho AL, Veeravagu A. Robotic-assisted spine surgery: history, efficacy, cost, and future trends. Robot Surg Res Rev. 2019;6:9–23.
9. Cianchetti M, Ranzani T, Gerboni G, Nanayakkara T, Althoefer K, Dasgupta P, et al. Soft robotics technologies to address shortcomings in today's minimally invasive surgery: the STIFF-FLOP approach. Soft Robot. 2014;1:122–31.
10. Grassmann R, Modes V, Burgner-Kahrs J. Learning the forward and inverse kinematics of a 6-DOF concentric tube continuum robot in SE(3). 2018 IEEERSJ Int Conf Intell Robots Syst IROS. Madrid: IEEE; 2018. p. 5125–32.
11. Watts T, Secoli R, Baena FR, y. A mechanics-based model for 3-D steering of programmable bevel-tip needles. IEEE Trans Robot. 2019;35:371–86.
12. Berthet-Rayne P, Gras G, Leibrandt K, Wisanuvej P, Schmitz A, Seneci CA, et al. The i2Snake robotic platform for endoscopic surgery. Ann Biomed Eng. 2018;46:1663–75.

13. Craig JJ. Introduction to robotics: mechanics and control. 4th ed. NY: Pearson; 2018.
14. Denavit J, Hertenberg RS. A kinematic notation for lower-pair mechanisms based on matrices. J Appl Mech. 1955:215–21.
15. Su H, Enayati N, Vantadori L, Spinoglio A, Ferrigno G, De Momi E. Online human-like redundancy optimization for tele-operated anthropomorphic manipulators. Int J Adv Robot Syst. 2018;15:172988141881469.
16. Merlet J-P, Gosselin C. Parallel mechanisms and robots. In: Siciliano B, Khatib O, editors. Springer handbook of robotics. Berlin, Heidelberg: Springer Berlin Heidelberg; 2008. p. 269–85.
17. Taylor RH, Funda J, Eldridge B, Gomory S, Gruben K, LaRose D, et al. A telerobotic assistant for laparoscopic surgery. IEEE Eng Med Biol Mag. 1995;14:279–88.
18. Taylor RH, Funda J, Grossman DD, Karidis JP, LaRose DA. Remote center-of-motion robot for surgery; 1995. https://patents.google.com/patent/US5397323A/en
19. Boctor EM, Webster RJ, Mathieu H, Okamura AM, Fichtinger G. Virtual remote center of motion control for needle placement robots. Comput Aided Surg. 2004;9:175–83.
20. Benabid AL, Hoffmann D, Seigneuret E, Chabardes S. Robotics in neurosurgery: which tools for what? Acta Neurochir Suppl. 2006;98:43–50.
21. Kurfess TR, editor. Robotics and automation handbook. Boca Raton: CRC Press; 2005.
22. Govers FX. Artificial intelligence for robotics. Build intelligent robots that perform human tasks using AI techniques. Birmingham: Packt Publishing; 2018.
23. Bholat OS, Haluck RS, Kutz RH, Gorman PJ, Krummel TM. Defining the role of haptic feedback in minimally invasive surgery. Stud Health Technol Inform. 1999;62:62–6.
24. Lécuyer A. Simulating haptic feedback using vision: a survey of research and applications of pseudo-haptic feedback. Presence. 2009;18:39–53.
25. Shettigar S, Yadav V, Kanase VG. An overview on the trends, features and applications of robotic surgery. Int J Pharm Sci Res. 2020;11(10):4794–804.
26. Nathoo N, Çavuşoğlu MC, Vogelbaum MA, Barnett GH. In touch with robotics: neurosurgery for the future. Neurosurgery. 2005;56:421–33.
27. Virdyawan V, Secoli R, Matheson E, Pinzi M, Watts T, Galvan S, et al. Supervisory-control robots. In: Marcus HJ, Payne CJ, editors. Neurosurgical robotics. New York, NY, Springer US; 2021. p. 35–47.
28. Jakopec M, Harris SJ, Rodriguez y Baena F, Gomes P, Davies BL. The Acrobot ® system for total knee replacement. Ind Robot Int J. 2003;30:61–6.
29. Vertut J, Coiffet P. Robot technology. Vol. 3A. Teleoperation and robotics: evolution and development. ETDEWEB; 1985.
30. Shahbazi M, Atashzar SF, Patel RV. A systematic review of multilateral teleoperation systems. IEEE Trans Haptics. 2018;11:338–56.
31. Schäfer MB, Stewart KW, Pott PP. Industrial robots for teleoperated surgery—a systematic review of existing approaches. Curr Dir Biomed Eng. 2019;5:153–6.
32. George EI, Brand TC, LaPorta A, Marescaux J, Satava RM. Origins of robotic surgery: from skepticism to standard of care. JSLS. 2018;22:e2018.00039.
33. Sutherland GR, Wolfsberger S, Lama S, Zarei-nia K. The evolution of neuroArm. Neurosurgery. 2013;72:A27–32.
34. Sheridan TB. Human supervisory control. In: Salvendy G, editor. Handbook of human factors and ergonomics. Hoboken, NJ: John Wiley & Sons, Inc.; 2012. p. 990–1015.
35. Attanasio A, Scaglioni B, Leonetti M, Frangi AF, Cross W, Biyani CS, et al. Autonomous tissue retraction in robotic assisted minimally invasive surgery—a feasibility study. IEEE Robot Autom Lett. 2020;5:6528–35.
36. Pedram SA, Ferguson PW, Shin C, Mehta A, Dutson EP, Alambeigi F, et al. Toward synergic learning for autonomous manipulation of deformable tissues via surgical robots: an approximate q-learning approach. 2020 8th IEEE RASEMBS Int Conf biomed robot biomechatronics BioRob. New York City: IEEE; 2020. p. 878–84.

37. Sen S, Garg A, Gealy DV, McKinley S, Jen Y, Goldberg K. Automating multi-throw multilateral surgical suturing with a mechanical needle guide and sequential convex optimization. 2016 IEEE int conf robot autom ICRA. Stockholm, Sweden: IEEE; 2016. p. 4178–85.
38. Varier VM, Rajamani DK, Goldfarb N, Tavakkolmoghaddam F, Munawar A, Fischer GS. Collaborative suturing: a reinforcement learning approach to automate hand-off task in suturing for surgical robots. 2020 29th IEEE int conf robot hum interact commun RO-MAN. Naples, Italy: IEEE; 2020. p. 1380–6.
39. Da Col TD, Mariani A, Deguet A, Menciassi A, Kazanzides P, De Momi E. SCAN: system for camera autonomous navigation in robotic-assisted surgery. 2020 IEEERSJ int conf intell robots syst IROS. Las Vegas, NV: IEEE; 2020. p. 2996–3002.
40. Faria C, Erlhagen W, Rito M, De Momi E, Ferrigno G, Bicho E. Review of robotic technology for stereotactic neurosurgery. IEEE Rev Biomed Eng. 2015;8:125–37.
41. Gildenberg P, Tasker R, Franklin P. The history of stereotactic and functional neurosurgery. In: Gildenberg P, Tasker R, editors. Textbook of stereotactic and functional neurosurgery. McGraw-Hill Companies; 1998. p. 5–19.
42. Huang M, Tetreault TA, Vaishnav A, York PJ, Staub BN. The current state of navigation in robotic spine surgery. Ann Transl Med. 2021;9:86.
43. Chen Y-W, Hanak BW, Yang T-C, Wilson TA, Hsia JM, Walsh HE, et al. Computer-assisted surgery in medical and dental applications. Expert Rev Med Devices. 2021:17434440.2021.1886075.
44. Wijsmuller AR, Romagnolo LGC, Consten E, Melani AEF, Marescaux J. Navigation and image-guided surgery. In: Atallah S, editor. Digit Surg. Cham: Springer International Publishing; 2021. p. 137–44.
45. Faraji-Dana Z, Mariampillai ALD, Standish BA, Yang VXD, Leung MKK. Machine-vision image-guided surgery for spinal and cranial procedures. In: Abedin-Nasab MH, editor. Handbook of robotic and image-guided surgery. Elsevier; 2020. p. 551–74.
46. Jin H, Liu J. Application of the hybrid operating room in surgery: a systematic review. J Investig Surg. 2020:1–12.
47. Cardinale F, Cossu M, Castana L, et al. Stereoelectroencephalography: surgical methodology, safety, and stereotactic application accuracy in 500 procedures. Neurosurgery. 2013;72(3):353–66.
48. Cardinale F, Rizzi M, d'Orio P, Casaceli G, Arnulfo G, Narizzano M, et al. A new tool for touch-free patient registration for robot-assisted intracranial surgery: application accuracy from a phantom study and a retrospective surgical series. Neurosurg Focus. 2017;42:E8.

Chapter 4
Image Guidance for Intracranial Surgery with Supervisory-Control Robots

Francesco Cardinale, Martina Revay, Piergiorgio d'Orio, Sergio Raspante, Lorenzo Maria Giuseppe Bianchi, Khalid Al Orabi, Luca Berta, and Giorgio Lo Russo

The original version of the chapter has been revised. A correction to this chapter can be found at https://doi.org/10.1007/978-3-031-08380-8_20

F. Cardinale (✉) · P. d'Orio
"Claudio Munari" Center for Epilepsy Surgery, Azienda Socio-Sanitaria Territoriale Grande Ospedale Metropolitano Niguarda, Milano, Italy

Department of Medicine and Surgery, Unit of Neuroscience, Università degli Studi di Parma, Parma, Italy
e-mail: francesco.cardinale@ospedaleniguarda.it; piergiorgio.dorio@ospedaleniguarda.it

M. Revay
"Claudio Munari" Center for Epilepsy Surgery, Azienda Socio-Sanitaria Territoriale Grande Ospedale Metropolitano Niguarda, Milano, Italy

Department of Biomedical and Clinical Sciences "L. Sacco", Università degli Studi di Milano, Milano, Italy
e-mail: martina.revay@ospedaleniguarda.it

S. Raspante
Department of Neuroradiology, Azienda Socio-Sanitaria Territoriale Grande Ospedale Metropolitano Niguarda, Milano, Italy
e-mail: sergio.raspante@ospedaleniguarda.it

L. M. G. Bianchi
Postgraduate School in Radiodiagnostics, Università degli Studi di Milano, Milano, Italy
e-mail: lorenzomaria.bianchi@unimi.it

K. Al Orabi
"Claudio Munari" Center for Epilepsy Surgery, Azienda Socio-Sanitaria Territoriale Grande Ospedale Metropolitano Niguarda, Milano, Italy

Department of Neurosurgery, King Abdullah Medical City, Al Mashair, Saudi Arabia
e-mail: al-orabi.k@kamc.med.sa

L. Berta
Department of Medical Physics, Azienda Socio-Sanitaria Territoriale Grande Ospedale Metropolitano Niguarda, Milano, Italy
e-mail: luca.berta@ospedaleniguarda.it

J. A. González Martínez, F. Cardinale (eds.), *Robotics in Neurosurgery*,
https://doi.org/10.1007/978-3-031-08380-8_4

G. L. Russo
"Claudio Munari" Center for Epilepsy Surgery, Azienda Socio-Sanitaria Territoriale Grande Ospedale Metropolitano Niguarda, Milano, Italy
e-mail: giorgio.lorusso@ospedaleniguarda.it

> "Sometimes doing your best is not good enough. Sometimes you must do what is required"—Winston Churchill

Introduction

Why would a surgeon like to use a robotic assistant?

According to Schweikard and Ernst, we can distinguish four goal-based scenarios [1]:

- Robots for navigation
- Robots for motion replication
- Robots for imaging
- Robots for rehabilitation and prosthetics

In the first scenario, "**robots for navigation**," the surgical device is positioned by the robotic arm in the surgical space, based on a stereotaxic planning.

In the second scenario, "**robots for motion replication**," the surgeon's hands motion is replicated by the robot via a dedicated interface. It is possible to downscale the motion and reduce the tremor, thus improving the dexterity and making easier the surgical movements in a context of minimally invasive surgery.

In the third scenario, "**robots for imaging**," two-dimensional (2D) or three-dimensional (3D) images are obtained by means of an imaging device mounted to a robotic machine.

In the fourth scenario, "**robots for rehabilitation and prosthetics**," mechatronic devices can support the movement of paralyzed segments of the body or fully replace missing parts, such as limb.

Robots for motion replication and for rehabilitation/prosthetics will be exhaustively illustrated in other chapters of the present textbook. In this chapter, we will essentially cover the topic of image-based planning of supervisory-control robotic assistance, out of doubt the most popular scenario in neurosurgery. Since most of the robot-assisted surgeries at our center ("Claudio Munari" center for Epilepsy Surgery) are performed in the context of StereoElectroEncephaloGraphy (SEEG) implantations, we will provide also an example of the use of a robotic mobile computed tomography (CT) scanner that is integrated in our workflow, thus briefly covering also the topic of robots for imaging.

The aim of this chapter is to provide the reader with the strategical and technical fundamentals of image-based navigated robotic surgery. Supervisory-control robots available on the medical market are wonderful devices able to assist the neurosurgeon in positioning intracranial probes along the vectors of planned trajectories. These high-cost machines are intrinsically accurate but are only a part of a complex procedural chain. In fact, "*the total clinically relevant error* ***(application accuracy)*** *comprises errors associated with each procedural step, including imaging, target selection, vector calculations, and the mechanical errors…*" [2]. In other words, to buy an expensive robot is not enough to guarantee an accurate, safe, and efficacious diagnostic or therapeutic stereotactic procedure. The neurosurgeon must understand what's before, behind and after the robot-assisted surgery. Most popular systems are versatile, offering different workflows and operating modalities. How to choose between CT and magnetic resonance (MR) datasets? And what about the choice between frame-based or frameless robotic procedures?[1] What are the best options for biopsy, deep brain stimulation (DBS), or SEEG surgeries?

Let's go back to the initial question, slightly modified for the context that now is more specific: why would a neurosurgeon like to use a supervisory-control robot instead of a more conventional frame-based non-robotic stereotactic equipment? A possible answer is "to save time and reduce the risk of procedural errors (especially in case of multiple trajectories), still guaranteeing an accuracy at least as high as with conventional frames." The reader could note that we repeatedly used the term "**accuracy"** and not "**precision**." It is important to understand that they are not synonyms, as it was clearly explained by Maciunas and coworkers who were inspired by a milestone textbook of biomedical statistics: "*…a clear distinction must be drawn between three commonly misused terms: 'unbiasedness' or lack of skew, 'precision,' and 'accuracy'. A series of observations that tend to the true value are 'unbiased' or without skew. If these observations have considerable spread, however, they lack 'precision'. A series of observations with little spread among them indicates precision, although they are biased or skewed if the observations tend to center at a value displaced from the true value. The term 'accuracy' encompasses both unbiasedness and precision: accurate measurements are both unbiased and precise, whereas inaccurate measurements may be biased, imprecise, or both* [2]." Looking at Fig. 4.1, it is easy to understand that we need accurate robots (and procedural robot-assisted workflows) because precision alone is not enough. For safety reasons, it is necessary to obtain the highest accuracy at the first attempt for every trajectory: both the neurosurgeon and, most important, the patient could have not a second chance.

The application accuracy of the stereotactic procedure is ultimately in charge of the neurosurgeon, as clearly stated by Bucholz (probably the true clinical father of modern optical-tracking navigation systems): "*Although consultation with a radiologist or a specialist in nuclear medicine is important in the interpretation of diagnostic images, the surgeon is ultimately responsible for the direction and conduct of surgery. As the surgeon relies on imaging to guide surgery during a stereotactic procedure, it is vitally important that the surgeon fully understand the basics of each imaging technique. Further, in a time of cost containment, the choice of imaging technology has to be based not only on clinical efficacy, but also on the risk to the patient, cost, and benefit gained. Therefore, the choice of imaging used for the guidance of surgery must be made by the surgeon, as only the surgeon knows what has to be avoided en route to what should be removed* [3]."

The setup of an appropriate workflow, optimizing the mandatory requirements with the available facilities and equipment, is therefore crucial to guarantee the

[1] This is not a mistake: a "robotic" procedure is not always "frame-less"!

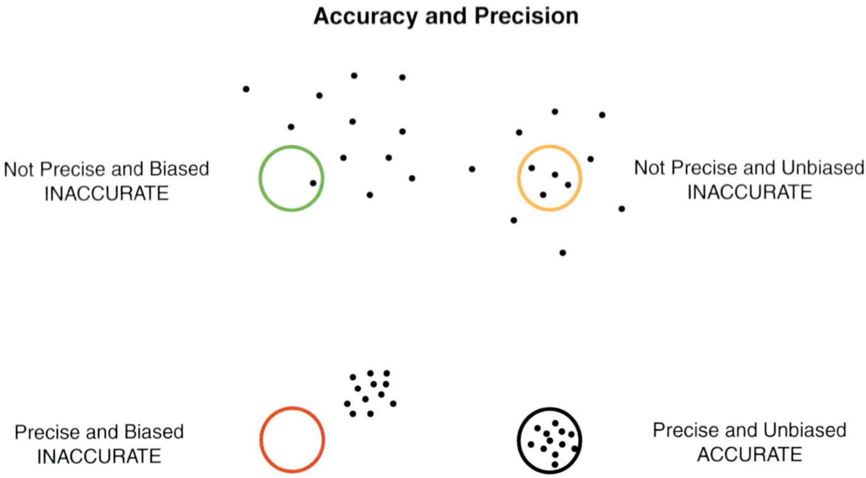

Fig. 4.1 Difference between accuracy and precision
In metrology, accuracy is closeness of repeated measurements to the true value. The circles in the figure represent the range of values approximating the true value sufficiently well. This range depends on the specific field of interest
A measuring device can be inaccurate because of random or systematic errors, leading to impreciseness or bias, respectively. A measurement device can be inaccurate because characterized only by impreciseness (orange circle), or only by bias (red circle), or both (green circle). It is important to emphasize that a precise system (all the measurements are close each other) can be inaccurate because of bias (all the measurements are far from the true value). It is also important to note that an unbiased system (the mean of the measurement is close to the true value) can be inaccurate because of impreciseness (the measurement values are too much spread). These concepts can be translated with slight modifications in other sciences such as statistics or robotics
In the field of neurosurgical robotics, especially when dealing with supervisory-control systems aimed at advancing a diagnostic or therapeutic probe into the intracranial space, the situations represented by the green and red circles are not acceptable because they do not tend do the true value (correct positioning), of course. It is important to understand that also the case represented by the orange circle is not acceptable. We cannot perform repeated procedures and then calculate the mean. We have to reach correctly the target (correct positioning of the probe) with the only chance we have. An incorrect stereotactic placement could lead to a severe bleeding or to the failure of the diagnostic procedure

needed accuracy. The following sections of the chapter are intended to help the neurosurgeon in embedding the chosen robotic assistant in a coherent workflow covering all the steps from the planning to the verification of the obtained result.

Strategical Planning

In most applications, the strategy of implantation, intended as the number and the position of targets to be reached by the implanted probes, is quite “simple.” Targets can be deep, as in case of tumors for biopsies and subthalamic nucleus (STN) or anterior nucleus of thalamus (ANT) for DBS (for the treatment of Parkinson disease or drug-resistant partial epilepsy, respectively). In these situations, no more than two trajectories are generally implemented, usually planned only on neuroimage datasets that could be co-registered with an atlas when targeting MR-not-visible deep nuclei. The case of SEEG is largely different. The study of an epileptogenic lesion (when present) and the 3D definition of the epileptogenic zone are the main aims of the investigation [4]. "*…we believe that the surgical therapeutic decision must be based on clinical, EEG and neuroradiological investigations* [5]." It is necessary to sample many deep or superficial cortical areas, as long as white matter bundles and mesial temporal lobe structures. An appropriate planning is based mostly on structural MR images, but also many other modalities are utilized such as functional MR (fMR), white matter bundles reconstructed from diffusion-weighted image (DWI) datasets, positron emission tomography (PET), single photon emission computed tomography (SPECT), and many others. Some software packages or pipelines can be also adopted to enhance the visualization of difficult-to-see epileptogenic lesions or epileptic networks [6–13]. Information provided by all these image modalities must be "co-registered" in the patient-specific intracranial space, ideally together with data coming from clinical history, neurological examination, neuropsychological testing, and interictal/ictal electroencephalography (EEG), often coupled with long-term video recording (video-EEG).

By means of registration techniques, multimodal information can be mapped into the individual intracranial space according to the method originally developed by Jean Talairach, the "*true father of what we now call image-guided stereotactic surgery* [14]." Horsley and Clarke, when first implanted an electrode in an animal [15], coined the term "**stereotaxic**," a composite word derived from the ancient Greek "stereos" (three-dimensional) and "taxic" (referring to an arrangement of data, as in taxonomy). The term "**stereotactic**" (from the Latin "tactus," to touch) was introduced years later to define the surgical advancement of a probe to a target (Fig. 4.2).

Therefore, every stereotactic procedure must be preceded by the stereotaxic mapping of multimodal information. In the context of SEEG, this way of working is particularly important because its goal is the 3D definition of the epileptogenic zone. "Stereo-EEG" means much more than "stereotactic EEG": the method is stereotaxic and three-dimensional, including a crucial stereotactic surgery. It is a big error to reduce conceptually the SEEG method to the simple implantation of intracerebral electrodes. The global strategy must be defined having in mind that its purpose is to test a patient-specific anatomo-electro-clinical hypothesis, based on clinical history, semiology, imaging, and video-EEG data [16]. It is also important to underline that the position of SEEG electrodes must be aimed not only at gray matter recordings. Electrical stimulations, performed with low-frequency or high-frequency modality, allow to induce seizures but also to map brain functions, probing both cortical areas and white-matter tracts [17, 18].

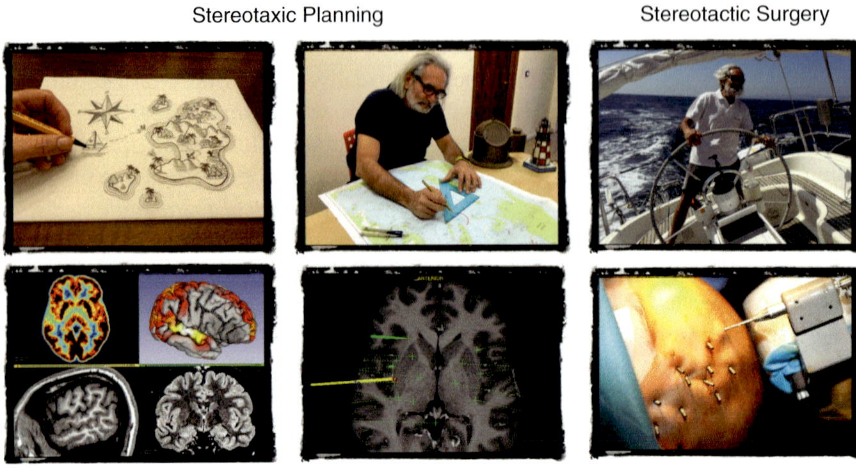

Fig. 4.2 Stereotaxic planning and stereotactic surgery
The stereotactic advancement of a probe to an intracranial target is performed after a stereotaxic planning has been done. Such planning includes the mapping of all information into the intracranial space, defined by a 3D coordinate system, and the use of the map to plan the trajectories

Principles and Terminology of Trajectory Planning

Even if the first stereotactic procedures in humans were performed at the end of the XIX century, the birth of modern stereotaxy is commonly localized around the middle of the XX century [19]. Ernest A. Spiegel and Henry T. Wycis first performed at the Temple Medical School in Philadelphia a number of lesioning procedures aimed at treating "*mental disorders, intractable pain, petit mal and extrapyramidal disorders* [20, 21]." All the targets were point-shaped and seated in deep brain structures. Thus, stereotactic trajectories started to be generally intended as rectilinear segments obviously defined by a target point and, unavoidably and only secondarily, by an entry point that had to be as safe as possible. Almost simultaneously, Jean Talairach, after his first period in psycho-surgery, moved his main focus of interest to epilepsy surgery co-working with Jean Bancaud and Gabor Szikla at another temple of stereotaxy, the Hôpital St. Anne in Paris [22, 23]. In 1980, Szikla reported the words written in a letter by Nicholas Zervas, neurosurgeon at the Massachusetts General Hospital, who had written "*…stereotaxis is at a dead end in this country…*," after the decreased number of indications determined by the advent of L-Dopa in the drug treatment of Parkinson disease. Szikla argued that stereotaxy was not dying and that it was rather increasing the area of interest. He schematized the evolution of the stereotaxy concept listing three fundamental points: "(1) *The target point became enlarged and transformed into the target volume; such is the case for epileptogenic cortical areas and even more for brain tumors* (2). *The field of application of stereotactic methods was progressively extended from some centrally located deep structures to the entire brain including the cortex* (3). *Multi-probe methods* *became available, allowing for safe simultaneous exploration of several brain structures* [24]."

Szikla perfectly analyzed the ongoing evolution and forecasted the future. Nowadays, the number of trajectories planned to reach a simple point-shaped target is very limited. Even in the cases of DBS or biopsies, the neurosurgeon needs to cover with the probe a deep-seated segment rather than a small spherical volume. The multi-lead stimulating probe implanted for DBS should be aligned with the major axis of the subthalamic nucleus and positioned according to its functional topography [25]. Similarly, even in the case of a stereotactic tumor biopsy, multiple points of interest can be targeted [26]. The neurosurgeon likely will want to cover more points along the trajectory in order to sample different parts of the lesion and the surrounding tissue as indicated by the images (the perilesional brain tissue, the transition zone between healthy and diseased tissue, the gadolinium-enhanced component, the necrotic part, etc.). In a recent retrospective study on 377 patients, the histo-molecular diagnosis of a diffuse glioma and the glioma grade were obtained in 98.7% and in 92.6% of patients, respectively, by means of multiple-bite robot-assisted biopsy [27]. Image guidance of stereotactic needle biopsies is important not only for an appropriate histological and molecular characterization, but also for safety. Since many tumors are highly vascularized and the procedure aims at sampling the lesional tissue with a cutting tool, bleedings are more frequent than in electrode implantation for DBS or SEEG. The robotic assistant can guarantee a high accuracy but the human planning, based on preoperative images, is crucial. Zanello and coworkers reported that in most cases complicated by intraoperative bleeding the reason lay in a non-completely appropriate planning rather than in device inaccuracies [28].

SEEG implantation is the best example of a procedure in which every implanted probe targets an intracerebral segment, aiming at sampling multiple electrical sources all along the planned trajectory. Moreover, the overall strategy of implantation guarantees a large, multifocal, and hypothesis-driven sampling of several cortical areas aimed at delineating the 3D shape of the epileptogenic zone. The aforementioned concept illustrated by Szikla and the St Anne school is now fulfilled.

Stated that the target of different stereotactic minimally invasive procedures is almost never point-shaped, we can specify that we will continue to use the terms "**entry point**" (EP) and "**target point**" (TP) to indicate the points that describe every trajectory. We will thus maintain the classical terminology of the scientific community, but now we are convinced that the readers can understand what we mean as "target."

On another terminological topic, we will not adopt the terms "depth electrodes" (DE) and "intracerebral electrodes" as synonyms in the field of stereoelectroencephalography. SEEG electrodes record the brain activity from every brain structure, including the crowns and the sulcal banks of gyri seated not only in the depth but also on the convexity of the hemispheres. The term DE should therefore be reserved to the electrodes that are aimed at recording only from deep structures [29–31], as typically in the case of bilateral hippocampal sampling for mesial temporal epilepsy lateralization. When only DE are implanted, the term SEEG is not appropriate even if a percutaneous technique is implemented.

Multimodal Image-Guided Trajectory Planning

Neuroimages contain the information needed for a safe and successful stereotactic procedure, and the trajectory planning for supervisory-control robotic assistants is therefore based on them. Image properties strongly affect both the diagnostic or therapeutic yield and the application accuracy.

The diagnostic information is almost always multimodal. The neurosurgeon must take the most useful data from every available image dataset, combining criteria for best diagnostic information and accurate 3D localization. As an example, when performing a DBS procedure aimed at implanting the stimulating electrode into the subthalamic nucleus, the best visualization of the target is commonly obtained with dedicated T2-weighted (T2W) MR sequences, but the best scan for a complete view of the head and its registration in the surgical space is generally a 3D T1-weighted (T1W) sequence. Thus, the neurosurgeon will want to bring the T2W-derived visualization of the subthalamic nucleus into the T1W image space, performing a registration process (Fig. 4.3). It is thus important that the neurosurgeon knows at least the basic principles of registrations in order to set a proper workflow.

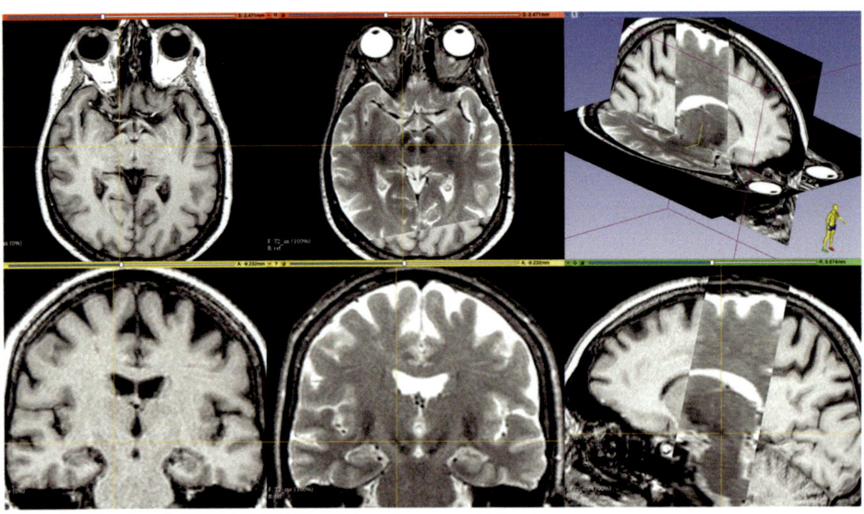

Fig. 4.3 Multimodal imaging
The subthalamic nucleus, the most common target of DBS procedures aimed at treating Parkinson disease, is not directly visible in 3D T1W images. Differently, it is well visible with T2W sequences. Registration guarantees the combination of the information in the same space

Coordinate Systems

The three-dimensional space can be described with different coordinate systems. René Descartes recognized that the position of a point in a plane can be defined with a simple graph comprising two perpendicular lines, the x and y axes, intersecting at the origin. Given a point on the plane, the distances from the origin along both the axes (x and y coordinates) define univocally its location. Indeed, the position of every point is uniquely defined by an ordered pair of numbers. The x,y coordinates of the origin are 0,0. Such Cartesian coordinate system may be extended to the third dimension, including a z axis, and can be therefore used to define and quantify every 3D space. It is the most popular coordinate system, and it is adopted in many image-guided-surgery (IGS) systems. Other coordinate systems can be used, such as the polar and the cylindric ones and coordinates can be converted from one system to another [32].

By medical convention, the **Cartesian coordinate system** is applied to human anatomy describing the positions along the right-left, the antero-posterior, and the cranio–caudal axes with x, y, *and* z coordinates, respectively. Every image or physical 3D space can be defined and quantified in this way.

Medical Images and 3D Localization of Anatomical Structures

Medical images, with the exception of very advanced techniques (immersive virtual reality, augmented reality, holograms), are generally reproduced on simple paper sheets, on printed films or, more modernly, on computer screens. They are 2D representations of data obtained from human anatomical structures by means of different scanners. In fact, whatever the 3D complexity of the represented object and its appearance, information must be mapped on a Cartesian plane (the paper, the film, or the computer screen).[2] It is thus important to understand how 3D coordinates can be managed to plan trajectories and drive robotic assistants.

Medical images for stereotaxic planning can be projective or stacks of slices.

X-ray 2D images are projective in nature. From a point-shaped source, a conic beam of X-rays is directed towards the region to be studied. The denser or the thicker the scanned object, the larger the absorption of X-ray quanta: this phenomenon is at the basis of final image appearance. It is important to understand that it is impossible to get tridimensional information from only one 2D projective image. In order to use 2D X-rays for stereotaxic planning and subsequent stereotactic

[2]The problem is not different with stereoscopic technologies, where a pair of slightly different 2D images (taken or reconstructed from different points of view) is presented to the user in a way that allows the perception of depth. These images are not really 3D: despite the illusion of three-dimensionality, the user cannot see the hidden face of the objects. Therefore, surgical microscopes, endoscopes, and otoscopes provide the neurosurgeon with a stereoscopic view of the surgical field, and the term 3D should not be considered appropriate even if it is very popular.

guidance, it is necessary to acquire at least two of them from different angles with dedicated localizers aimed at registering the 3D image space with the stereotactic space (see below).

On the other hand, conventional **CT** datasets provide a volumetric representation of the scanned objects, not its 2D projection. Classically and schematically, a highly collimated beam of X-rays is directed towards the head of the patient while an emitter/detector system rotates around it acquiring a slice-shaped volume. After an image has been obtained, the bed is moved and another image is acquired. The whole dataset is thus made of a stack of sliced images, each one of them computed applying the Radon Transform to the intensity profile detected throughout the 360-degrees rotation. Besides the higher sensitivity and the possibility of quantitative measurements, the most important advantage of CT versus projective X-ray images is the possibility of localizing anatomical structures. In fact, CT records X-ray attenuation for small volumetric elements (the slices) independently. Differently, X-ray images superimpose the X-ray absorption values of a number of tissues along a ray [33]. The spatial resolution of a CT dataset is essential for accurate 3D localization of scanned objects and crucially affects the final application accuracy of every stereotactic procedure. It is defined by the parameters of CT scanning: the "image matrix" (the number of pixels per slice, e.g., 512 × 512), the size of the pixels (e.g., 0.5 × 0.5 mm^2), the number of slices (e.g., 200), and the slice thickness (e.g., 1 mm). With the above reported example parameters, the reconstructed 3D field of view (FOV) of a typical axial acquisition is 256 × 256 × 200 mm^3, being the voxel size (voxel = pixel extended to the third dimension) 0.5 × 0.5 × 1 mm^3. It appears obvious that the higher the spatial resolution, the more accurate the localization of the objects. Anyway, the thinner the slice, the lower the signal/noise ratio. The accuracy of 3D localization and the image diagnostic quality are therefore inversely proportional. The best balance between quality of the images, accuracy of localization, and radiation protection must be tuned based on patient- and procedure-specific clinical needs.

Even if some correction algorithms are available with modern equipment and software, to acquire CT dataset with a gantry tilt is not advisable because the compensation warping could be not appropriately managed by the planning software. Also, the use of a dataset with scanning parameters that are not identical for all the slices (e.g., when the slice thickness is different between cranial and caudal slices) must be absolutely avoided because the 3D reconstruction would be incorrect. On the other side, it is not mandatory to use isotropic voxels and this important because most CT scanners output datasets with non-isotropic voxels. A slice thickness larger than planar pixel size can be advantageous to increase the signal-to-noise ratio, without affecting the correctness of 3D reconstruction. The uncertainty (see below) along the z axis will be increased, but if the thickness is not larger than 1 mm, the planning inaccuracy will be clinically irrelevant in most situations.

The **uncertainty** of measurements and localization is strictly related to pixel/voxel size. When the neurosurgeon selects a point on the computer screen with the mouse, the visual target is located "somewhere" in the pixel space, and the uncertainty of the position selection is half of the voxel spacing (e.g., it is 0.25 mm if the pixel size is 0.5 mm). Similarly, the uncertainty along the z axis for axial datasets is half the slice thickness. Since a distance is measured between two selected points, the uncertainty of the measure is double than that of a single point selection [34]. Last but not least, the accuracy of point selection on the computer monitor is related also to the pointer (usually a mouse or a trackpad) and to the screen resolution. Zooming in the images is a useful trick to mitigate these sources of inaccuracy.

Of note, modern CT scanners acquire images in a much more complex way than above schematically described. However, modern improvements (multi-slice, helical or spiral, etc.) have largely improved the quality of images and reduced the time of acquisition but the features of the datasets relative to planning principles remain essentially unmodified.

The above-mentioned CT scanners are essentially based on fan-shaped beams of X-rays. Using different back-projection algorithms of reconstruction, it is possible to acquire several 2D images obtained with cone-shaped beams of X-rays while the system emitter/detector rotates around the head of patient. The output is a dataset with the same properties of conventional CT scanners that can be similarly used for stereotaxic planning. Such Cone-Beam CT (**CBCT**) scanners are often designed for intraoperative imaging. Two popular examples are the O-arm® (Medtronic; Minneapolis, Minnesota, USA) and the Loop-X® ((Brainlab AG, München, Germany) systems. These O-ring mobile scanners are robotized, thus pertaining to the third category of robots as classified at the beginning of the present chapter. In fact, different positions of the emitter/detector system and of the whole gantry can be memorized and replicated thanks to their robotic features, providing both 2D projective images and 3D datasets. Of note, with such systems, the gantry can be tilted without adding any geometrical inaccuracy.

Modern angiographic equipment offer a similar modality, called **Rotational Angiography**, obtained rotating the C-arm around the head of the patient [35, 36]. Again, the output dataset is very similar to conventional CT ones and can be used for stereotaxic planning under the same principles. However, particular attention must be paid to distortion artifacts. The "pincushion" distortion is a typical artifact occurring with X-ray image intensifiers. A source of such pincushion effect is the deflection of electrons in the earth's magnetic field, continuously changing during the rotational acquisition. This artifact can be corrected using a rectilinear grid of small steel beads and performing a subsequent calibration procedure. Of note, this crucial calibration cannot be handled by the user, and therefore periodic maintenance and quality check must be rigorously scheduled. Thanks to this calibration, also other causes of distortion (much more relevant with present flat-panel technology) can be mitigated, as deviations from a perfect circular trajectory of rotation.

Magnetic resonance is the "king" of modern diagnostic modalities. Its sensitivity to tissue properties and a large variety of available sequences allow to discriminate the three main tissue classes: gray matter, white matter, and cerebrospinal fluid. Therefore, the planning of stereotactic trajectories will be mainly guided by MR imaging (MRI). To describe the main physical principles of MRI is out of the scopes of the present chapter.

From the planning point of view, also MR datasets are made of multi-slice volumetric data with the same properties described for CT (orientation, localization, etc.). The ability of discriminating soft-tissues make MRI the best modality for neurological diagnosis and optimal planning in most cases. 3D T1W sequence is used at most centers. It serves efficiently as anatomical base for stereotactic planning because of its low geometrical distortion and good gray/white matter discrimination. FLuid Attenuation Inversion Recovery (FLAIR) sequences are also frequently used because they are more sensitive to abnormal tissue, but their use in children younger than 3 years should be considered with caution for the lower diagnostic yield due to incomplete myelination. It must be underlined that even if MR is superior for soft-tissue, CT remains advantageous for hard tissues and objects, such as bone or metal probes. Thus, when it is necessary to get detailed information about the skull, a high-resolution CT dataset must be used besides MR. This is the case of many SEEG trajectories, when the neurosurgeon wants to check that the bony entry point is not at the level of para-nasal cavities or if the skull is thick enough to hold the guiding screw.

Compared to CT scans, MR images are much more informative but are also more insidious for stereotaxic planning. Distortion is a not negligible source of stereotactic error. Balachandran and coworkers have studied the stereotactic localization error due to MRI distortion in DBS procedures. With a clinical 3 T MR scanner, "*mean targeting error due to MR distortion in T2 was found to be 0.07 ± 0.025 mm with a maximum of 0.13 mm over 12 targets; error in the T1 images was smaller by 4%.*" The reported error was thus found small, likely negligible for stereotaxic planning [37]. Anyway, the situation can be much more dangerous, in particular when metal artifacts are present. Hardy and Barnett reported a targeting error of more than 2 cm in a stereotactic procedure in a patient with dental braces [38]. Modern correction algorithms can mitigate these errors but the neurosurgeon has to pay attention to this kind of error sources. Indeed, metal artifacts can affect the accuracy of both the image-to-patient registration and the planning of the trajectories. Moreover, also the maintenance and the quality check of MRI equipment must be periodically and rigorously performed in order to guarantee inherent errors as small as possible.

Of note, distortion is larger with very fast MR acquisition techniques. This means that image datasets such as the echo-planar images (EPI), commonly acquired for functional MR, are the most distorted and this should be considered.

All other volumetric datasets, such **PET** and **SPECT** ones, can be considered similar to CT and MR ones for the aspects pertaining to stereotactic planning and localization. We invite the reader to consult more specific textbooks for the technical specificities.

Up to 20 or even more multi-lead electrodes per SEEG investigation are implanted at many centers [29]. Since the surgical technique of implantation is percutaneous, preoperative image-based visualization of brain vasculature is crucial to avoid intracranial bleeding. Several angiographic modalities are available, and an appropriate choice can lead to safer procedures. In the first decades of SEEG, catheter angiography obtained in tele-stereoscopic-stereotaxic framed conditions was the only available modality. See references by Musolino et al. and Benabid et al. for technical details [39, 40]. Actually, as far as we know, the use of 3D angiographic datasets has completely replaced framed 2D X-rays. MR angiography with gadolinium-enhanced 3D T1W sequence is used at most centers where new SEEG programs have been started in the last decade [29]. Minkin et al. have also proposed a modified gadolinium-enhanced MR venography protocol with a short acquisition delay, allowing simultaneous arterial and venous visualization [41]. Anyway, the team of Cleveland Clinic Foundation has recently "*identified MRI as the vascular imaging modality leading to higher hemorrhage and symptomatic hemorrhage rates,*" based on cumulative sum analysis [42]. This finding sounds coherent with the paper published by the researchers working at University College of London, who reported that "vascular segmentation from DSA images was significantly more sensitive than T1 + gadolinium or magnetic resonance venography (MRV) images" (DSA = digital subtraction angiography) [43]. Therefore, MR angiographic modalities should be considered potentially less safe than CT ones, likely due to higher distortions. Some teams are therefore replacing MR- with CT-angiography. Its most popular implementation is done with conventional fan-beam CT scanners with peripheral injection of iodinate contrast medium. The preliminary acquisition of a non-contrasted bone mask permits also to subtract hard tissue for better segmentation and visualization of brain vasculature.

At "Claudio Munari" center, we developed a similar technique based on the use of O-arm, a robotized mobile O-ring CBCT scanner [44]. The preliminary acquisition of a bone mask permits the bone tissue subtraction, in this case even more efficient because O-arm vascular images are more contrasted (soft-tissue is only mildly visualized). The main difference is that our technique is based on selective catheter injection of contrast medium in the internal carotid artery (and also in the vertebral one when necessary). Since the extra-cerebral vasculature is not enhanced, the visualization and gray-scale thresholding segmentation of brain vessels are more efficient, as clearly visible in the pictures we have already published [44]. It could be argued that catheter angiography is invasive and thus inherently dangerous. Anyway, as far as we know, older age (>54 years) and cardiovascular disease were the only patient-related predictors of adverse effect occurrence in a very large study [45]. Since candidates for SEEG are generally younger and free of comorbidities, the rate of complications occurring with our 3D CBCT DSA technique resulted extremely low [46].

3D Visualization

Interactive 3D visualization, namely **volume rendering**, is very helpful for surgical planning. The description of the different techniques that can be adopted to render the three-dimensionality of anatomical structures is out of the scopes of the present chapter. Anyway, we like to stress that 3D interactive visualization (the position of the object can be changed relative to the point of view of the user) is crucial for optimal planning. Since brain anatomy is extremely variable and complex, it is

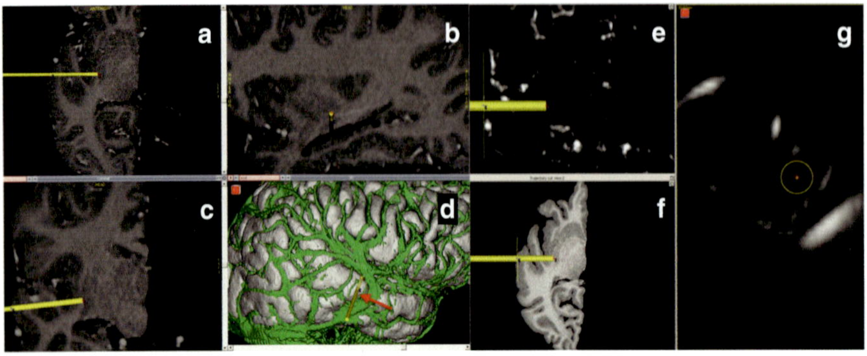

Fig. 4.4 Planning with multiplanar reconstructions, 3D rendering, trajectory cuts, and probe's eye view
In panels a, b and c axial, sagittal, and coronal 2D reconstructions are depicted, 50% faded between 3D T1W and 3D CBCT angiography. The projection of an SEEG trajectory, planned to sample the posterior part of the superior temporal gyrus, the Heschl gyrus and the posterior long gyrus of the insular lobe, is visible. The yellow shaft of the virtual probe is represented also on the 3D volume rendering of the brain surface and vasculature, closely posterior to the Labbé vein (panel d, red arrow). In panels e and f, the trajectory (not its projection) is fully represented in two trajectory cuts, one coronal (with only angiographic data) and one axial (with only MR data), respectively. In panel g, the probe's eye view is visible at the cortical entry point with the diameter of the virtual probe set at 5 mm. The same vessels depicted in the 3D view are recognizable around the cortical entry point

often too difficult to mentally imagine the three-dimensionality of interesting structures without the aid of volume rendering. On the other side, details that are "hidden" under the brain surface can be better investigated with multiplanar 2D reconstructions, being the details explorable pixel by pixel. Therefore, it is advisable to combine 2D and 3D visualization side by side. It is also possible to combine 2D and 3D information visualizing the intersection of a 3D segmented model and 2D slices or, vice versa, showing 2D slices in a 3D scene (Fig. 4.4).

3D visualization is helpful not only for optimal trajectory planning. Since brain anatomy is highly convoluted, the 3D estimation and rendering of brain surface can be helpful for the identification of abnormal gyral/sulcal patterns often related to difficult-to-see focal cortical dysplasias associated with drug-resistant epilepsy. Indeed, such 3D reconstructions increase the diagnostic yield when a small cortical malformation is not obvious at visual inspection of 2D slices [47–50].

Registrations

Multimodal image is based on image-to-image registrations, while the image guidance of stereotactic surgical procedures is based on image-to-patient registration, being the head of the patient in the robotic dexterous workspace.

Registration can be defined as "*...the determination of a one-to-one mapping between the coordinates in one space and those in another, such that points in the two spaces that correspond to the same anatomic point are mapped to each other* [51]."

Image-to-Image Registration

To align two image datasets is the goal of image-to-image registration. This a process between two (and only two) datasets: the **fixed (or reference)** dataset and the **moving (or input) dataset**. The moving dataset is registered to the fixed one. Registration between multiple spaces (e.g., from a FLAIR to a 3D T1W sequence, and then to an angiographic CT scan) can be obtained by concatenating several one-to-one registrations in a global multi-stage workflow.

The registration process includes **two sequential steps** (Fig. 4.5). First, a **transformation** must be applied to all voxels of the moving dataset to compute the new 3D coordinates of every voxel. Subsequently, a new intensity value must be assigned to every voxel based on an **interpolation** process.

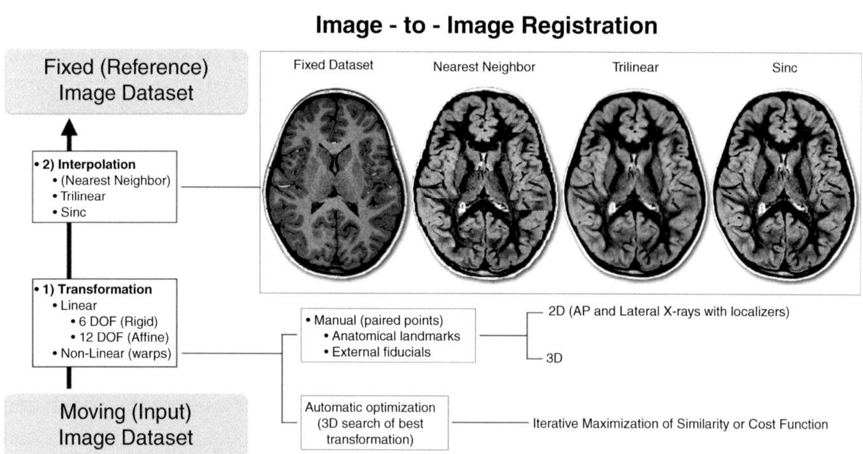

Fig. 4.5 Image-to-image registration
The main steps and options of an image-to-image registration process are depicted in the figure. Since the fixed dataset is not modified at all (neither translated, rotated, scaled, sheared or warped, nor interpolated), the reference dataset is typically the one carrying information about the brain vasculature (3D CBCT, 3D conventional angio-CT, angio-MR with or without contrast enhancement) in the context of intracranial stereotaxic planning. In fact, the interpolation, whatever the quality of the used algorithm, induces a degradation of the original information, albeit a minimal one. After a rigid transformation to a 3D T1W dataset has been applied, a 2D FLAIR dataset has been interpolated with three different algorithms available in FLIRT software package [52]. Nearest neighbor, trilinear and sinc algorithms have been applied, taking 25 s, 39 s, and more than 5 min, respectively, in our experiment. It is appreciable that the preservation of original information is proportional to the taken time. Of note, nearest neighbor algorithm gives often non optimal results because it produces artificially non-smooth boundaries, as in the depicted case. Despite its speed, it should be therefore avoided

A spatial transformation can be linear or not linear and is described with 4x4 matrices in computer graphics [53]. When a **linear transformation** is applied to the moving dataset, all voxels are moved to their new coordinates in the same way (e.g., all voxels are translated along the *x* axis by n pixels towards left). A linear transformation can have up to 12 parameters: 3 translation, 3 rotation, 3 scaling, and 3 shearing parameters, each of one can be named also as degree-of-freedom (DOF). All these separate parameters can be differently combined. The most commonly used linear transformation is called "Rigid" because it includes only 3 translation (along *x*, *y*, and *z* axes) and 3 rotation (about *x*, *y*, and *z* axes) parameters. Since every object in the image dataset is only moved in the 3D space without applying any shape modification (neither scaling nor shearing), it is clear why the term "**rigid transformation"**" is used. Such 6-DOF transformation is the best choice when it is assumed that the size and the shape of the objects represented in both images are constant. This is the case of the same brain acquired two times in different MR studies (split sessions) when the temporal gap is negligible and the position of the patient (usually supine) is similar. When the correction of MR eddy currents [54] is required, it can be advisable to add some more parameters. Therefore, when linear shape modifications must be allowed, it is possible to use "**affine transformations**," including up to 12 DOF (3 translations, 3 rotations, 3 scales, and 3 shears in the three dimensions) (Figs. 4.6 and 4.7).

When "different brains" must be co-registered, **non-linear transformations** can be used. They are known also as warps or elastic registrations and can have anything from tens to millions of DOFs. Warps can be advisable when we want to co-register pre- and post-resection datasets, or when the temporal gap between the two exams is long, or when large pathology modifications occurred, or even when we want to find a best inter-subject spatial correlation. The latter is the case of population studies where it is necessary to collect image data from different subjects in a unique template (e.g., fMRI studies), or the case of registration to an atlas (that must be intended as a different subject).[3]

It must be clear that "rigid" and "linear" are not synonyms. Rigid, 6-DOF transformations are a subset of affine, 12-DOF transformations. After the application of a rigid transformation, all the structures are only moved, remaining their shape and size preserved. When affine, 12-DOF registrations are applied, shapes and sizes can be changed but, analogously to rigid transformations, three points of the moving dataset that were on a same line before the application of the transformation continue to be on a same line after the image has been transformed. This is practically understandable because the same transformation has been applied to the coordinates of all voxels. On the opposite, when non-linear transformations are applied, the coordinates of each voxel are differently modified.

---

[3]A patient-to-atlas registration is common when a target is not directly visible in the patient images, as in the case of some DBS procedures. Other types of inter-subject registrations are never performed in surgical planning, but only in research studies registering different subjects to a common template.

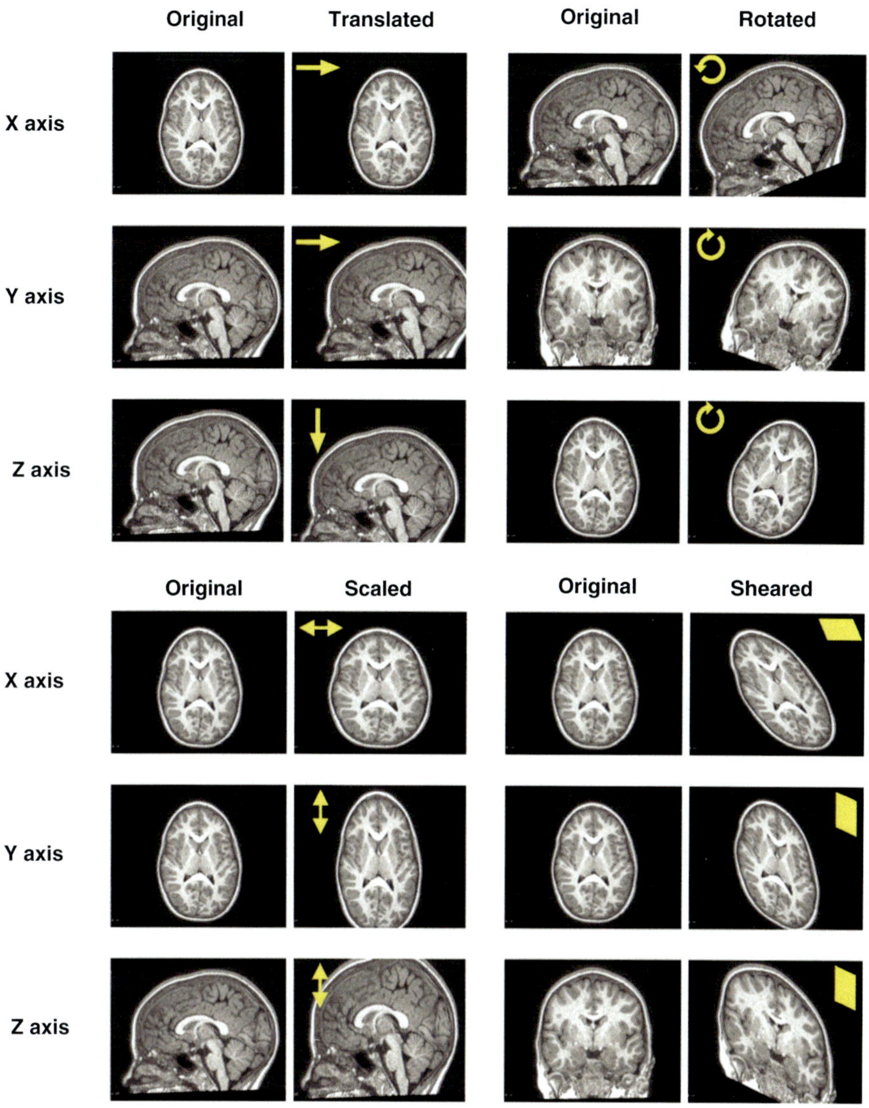

Fig. 4.6 Affine transformations (12 DOF)
Translations, rotations, scales, and shears along or about x, y, and z axes are represented. The effect of the transform application is represented for each parameter comparing the original image with the transformed one with convenient 2D images (axial, coronal, or sagittal)

Once the most appropriate type of linear transformation has been chosen accordingly to theoretical assumptions, up to 12 parameters must be computed.[4] The simplest case is that of a **manual alignment** obtained selecting some pairs of points

[4] Non-linear transformations are rarely adopted in the context of intracranial stereotaxic planning.

Translation

$$T = \begin{bmatrix} 1 & 0 & 0 & t_x \\ 0 & 1 & 0 & t_y \\ 0 & 0 & 1 & t_z \\ 0 & 0 & 0 & 1 \end{bmatrix}$$

Rotation about *x* axis

$$R_x(\theta) = \begin{bmatrix} 1 & 0 & 0 & 0 \\ 0 & cos\theta & -sin\theta & 0 \\ 0 & sin\theta & cos\theta & 0 \\ 0 & 0 & 0 & 1 \end{bmatrix}$$

$$identity = \begin{bmatrix} 1 & 0 & 0 & 0 \\ 0 & 1 & 0 & 0 \\ 0 & 0 & 1 & 0 \\ 0 & 0 & 0 & 1 \end{bmatrix}$$

Scaling

$$S = \begin{bmatrix} S_x & 0 & 0 & 0 \\ 0 & S_y & 0 & 0 \\ 0 & 0 & S_z & 0 \\ 0 & 0 & 0 & 1 \end{bmatrix}$$

Rotation about *y* axis

$$R_y(\theta) = \begin{bmatrix} cos\theta & 0 & sin\theta & 0 \\ 0 & 1 & 0 & 0 \\ -sin\theta & 0 & cos\theta & 0 \\ 0 & 0 & 0 & 1 \end{bmatrix}$$

$$M = \begin{bmatrix} 1.00 & 0.00 & 0.00 & 5.00 \\ 0.00 & 0.98 & -0.17 & 0.00 \\ 0.00 & 0.17 & 0.98 & -10.00 \\ 0.00 & 0.00 & 0.00 & 1.00 \end{bmatrix}$$

Shear

$$Sh = \begin{bmatrix} 1 & sh_x^y & sh_x^z & 0 \\ sh_y^x & 1 & sh_y^z & 0 \\ sh_z^x & sh_z^y & 1 & 0 \\ 0 & 0 & 0 & 1 \end{bmatrix}$$

Rotation about *z* axis

$$R_y(\theta) = \begin{bmatrix} cos\theta & -sin\theta & 0 & 0 \\ sin\theta & cos\theta & 0 & 0 \\ 0 & 0 & 1 & 0 \\ 0 & 0 & 0 & 1 \end{bmatrix}$$

Fig. 4.7 4 × 4 transformation matrices
The coordinates of every voxel in the moving dataset are multiplied by a matrix with $n \times m$ dimensions. T is a transformation that describes three translations, along x, y, and z axes, reported in the cells with tx, ty, and tz values, respectively. S describes three scales along x, y, and z axes, reported on the main diagonal of the matrix. Sh is the transformation describing the shears. Three transformations, describing the $\boldsymbol{\theta}$ rotation about x, y, and z axes, are reported in the central column of the picture. All translation, rotation, scaling, and shear matrices can be multiplied, obtaining a unique 4 × 4 matrix containing all the 12 parameters. M is an example of a 4 × 4 matrix written with 3D Slicer software that will translate all the voxels of the moving dataset by 5 mm towards right (red oval) and 10 mm upward (green oval) and will also rotate the dataset 10° about the x axis (light blue oval). Identity matrix, characterized by 1 numbers all along the main diagonal and zeros in all other cells, has no effect when multiplied with voxel coordinates

that are visually recognizable on both the image datasets. Once an adequate number of point pairs have been selected, the computation of the transformation matrix is fast and simple. The mathematics of this computation is out of the scopes of the present chapter, but it is important to know that a minimum of three non-colinear point pairs is required and best results are obtained with up to 6 pairs.

Points can be **anatomical landmarks** as sulcal or vascular bifurcations (intrinsic fiducials, based on patient-generated image content only). Anyway, such anatomical landmarks are not exactly point shaped. When **external fiducials**, usually spherical, are fixed to the patient's head, their center can be more easily and reproducibly recognized and selected. This is typically the case of fiducials used for the subsequent intraoperative image-to-patient transformation (extrinsic fiducials that are foreign objects introduced into the imaged space) [55].

The manual point-to-point definition of landmarks preliminary to the computation of the transformation matrix is very intuitive. Nonetheless, the accuracy of manual registrations is strictly operator-dependent and user's inexperience can be detrimental to its accuracy. Moreover, the selection of anatomical landmarks can be tricky and time consuming. External fiducials, fixed to the head of the patient (better if trans-osseous) or provided by a stereotactic frame, are easier to use and more accurate than anatomical landmarks, but they are usually not yet available when advanced multimodal diagnostics must be performed preliminary to the definitive planning. Multimodal imaging is therefore mainly based on an automatic search of the transformation that will guarantee the best fit of the moving dataset to the fixed one (**automatic registration**). The most common strategy adopted to find the best transformation is to measure iteratively the similarity or the dissimilarity between moving and fixed datasets after a number of transformations have been applied. The highest value of a similarity function or of a cost (dissimilarity) function is searched through an iterative series of trials. The most common similarity function is **Mutual Information**, based on the measurement of joint entropy [56, 57]. Since entropy is a measure of disorder, the lower it is, the higher is the value of the function and the better is the fit between the co-registered datasets. During the optimization process, the global maximum of the similarity function can be searched about every 3D axis. **Correlation Ratio** is another popular similarity function [58]. Some comprehensive overviews about the numerous optimization strategies are available in the literature [53–55, 59–64].

The lower the number of DOF, the faster and reliable is the registration. Conversely, the final fit can be better with more DOF. In fact, affine transformations often guarantee a better fit when slight distortions, or brain shape modifications or motion artifacts occur. Requested time is a bit higher, but the true problem is that sometimes the final fit can be paradoxically totally invalid (post-registration misalignment). When large local differences between the two brains to be registered exist (surgeries, modifications of structural lesions), non-linear registrations can be preferred. Anyway, warps are extremely time consuming (and more complex to be managed). While linear registrations take from some seconds to few minutes, non-linear registrations can take from tens of minutes up to a few days when millions of DOF are allowed with normally available computers.

Some important and practical suggestions can be resumed for the young readers[5]:

- The dataset that is most critical for the patient's safety should be used as the reference space. Especially when a percutaneous implantation of the probes must be performed, as in SEEG procedures, the less distorted dataset providing the crucial information for safety (usually brain vasculature) should be chosen as the reference dataset.
- After the best transformation has been found and applied, the moving dataset is interpolated and resampled, "acquiring" the geometric properties of the fixed datasets. This means that registering the lower resolution dataset (moving) to the higher resolution one (fixed) is always advisable. Vice versa, the details and the diagnostic yield of the high-resolution dataset will be irremediably lost.

[5] Many and more complex aspects of image registrations should be covered for special processing workflows such as the ones to estimate activations with functional MRI or white matter tracts from diffusion-weighted images datasets, but this is out of the scopes of the present chapter. Here we want to remain in the context of image registrations in the last mile of surgical planning.

- The automatic optimization step is aimed at finding the transformation that guarantees the best fit of the two datasets maximizing their similarity through a process of repeat trials and estimations, iteratively changing the matrix parameters according to allowed DOF. Simplifying, the search goes on until the similarity function value increases significantly and stops when further modifications of the moving dataset do not add any significant improvements. This implies that if the two datasets do not match at all at the beginning of the search process, or match too few, the registration will fail. When the initial position is not similar, as in the case of two datasets obtained in different studies, it is always advisable to start from an approximate global fitting that can be obtained by a rough manual alignment in many software packages.
- Best choice of cost function can be guided by simple criteria [54]. The two most common and successful choices are Mutual Information or Normalized Mutual Information for any two image datasets (e.g., T1W to CT) and Correlation Ratio for any two MR modalities (e.g., FLAIR to T1W).
- The basic assumption of linear registrations is that the content of the image datasets has not been modified between the two scanning sessions. This is approximately true for the brain whose movements in the intracranial space are negligible if both studies have been conducted in supine position but it is not true for mobile anatomical structures that are included in the image space such as the jaw or the neck. It is strongly advisable not to include these parts in the scanning FOV or, alternatively, to exclude them by manual cropping before running the automatic registration. If most of the air around the head will be also cropped, a rough initial alignment will be also guaranteed (see previous point). When cropping is not possible and the success of the registration is compromised by different positions of the mobile anatomical structures, a manual point-to-point registration is the only possible way to align the two brains.
- Unfortunately, most registration options are available only with free software developed at high level centers and "intended for research," such as 3D Slicer [65], Freesurfer [66], FSL [67], and SPM [68]. Commercially available IGS workstations rarely provide the neurosurgeon with details about the implemented algorithms for automatic search of the best fit. Likely, applying a rigid transformation is the most common choice to run a "fusion tool," but the user does not fully know what she/he is doing most of the times. Anyway, even if such algorithms cannot be chosen with most commercially available software, it is still important to understand which are the limits of the used devices and technologies. At meeting discussions, we have heard many times something sounding like "I correct MR distortions fusing T2W dataset with CT!" Only if the metrics of the transformation is affine (12 DOF), this assertion could be considered valid at least for linear sources of error, but most MR distortions (e.g., metal artifacts) are non-linear and cannot be compensated by means of linear transformations. The correction of major MR distortions by "fusing the dataset with a CT scan" is likely only an erroneous myth, at least for most IGS planning workstations. And, anyway, who knows? Implemented algorithms are almost always patent-protected and neither national, nor international regulatory medical authorities

deal with such fundamental aspects of the commercialized devices. Nonetheless, a certain level of intervention is still in the hands of the neurosurgeon even when only commercial software are used: the choice of most appropriate scans and of the best reference dataset, the scanning parameters (essentially the spatial resolution with the consequent uncertainty), the cropping (during the scanning session or later on, limiting the number of imported axial slices), the number of optimization iterations (even if it is not explicitly settable, the registration process can be often repeated starting from the results of the previous run, thus increasing the total number of iterations until the registrations looks satisfactory), etc.

- Manual registrations are operator-dependent, and inexperience can lead to low reproducibility. Anyway, expert users guarantee affordable results that can be considered as gold standard when external fiducials are used [64]. On the opposite, automatic registrations are perfectly reproducible when transformation metrics and optimization algorithms are fixed. Nonetheless, automatic registration can give even completely wrong results. In fact, it must be finally understood that it is impossible to be informed by a software package that the performed registration is accurate enough for the clinical goals. According to the above-mentioned principles of the optimization, an automatic registration can be stopped very far from finding the transformation that would guarantee the best fit, without any warning. **Accurate visual inspection of the two datasets, overlaid or side by side, is the only way to assess the correctness of the registration** [53, 63]. In other words, experimental results indicate that automatic registration "*techniques have the potential to produce satisfactory results much of the time, but that visual inspection is necessary to guard against large errors* [64]."

Image-to-Patient Registration

The topic of image-to-image registrations for multimodal diagnostics and stereotaxic planning has been briefly covered in the previous section of the present chapter. In that context, we have used the term "coordinates" referring to "**voxel coordinates**," used to specify the location of every voxel within an image dataset. Such coordinates just indicate the offset from a corner of the image, expressed as integer of pixels. The origin of the coordinates (0, 0, 0, or 1, 1, 1) is seated at a corner of the image space, and all other coordinates are defined only by positive values. Unfortunately, conventions for voxel coordinates are not standardized. With a certain software package, an x coordinate of 35 can indicate the position of the voxel along the latero-lateral axis starting from left, but it could be the opposite with another software tool, starting from right. Therefore, to deal with coordinates provided by different packages (included the commercial ones) is very complex, and the neurosurgeon must be helped by biomedical engineers or physicists if it is necessary to move coordinates from a package to another. The space defined by planning software, such the ones provided with robotic assistants, is defined by "**world coordinates**." It is obviously related to the surgical space, in which the patient's head is positioned and every point can be efficiently reached by the end effector attached to the extremity of the robotic arm (the dexterous robotic space). Differently from image space, that is discretized in a 3D grid of voxels and described by integer coordinates, the surgical space is described by world coordinates that are expressed in millimeters. Floating point values are used because the world space is not discretized. The way in which voxel coordinates are converted when image datasets are imported in the planning software is unpredictable. The position of a certain point is often expressed with both voxel and world coordinates, and the neurosurgeon must understand very well the difference between these two systems of coordinates. It must be understood that if the neurosurgeon wants to target a voxel that has been already chosen on a diagnostic image viewer, it is not enough to copy its voxel coordinates into the planning software. This simple operation can be done only if the planning software clearly uses different editable fields or tools to input the coordinates of entry and target points.

Once a trajectory has been defined in the planning software, the voxel coordinates of both the entry and the target point must be transferred to the world coordinates of the patient's head positioned in the stereotactic space. Analogously to simpler and most common image-to-image registrations, a rigid transformation will serve as a "coordinate mover" (image-to-patient registration). A point-to-point strategy can be simply adopted, based on the selection of an adequate number (not less than three) intrinsic or extrinsic fiducials. Anatomical landmarks cannot be fully adequate when high stereotactic accuracy is required. In fact, anatomical features as tragus or lateral canthi cannot be as discrete as many intracranial landmarks. Extrinsic fiducials, visible in the planning image dataset and localizable in the stereotactic space, can guarantee higher accuracy.

Image-to-patient scenario 1. We can now describe a **frameless workflow**, conceptually similar to the marker-based registration preliminary to a navigation procedure in which some head-attached fiducials are selected with a tracked pointer. First, some dedicated **bone markers** are fixed percutaneously to the skull with a minimally invasive procedure. Second, a contrasted 3D CT scan is obtained inside or outside the operating room. Third, the patient's head is fixed with a rigid holder that will guarantee a constant spatial relationship with the robotic space. Fourth, this image dataset is imported in the world space of the planning software and the center of each fiducial (usually spherical) is easily selected, thus defining its world coordinates. Fifth, the bone markers are physically touched with a dedicated probe attached to a robotic arm with haptic movement capabilities, as the one of the ROSA system (Zimmer Biomet, Warsaw, Indiana) in shared-controlled mode. By means of this step, the world coordinates of the bone fiducials are selected in the robotic space and the image-to-patient registration is completed.[6] Sixth, the trajectory is planned in the actual image dataset, registered to the patient, and the robotic arm can align the tool holder with the vector of the planned trajectory [69]. When the target of the procedure is not directly visible in the actual dataset, or when a high number of

[6] Differently from image-to-image registrations, an image-to-patient registration includes only the computation of a rigid transformation. In fact, the surgical space is physical, it is not a discretized image space and no interpolation is required.

trajectories and multimodal complex planning would take too long to be managed intraoperatively, trajectories can be planned some days in advance. The day of the stereotactic implantation, once the image-to-patient registration has been completed, the planning dataset can be imported into the planning software and registered manually or automatically to the actual dataset. Finally, the transformation of the latter registration is applied at both EP and TP of all the planned trajectories and the robotic arm can be moved sequentially in supervisory controlled mode assisting all the implantations, one by one.

Image-to-patient scenario 2. A similar frameless strategy can be implemented with **Neurolocate**®, a touch-less registration tool provided with Neuromate® robotic assistant (Renishaw, Wotton-under-Edge, UK). It is a tool with five spherical fiducials attached to carbon-fiber rods that must be fixed as an end effector to the robotic arm (Fig. 4.8).

Once the head of the patient is fixed in the robotic space with a rigid holder, the robotic arm is moved with a special remote control to approach the Neurolocate fiducials very close to the scalp. Next, a 3D CBCT dataset is obtained intraoperatively with O-arm system, a mobile scanner that is spatially compatible with Neuromate shape and size. This dataset is then imported in the planning software, and the coordinates of the five fiducials are selected with a semi-automated procedure. Since the coordinates of the fiducials in the robotic space are already known because Neurolocate's geometry is fixed and it is attached to the robotic arm, the rigid transformation is easily computed. Similar to the previous example, trajectories can be imported from a planning dataset automatically registered to the actual one scanned with O-arm and the robotic arm can then be moved [70]. Compared to the above-described ROSA-based workflow, the main advantage is that the invasive fixation of bone markers is not necessary. Conversely, the image dataset can be acquired only when the patient's head is already fixed in the robotic space and an expensive intraoperative CT scanner is required. On the other side, if such a scanner

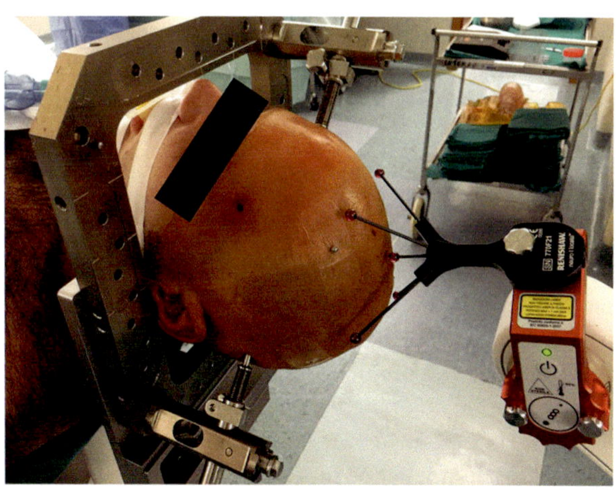

Fig. 4.8 Neurolocate Neurolocate is attached as an end effector to the robotic arm and provides five extrinsic fiducials that must be approached very close to the patients head in order to be included in 3D CBCT for image-to-patient registration

is available, the correct probe positioning can be intraoperatively assessed and it is not necessary to go outside the operating room for the final check.

Image-to-patient scenario 3. Another device is available with Neuromate for point-to-point image-to-patient registration, based on ultra-sound (**US**). A localizer with five CT- or MR-visible fiducials is fixed to the skull and an appropriate image dataset is acquired. In the operating room, the localizer is substituted with a similar tool that positions five US microphones at the same places of the image-visible fiducials. Their location in the robotic space is then automatically assessed activating an US emitter as end effector [71]. The use of this registration device is quite simple but it requires an invasive fixation onto the patient's head and the guaranteed accuracy is lower than with Neurolocate or with a frame-based technique [72].

A frameless image-to-patient registration procedure can be differently based on a surface matching strategy [73] "*in which unordered sets of points may be used, as in matching the surface of the head as imaged by CT or MRI … with the surface of the scalp as digitized in the operating room. This surface-to-surface matching has the advantage of using a natural feature of the head … whose segmentation can be automated* [32]." This technique is similar to a **surface registration** preliminary to navigation in which a tracked pointer is slithered on the scalp to generate a cloud of points. The ROSA system can use a 3D laser scanner as an end effector aimed at digitizing the face and the forehead of the patient. The scalp surface is automatically modelled exploiting the clear-cut interface between skin and air in the planning dataset, and a surface-to-surface matching can be computed [74]. This registration method is procedurally easy and semi-automatic, but it guarantees an accuracy slightly lower if compared with the use of bone markers, especially for posterior targets because the centroid of the registration plane is more distant from intracranial targets [75]. In fact, the longer the distance between the registration volume (where the fiducials or a cloud of surface points are positioned) and the target, the lower the targeting accuracy.

Image-to-patient scenario 4. Robotic assistants can be used also in **frame-based mode**, with 3D or 2D images. With 3D images, similar to framed navigation procedures, the planning dataset is scanned after the head of the patient has been fixed in a stereotactic frame with a localizer mounted on it. Such localizer provides four fiducials (anterior, posterior, left, right), radio-opaque for CT or fillable with copper-sulfate for MR. These **V-, N-, or Z-shaped fiducials** appear as lines of two or three dots all around the head in axial slices, and their coordinates can be easily selected manually or, more modernly, with an affordable and semi-automatic procedure that is commonly available on the planning software of most popular frames. The definition of the fiducial coordinates guarantees the registration between the image space and the stereotactic space as defined by the world coordinate system of the frame [76]. In the operating room, the frame is fixed to the robot base with a frame-specific rigid adapter. The final registration, from the frame space to the robotic space is computed in advance by means of a calibration procedure. The transformation computed during such calibration is not procedure-specific because the frame is well fixed every time in the same position relative to the robot. Anyway, such calibration must be repeated during maintenances (usually every 3–4 months) to guarantee a constant accuracy. 3D frame-based registrations are highly accurate. The main disadvantage is that the frame must be maintained fixed to the patient in the period occurring between image acquisition and surgical implantation.

Image-to-patient scenario 5. Last, a **2D frame-based registration** can be obtained also with a pair of X-rays and dedicated localizers [77]. Four plastic, radiolucent plates are fixed to the frame, each one providing four radio-opaque fiducials perfectly corresponding to the position of the analogous ones on the opposite plate (Fig. 4.9).

Two projective X-rays are obtained intraoperatively from two different perspectives, approximately antero-posterior and lateral. Eight fiducials are visible in each one of these two images because their distance from the source of the conic X-ray is different for anterior-posterior and left-right pairs of plates. Once the images are imported in the planning software, the neurosurgeon selects the center of the eight fiducials visible in both projections, and the pair of images is 3D registered [76]. The coordinates of every point in the frame space are selectable clicking with the mouse on both images: the selection of a point on the lateral image defines y and z coordinates, and the selection of a point on the AP image defines x and z coordinates. Thus, the combined selection of a point in both projections defines all the 3D coordinates. Any 3D dataset, obtained preoperatively, can be then registered to these stereotactically paired 2D images if an adequate number of fiducials (intrinsic or extrinsic) are visible in both modalities. Such 2D frame-based registration

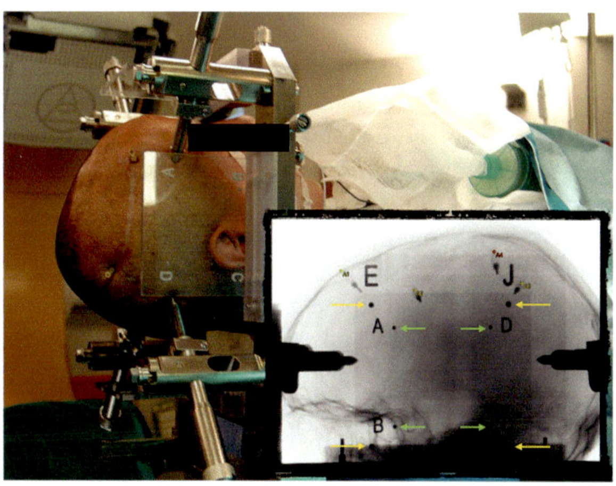

Fig. 4.9 2D frame-based localizers
The plastic plates holding the fiducials for 2D X-rays are mounted onto the base of Talairach frame. For every pair of plates (anterior and posterior; left and right), eight fiducials (arrows in the picture) are visible in the X-rays because the distance of every plate from the X-ray source is different and beams are not parallel. Bone markers are also visible in the picture, both in the patient's photo and in the radiograph. They were used in the past at "Claudio Munari" center to register the 3D image space (MR, CT, PET) to the frame space for using the robot in frame-based modality. At present, Neurolocate-based frameless modality has replaced this method at our center

procedure is time expensive and a bit tricky: "… *the accuracy of the registration process will depend on the accuracy of the estimates of the projection parameters, which in turn is a function of the accuracy of the fiducial markers localization… in order to achieve a registration accuracy better than 1 mm, the fiducial markers have to be located with an accuracy better than 150μm* [78]." The main advantage of this registration technique is that it can be completed with a simple C-arm.

We would like to finish this very brief overview of main image-to-patient registration strategy highlighting the geniality of Talairach stereotactic method (and similar systems). The complexity of transformations was extremely reduced in practice when computers were not available and only 2D X-rays could be obtained. The use of teleradiographs, with the X-ray source well aligned with the frame's center and 5 meters far from it, guaranteed images obtained by means of X-rays that could be approximated as parallel. Thanks to this, the mathematics of transformations was simplified reducing to the three DOF to deal with, only translations along x, y, and x axes [32].

Intra- and Postoperative Verification of Probe Positioning

Once the probes have been advanced into the intracranial space, the verification of the positioning accuracy is crucial. Intraoperative imaging can be 2D or 3D. As already summarized, in case of two-dimensional images, two radiographs (usually in lateral and antero-posterior projections, orthogonal each other) are obtained with a dedicated localizer often mounted on a stereotactic frame. Alternatively, a three-dimensional dataset can be obtained with an intraoperative CT scanner. Some pros and cons exist with both the techniques. The 2D images can be obtained with conventional c-arm equipment, often available in the operating room. The X-ray dose is very low, thus these images are especially indicated when multiple checks are requested throughout the execution of the procedure, as in the case of multiple-bite biopsies [27] or DBS with micro-electrode recordings. On the other side, every pair of 2D images must be registered to the 3D planning dataset (CT or MR) with a manual procedure that takes some minutes, as previously described. Differently, a 3D CT dataset can be easily and quickly registered to the planning images in a fully automatic fashion, but the X-ray dose is higher than with 2D images. 3D datasets are therefore usually obtained for the final assessment of the probe position.

When a stereotactic biopsy is performed, the evidence of neoplastic tissue at immediate histologic examination can be not enough to assess the correctness of the procedure. If the tumor appears heterogeneous at diagnostic imaging, it is advisable to sample different parts of the lesional and perilesional tissue. Therefore, it is important to verify that all the tissue samples have been obtained according to the stereotaxic planning, guaranteeing a higher diagnostic yield with multiple bites [27, 79, 80]. The correctness of the stereotactic procedure can be assessed with the probe in situ and intraoperative images or postoperatively, determining the position of air bubbles or canals [81, 82].

The correct positioning of the stimulating electrode is crucial also in DBS procedures. The visualization of the implanted probe can be assessed with CT or MR. Such intraoperative check is often performed by means of the O-arm system [69, 83–88].

Intracranial bending of the probes can occur in SEEG more easily than in DBS or biopsies because proper electrodes are semi-rigid, do not have a stylet inside, and are not guided by an external rigid cannula. Therefore, cerebral sulci can induce deviations from the planned trajectory. At "Claudio Munari" center, we first introduced the use of O-arm scanner in our workflow to perform pre-implantation 3D CBCT DSA, to register the head of the patient to the robotic space, to assist the intracranial advancement of the probes under X-ray control and to obtain a final 3D dataset with the implanted electrode [44, 70, 77, 89–91]. When an electrode is bended, or when it is advanced less or more than planned, its position can be often corrected thanks to intraoperative imaging. Once the implantation has been completed, the assessment of the position of every single recording lead allows to understand where SEEG traces come from and which anatomical structures are stimulated in order to induce seizures and map brain

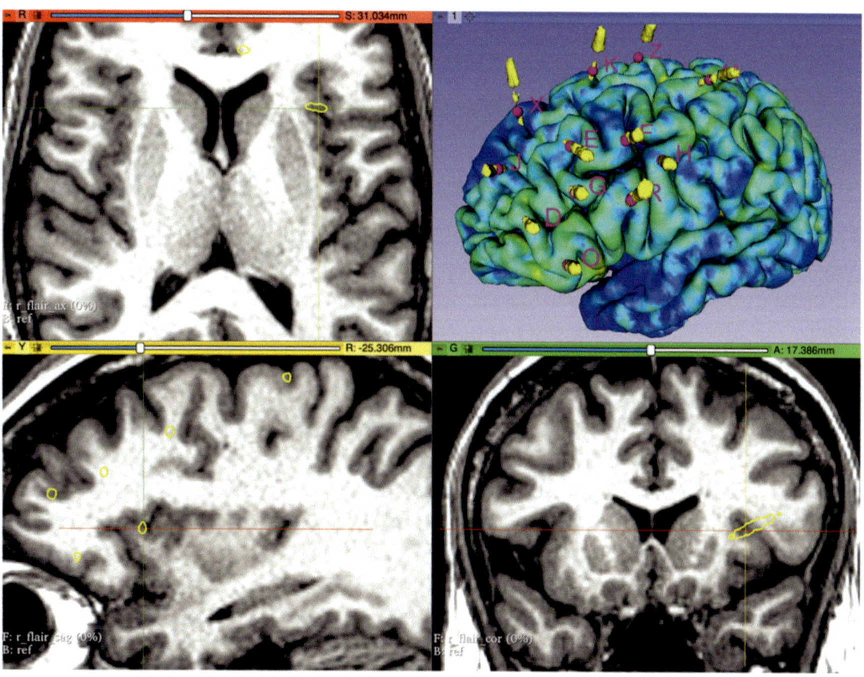

Fig. 4.10 Multimodal post-SEEG implantation scene
Once electrodes have been implanted, multimodal scene can be built to guide the interpretation of SEEG findings and the planning of subsequent treatment. The model of the electrodes is represented in yellow and it is rendered in 3D view. Moreover, its intersections with 2D slices are visible in multiplanar reconstructions. Brain surface is "painted"' with cortical metabolic information obtained from 2-deoxy-2-[fluorine-18]fluoro-D-glucose (^{18}F-FDG PET)

functions. We register the postimplantation CBCT to preoperative MR and collect all image data in a multimodal scene with 3D Slicer software package (Fig. 4.10).

The sources of intracerebral EEG signals can be visualized with 2D multiplanar reconstructions and with the 3D brain surfaces as estimated by FreeSurfer software package. Since the number of recording leads is very high (often more than 200), the manual positioning of a mark-up for each one of them is very time consuming. We therefore use SEEG-A (**SEEG Assistant**), a dedicated 3D Slicer plug-in able to automatically put a mark-up in correspondence of lead centroids and estimate the sampled brain structure according to Desikan-Killiany or Destrieux atlas [92–95]. This workflow, partially or fully adopted, is gaining popularity and similar multimodal 3D scenes are now built at many centers [41, 49, 96–98]. Moreover, a number of packages with functionalities similar to the ones included in SEEG-A are now freely available, such as BrainNetworks [99], EpiNav [100], EpiTools [101], iEEGView [102], iElectrodes [103], IntraAnat Electrodes [104], and Sylvius [105]. Another software package, able to classify the SEEG contacts as gray- or white-matter recording only on the basis of electrical signals (thus ignoring imaging) has been recently developed [106].

Accurate detection and segmentation of intracerebral electrodes are crucial not only for the best interpretation of SEEG traces and planning of subsequent treatment, but also for the countless research studies in the field of basic and clinical neurosciences [107–116].

Application Accuracy

The postimplantation imaging allows also the assessment of the application accuracy. Usually, the postoperative dataset is registered to the planning dataset, and different distances can be measured comparing the plans with actual position of the probes. As already stressed, the application accuracy of robot-based workflows is determined not only by the intrinsic mechanical accuracy of the robotic assistant. Many other variables crucially affect the total accuracy, such as the resolution of image datasets, the quality of registrations, and the rigidity of the head holder. It is important to highlight that when it is necessary to evaluate the accuracy of the robot (or, more generally, of the stereotactic device), it is better to look at the accuracy at the EP, thus avoiding to add intracranial deviations of the implanted probe to all other sources of error. The results of a narrative review of the literature are reported in Table 4.1 [70, 71, 74, 77, 96, 98, 117–128]. Only the articles reporting accuracy as Euclidean distance between planned and actual probe positions have been selected. It can be noted that different accuracy can be obtained with the same robot, ultimately suggesting the importance of the other components of the adopted workflow.

Some papers reporting the comparison between different registration tools can be of particular interest for all the neurosurgeon who are setting their workflow [70, 75, 117]

Table 4.1 Narrative review of articles reporting the application accuracy of robotic procedures as Euclidean distance. Rows have been ordered for procedure type, EPLE and TPLE. Distances are reported in millimeters (mm). Abbreviations: *EPLE* Entry point localization error, *TPLE* Target point localization error, *SD* Standard deviation, *IQR* Inter-quartile range, *NA* Not available

Bibliographic reference	Procedure	Cases	Frame coordinate system	Head-holder	Robotic assistant	Registration device	Fiducial type	Fiducial fixation	Verified trajectories	EPLE	TPLE
Lefranc et al. (2014)	Biopsy	3	Frameless	Three pin-points clamp	ROSA	Robotic-arm-mounted touching probe	Bone markers	Invasive	3	NA	0.42 (SD: 0.2)
Lefranc et al. (2014)	Biopsy	4	Frameless	Three pin-points clamp	ROSA	Robotic-arm-mounted touching probe	Skin markers	Non-invasive	4	NA	0.94 (SD: 0.4)
Lefranc et al. (2014)	Biopsy	24	Frameless	Three pin-points clamp	ROSA	Robotic-arm-mounted laser scanner	Scalp point cloud	Non-invasive	24	NA	1.22 (SD: 0.73)
Varma et al. (2006)	Biopsy	19	Frameless	Sugita-like	Neuromate	Head-mounted US device	Head-mounted US device	Invasive	22	NA	2.9 (SD: NA)
Moran et al. (2020)	DBS	113	Frameless	Leksell	Neuromate	Neurolocate-to-robot calibration	Robotic-arm-mounted fiducials (Neurolocate)	Non-invasive	226	NA	0.78 (SD: 0.37)
Lefranc et al. (2014)	DBS	27	Leksell	Leksell	ROSA	Frame-to-robot calibration	Frame-mounted 3D localizer	Non-invasive	52	NA	0.81 (SD: 0.39)
De Benedictis et al. (2017)	DBS	3	Frameless	Three pin-points clamp	ROSA	Robotic-arm-mounted laser scanner	Scalp point cloud	Non-invasive	6	NA	1.56 (SD: 0.35)
De Benedictis et al. (2017)	Pallidotomy	12	Frameless	Three pin-points clamp	ROSA	Robotic-arm-mounted laser scanner	Scalp point cloud	Non-invasive	12	NA	1.45 (SD: 0.32)

(continued)

Table 4.1 (continued)

Bibliographic reference	Procedure	Cases	Frame coordinate system	Head-holder	Robotic assistant	Registration device	Fiducial type	Fiducial fixation	Verified trajectories	EPLE	TPLE
Cardinale et al. (2017)	SEEG	8	Frameless	Talairach	Neuromate	Neurolocate-to-robot calibration	Robotic-arm-mounted fiducials (Neurolocate)	Non-invasive	127	0.59 (IQR: 0.25–0.88)	1.49 (IQR: 1.06–2.4)
Sharma et al. (2019)	SEEG	14	Leksell	Leksell	Neuromate	Frame-to-robot calibration	Frame-mounted 3D localizer	Non-invasive	218	0.71 (IQR: 0.47–1.03)	1.07 (IQR: 0.71–1.59)
Cardinale et al. (2013)	SEEG	81	Talairach	Talairach	Neuromate	Frame-to-robot calibration	Frame-mounted 2D localizer	Non-invasive	1050	0.78 (IQR: 0.49–1.08)	1.77 (IQR: 1.25–2.51)
Gonzalez-Martinez et al. (2016)	SEEG	46	Frameless	Leksell	ROSA	Robotic-arm-mounted laser scanner	Scalp point cloud	Non-invasive	500	1.2 (IQR: 0.78–1.83)	1.7 (IQR: 1.2–2.3)
Dorfer et al. (2017)	SEEG	16	Frameless	Three pin-points clamp	iSys1 (StealthGuide)	Navigation system (stealth)	Bone markers	Invasive	93	1.3 (IQR: NA)	1.5 (IQR: NA)
Zheng et al. (2021)	SEEG	19	Frameless	Three pin-points clamp	SINO	Robotic-arm-mounted touching probe	Bone markers	Invasive	230	1.39 (SD: 0.48)	1.54 (SD: 0.43)
Kim et al. (2020)	SEEG	25	Frameless	Three pin-points clamp	ROSA	Robotic-arm-mounted touching probe	Bone markers	Invasive	257	1.39 (SD: 0.75)	3.05 (SD: 2.02)
Rollo et al. (2021)	SEEG	150	Frameless	Three pin-points clamp	ROSA	Robotic-arm-mounted touching probe	Bone markers	Invasive	2040	1.45 (SD: 1.02)	1.8 (SD: 2.06)
Bottan et al.	SEEG	41	Leksell	Leksell	Neuromate	Frame-to-robot calibration	Frame-mounted 3D localizer	Non-invasive	98	1.5 (SD: 1.24)	2.3 (SD: 1.47)

Zheng et al. (2021)	SEEG	14	Frameless	Leksell	SINO	Robotic-arm-mounted touching probe	Bone markers	Invasive	90	1.51 (SD: 0.53)	1.59 (SD: 0.71)
Candela-Cantò et al. (2018)	SEEG	14	Frameless	Sugita-like	Neuromate	Head-mounted US device	Head-mounted US device	Invasive	164	1.57 (IQR: 1–2.25)	1.77 (IQR: 1.2–2.6)
De Benedictis et al. (2017)	SEEG	36	Frameless	Three pin-points clamp	ROSA	Robotic-arm-mounted laser scanner	Scalp point cloud	Non-invasive	386	1.59 (SD: 1.1)	2.22 (SD: 1.71)
Ollivier et al. (2017)	SEEG	66	Frameless	Three pin-points clamp	ROSA	Robotic-arm-mounted laser scanner	Scalp point cloud	Non-invasive	857	1.62 (SD: 1.8)	2.66 (SD: 2.3)
Spyrantis et al. (2018)	SEEG	5	Frameless	Three pin-points clamp	ROSA	Robotic-arm-mounted laser scanner	Scalp point cloud	Non-invasive	40	2.53 (SD: 0.24)	2.96 (SD: 0.24)
Bourdillon et al. (2019)	SEEG	50	Leksell	Leksell	Neuromate	Frame-to-robot calibration	Frame-mounted 3D localizer	Non-invasive	565	NA	1.15 (SD: 0.36)
Ho et al. (2018)	SEEG	20	Frameless	Three pin-points clamp	ROSA	Robotic-arm-mounted laser scanner	Scalp point cloud	Non-invasive	222	NA	3.39 (SD: 1.08)

Future Perspectives

Automated trajectory planning is one of the most promising directions for present and future development in the field. It is important to stress that the output of automated planning algorithms must be considered only as a proposal: the responsibility of the planning is still in charge of the neurosurgeon! The difference is that she/he starts the planning not from zero but from some pre-planned trajectories, evaluating on her/his own risks and benefits.

Since SEEG implies the implantation of a large number of electrodes, **automated procedures** can be indicated to reduce the planning time optimizing the number of probes according to the general strategy of investigation and reducing both the risk of intracranial bleeding and electrode deviation from the planned trajectory. The computation of a cumulative risk score based on vessel distance all along the trajectory is a common approach to minimize the chance of hemorrhagic complications, and the angle at the bone surface is often optimized to reduce the risk of drill skiving and the consequent electrode misplacement [129]. The segmentation of brain vasculature is particularly important for optimal risk assessment, of course [43, 130–133]. Automatic lesion detection can also be included in the algorithm of automated planning [134]. Different strategies have been proposed to generate the best set of electrodes covering the needed epileptological strategy [135–137]. A data-based solution able to exploit the knowledge extracted by past cases has been proposed [138]. The use of **artificial intelligence** algorithms has been also advocated [139]. Automated planning of SEEG trajectories has given optimal results, comparable (if not better) to human manual planning [132, 136, 140–143].

Automated planning has been proposed also for DBS [144–148] and, very recently, for biopsies [149]. A novel approach for automated steerable path planning is of particular interest: it has been proposed for DBS but could be adopted also in other fields for both targeting optimization and risk reduction [150].

For a comprehensive overview of the literature concerning the automated planning of percutaneous trajectories, including neurosurgical procedures, see two recent systematic reviews [151, 152].

Conclusion

Robotic assistance for minimally invasive intracranial surgeries is the natural evolution of non-robotized framed systems, as perfectly foreseen by Benabid and coworkers 30 years ago [153]. The advent of powerful computers and 3D imaging led neurosurgical robotics from a pioneering era to daily routine at many centers worldwide. However, it must be well understood that accurate machines are not enough. A lack of proper strategy or insufficient application accuracy may lead to unsatisfactory diagnostic yield, unsuccessful treatment, or severe complications. When a new robot-based neurosurgery program is going to be started, the whole workflow must be carefully designed, understanding that the robotic assistant is crucial, but also that it is only a ring of a long chain.

Acknowledgements We like to express or gratitude to all our coworkers from the teams of "Claudio Munari Center," "Neuroradiology," "Anesthesiology," "Pediatrics," "Pathology," "Medical Physics," "Clinical Engineering," and "Information Technology" departments at Niguarda Hospital.

We would like to thank Gloria Innocenti for her contribution to bibliographic research and document retrieval, and all our friends from Politecnico di Milano and University of Genova for their constant collaboration and help in the field of biomedical engineering.

We want to thank also our close friends, Angela Catapano and Umberto Piccolo, for providing us with the drawing and the photos included in Fig. 4.2.

Finally, and most important, we would like to thank Claudio Munari, our mentor, who taught us mainly the value of team working among innumerable other things.

References

1. Schweikard A, Ernst F. Introduction. In: Schweikard A, Ernst F, editors. Medical robotics. Springer International Publishing Switzerland; 2015. p. 1–27.
2. Maciunas RJ, Galloway RL, Latimer J. The application accuracy of stereotactic frames. Neurosurgery. 1994;35:682–94.
3. Bucholz RD, Sturm CD, Hogan RE. The use of three-dimensional images in stereotactic neurosurgery. In: Gildenberg PL, Tasker RR, editors. Textbook of stereotactic and functional neurosurgery. New York: McGraw-Hill; 1998. p. 337–49.
4. Lo Russo G, Tassi L, Cossu M, Cardinale F, Mai R, Castana L, et al. Focal cortical resection in malformations of cortical development. Epileptic Disord. 2003;5:S115–23.
5. Bancaud J. Surgery of epilepsy based on stereotactic investigations—the plan of the SEEG investigation. In: Gillingham F, Gybels J, Hitchcock E, Rossi G, Szikla G, editors. Advanced stereotactic and functional neurosurgery 4. Acta Neurochirurgica Supplementum, vol. 30. Vienna: Springer; 1980. p. 25–34.
6. Cardinale F, Francione S, Gennari L, Citterio A, Sberna M, Tassi L, et al. SUrface-PRojected FLAIR analysis: a novel tool for advanced imaging of epilepsy. World Neurosurg. 2017;98:715–26.
7. Duncan JS, Winston GP, Koepp MJ, Ourselin S. Brain imaging in the assessment for epilepsy surgery. Lancet Neurol. 2016;4422:1–14.
8. Focke NK, Bonelli SB, Yogarajah M, Scott C, Symms MR, Duncan JS. Automated normalized FLAIR imaging in MRI-negative patients with refractory focal epilepsy. Epilepsia. 2009;50:1484–90.
9. Huppertz H-J, Grimm C, Fauser S, Kassubek J, Mader I, Hochmuth A, et al. Enhanced visualization of blurred gray-white matter junctions in focal cortical dysplasia by voxel-based 3D MRI analysis. Epilepsy Res. 2005;67:35–50.
10. Kassubek J, Huppertz H-J, Spreer J, Schulze-Bonhage A. Detection and localization of focal cortical dysplasia by voxel-based 3-D MRI analysis. Epilepsia. 2002;43:596–602.
11. Sulc V, Stykel S, Hanson DP, Brinkmann BH, Jones DT, Holmes DR, et al. Statistical SPECT processing in MRI-negative epilepsy surgery. Neurology. 2014;82:932–9.
12. Wagner J, Weber B, Urbach H, Elger CE, Huppertz H-J. Morphometric MRI analysis improves detection of focal cortical dysplasia type II. Brain. 2011;134:2844–54.
13. Wang ZI, Jones SE, Jaisani Z, Najm IM, Prayson RA, Burgess RC, et al. Voxel-based morphometric magnetic resonance imaging (MRI) postprocessing in MRI-negative epilepsies. Ann Neurol. 2015;77:1060–75.

14. Kelly PJ. Stereotactic navigation, Jean Talairach, and I. Neurosurgery. 2004;54:454–64.
15. Horsley V, Clarke R. The structure and functions of the cerebellum examined by a new method. Brain. 1908;31:45–124.
16. Chabardès S, Abel TJ, Cardinale F, Kahane P. Commentary: understanding stereoelectroencephalography: what's next? Neurosurgery. 2017;82:E15–6.
17. Trébuchon A, Chauvel P. Electrical stimulation for seizure induction and functional mapping in stereoelectroencephalography. J Clin Neurophysiol. 2016;33:511–21.
18. Trébuchon A, Racilia R, Cardinale F, Lagarde S, McGonigal A, Lo Russo G, et al. Electrical stimulation for seizure induction during SEEG exploration: a useful predictor of post-surgical seizure recurrence? J Neurol Neurosurg Psychiatry. 2021;92:22–6.
19. Bourdillon P, Apra C, Lévêque M. First clinical use of stereotaxy in humans: the key role of x-ray localization discovered by Gaston Contremoulins. J Neurosurg. 2018;128:932–7.
20. Spiegel EA, Wycis HT, Marks M, Lee A. Stereotaxic apparatus for operations on the human brain. Science. 1947;106:349–50.
21. Spiegel EA, Wycis HT, Thur C. The stereoencephalotome (model III of our stereotaxic apparatus for operations on the human brain). J Neurosurg. 1951;8:452–3.
22. Benabid AL, Chabardès S, Seigneuret E. History of stereotactic surgery in France. In: Lozano AM, Gildenberg PL, Tasker RR, editors. Textbook of stereotactic and functional neurosurgery. 2nd ed. Berlin: Springer-Verlag; 2009.
23. Chauvel P. Contributions of Jean Talairach and Jean Bancaud to epilepsy surgery. In: Lüders HO, Comair YG, editors. Epilepsy surgery. 2nd ed. Philadelphia: Lippincott Williams & Wilkins; 2001. p. 35–41.
24. Szikla G. Target point, target volume, "whole brain" stereotaxis: remarks on some present trends of evolution in stereotactic neurosurgery. In: Gillingham F, Gybels J, Hitchcock E, Rossi G, Szikla G, editors. Advanced stereotactic and functional neurosurgery 4. Acta Neurochirurgica Supplementum, vol. 30. Vienna: Springer; 1980. p. 1–3.
25. Benabid AL, Mitrofanis J, Chabardès S, Seigneuret E, Torres N, Piallat B, et al. Subthalamic nucleus stimulation for Parkinson's disease. In: Lozano AM, Gildenberg PL, Tasker RR, editors. Textbook of stereotactic and functional neurosurgery. 2nd ed. Berlin: Springer-Verlag; 2009. p. 1603–30.
26. Rachinger W, Grau S, Holtmannspötter M, Herms J, Tonn J, Kreth F. Serial stereotactic biopsy of brainstem lesions in adults improves diagnostic accuracy compared with MRI only. J Neurol Neurosurg Psychiatry. 2009;80:1134–9.
27. Zanello M, Roux A, Senova S, Peeters S, Edjlali M, Taauziede-Espariat A, et al. Robot-assisted stereotactic biopsies in 377 consecutive adult patients with supratentorial diffuse gliomas: diagnostic yield, safety and postoperative outcomes. World Neurosurg. 2021;148:e310–3.
28. Zanello M, Roux A, Debacker C, Peeters S, Edjlali-Goujon M, Dhermain F, et al. Postoperative intracerebral hematomas following stereotactic biopsies: poor planning or poor execution? Int J Med Robot. 2021;17:e2211.
29. Cardinale F, Casaceli G, Raneri F, Miller JP, Lo RG. Implantation of StereoElectroEncephaloGraphy (SEEG) electrodes: a systematic review. J Clin Neurophysiol. 2016;33:490–502.
30. Munari C, Hoffmann D, Francione S, Kahane P, Tassi L, Lo Russo G, et al. Stereo-electroencephalography methodology: advantages and limits. Acta Neurol Scand. 1994;89:56–67.
31. Olivier A. Diagnostic operative techniques in the treatment of epilepsy: depth electrodes. In: Schmidek HH, Sweet WH, editors. Schmidek & sweet operative neurosurgical techniques: indications, methods, and results. 3rd ed. Philadelphia: Saunders Company; 1995. p. 1271–85.
32. Roberts DW. Fundamentals of registration. In: Barnett GH, Maciunas RJ, Roberts DW, editors. Computer assisted neurosurgery. New York: Taylor & Francis Group; 2006. p. 3–17.

33. Preim B, Bartz D. Acquisition of medical image data. In: Preim B, Bartz D, editors. Visualization in medicine. Burlington, MA: Morgan Kaufmann Publishers, Inc.; 2007. p. 35–64.
34. Preim B, Bartz D. Measurements in medical visualization. In: Preim B, Bartz D, editors. Visualization in medicine. Burlington, MA: Morgan Kaufmann Publishers, Inc.; 2007. p. 313–39.
35. Fahrig R, Fox A, Holdsworth DW. Characterization of a C-arm mounted XRII for 3D image reconstruction during interventional neuroradiology. Proc SPIE. 1996;2708:351–60.
36. Fahrig R, Fox A, Lownie SP, Holdsworth DW. Use of a C-arm system to generate true three-dimensional computed rotational angiograms: preliminary in vitro and in vivo results. Am J Neuroradiol. 1997;18(8):1507–14.
37. Balachandran R, Welch EB, Dawant BM, Fitzpatrick MJ. Effect of MR distortion on targeting for deep-brain stimulation. IEEE Trans Biomed Eng. 2010;57(7):1729–35.
38. Hardy PA, Barnett GH. Spatial distortion in magnetic resonance imaging: impact on stereotactic localization. In: Gildenberg PL, Tasker RR, editors. Textbook of stereotactic and functional neurosurgery. New York: McGraw-Hill; 1998. p. 271–80.
39. Musolino A, Tournoux P, Missir O, Talairach J. Methodology of "in vivo" anatomical study and stereo-electroencephalographic exploration in brain surgery for epilepsy. J Neuroradiol. 1990;17(2):67–102.
40. Benabid AL, Chabardès S, Seigneuret E, Hoffmann D, LeBas JF. The Talairach stereotactic system. In: Lozano AM, Gildenberg PL, Tasker RR, editors. Textbook of stereotactic and functional neurosurgery. 2nd ed. Berlin: Springer-Verlag; 2009. p. 495–509.
41. Minkin K, Gabrowsky K, Penkov M, Todorov Y, Tanova R, Milenova Y, et al. Stereoelectroencephalography using magnetic resonance angiography for avascular trajectory planning: technical report. Neurosurgery. 2017;81:688–95.
42. McGovern RA, Butler RS, Bena J, Gonzalez-Martinez JA. Incorporating new technology into a surgical technique: the learning curve of a single surgeon's stereo-electroencephalography experience. Neurosurgery. 2020;86(3):E281–9.
43. Li K, Vakharia VN, Sparks R, Rodionov R, Vos SB, McEvoy AW, et al. Stereoelectroencephalography electrode placement: detection of blood vessel conflicts. Epilepsia. 2019;60:1942–8.
44. Cardinale F, Pero G, Quilici L, Piano M, Colombo PE, Moscato A, et al. Cerebral angiography for multimodal surgical planning in epilepsy surgery: description of a new three-dimensional technique and literature review. World Neurosurg. 2015;84:358–67.
45. Willinsky RA, Taylor SM, TerBrugge K, Farb RI, Tomlinson G, Montanera W. Neurologic complications of cerebral angiography: prospective analysis of 2,899 procedures and review of the literature. Radiology. 2003;227(2):522–8.
46. Cardinale F, Rizzi M, Vignati E, Cossu M, Castana L, D'Orio P, et al. Stereoelectroencephalography: retrospective analysis of 742 procedures in a single Centre. Brain. 2019;142:2688–704.
47. Mellerio C, Roca P, Chassoux F, Danière F, Cachia A, Lion S, et al. The power button sign: a newly described central sulcal pattern on surface rendering MR images of type 2 focal cortical dysplasia. Radiology. 2015;274(2):500–7.
48. Minkin K, Gabrowsky K, Sirakov S, Penkov M, Todorov Y, Karakostov V, et al. Three-dimensional neuronavigation in SEEG-guided epilepsy surgery. Acta Neurochir. 2019;161:917–23.
49. Nowell M, Rodionov R, Zombori G, Sparks R, Winston GP, Kinghorn J, et al. Utility of 3D multimodality imaging in the implantation of intracranial electrodes in epilepsy. Epilepsia. 2015;56(3):403–13.
50. Régis J, Tamura M, Park MC, McGonigal A, Rivière D, Coulon O, et al. Subclinical abnormal gyration pattern, a potential anatomic marker of epileptogenic zone in patients with magnetic resonance imaging-negative frontal lobe epilepsy. Neurosurgery. 2011;69(1):80–94.

51. Maurer CRJ, Fitzpatrick MJ. A review of medical image registration. In: Maciunas RJ, editor. Interactive image-guided neurosurgery. AANS; 1993. p. 17–44.
52. Jenkinson M, Bannister PR, Brady JM, Smith SM. Improved optimization for the robust and accurate linear registration and motion correction of brain images. NeuroImage. 2002;17(2):825–41.
53. Jenkinson M. Registration, atlases and cortical flattening. In: Jezzard P, Matthews PM, Smith SM, editors. Functional MRI an introduction to methods. Oxford: Oxford University Press, Inc.; 2001. p. 271–93.
54. Jenkinson M, Chappell M. Registration. In: Jenkinson M, Chappell M, editors. Introduction to neuroimaging analysis. Oxford: Oxford University Press, Inc.; 2018. p. 210–63.
55. Maintz JA, Viergever MA. A survey of medical image registration. Med Image Anal. 1998;2(1):1–36.
56. Maes F, Collignon A, Vandermeulen D, Marchal G, Suetens P. Multimodality image registration by maximization of mutual information. IEEE Trans Med Imaging. 1997;16(2):187–98.
57. Viola P, Wells WMI. Alignment by maximization of mutual information. Int J Comput Vis. 1997;24(2):137–54.
58. Roche A, Malandain G, Pennec X, Ayache N. The correlation ratio as a new similarity measure for multimodal image registration. Lect Notes Comput Sci (Including Subser Lect Notes Artif Intell Lect Notes Bioinformatics). 1998;1496:1115–24.
59. Aladl UE, Peters T. Medical image registration. In: El-Baz A, Laine AF, Acharya R, Suri JS, editors. Multi-modality state-of-the-art medical image segmentation and registration methodologies, vol. II. New York: Springer; 2011. p. 227–45.
60. Hermosillo G, Chefd'hotel C, Herrmann K, Bousquet G, Bogoni L, Chaudhuri K, et al. Image registration in medical imaging: applications, methods, and clinical evaluation Gerardo. In: El-Baz A, Laine AF, Acharya R, Suri JS, editors. Multi modality state-of-the-art medical image segmentation and registration methodologies, vol. II. New York: Springer; 2011. p. 263–313.
61. Studholme C, Hill DL, Hawkes DJ. Automated 3-D registration of MR and CT images of the head. Med Image Anal. 1996;1(2):163–75.
62. van den Elsen PA, Evert-Jan DP, Viergever MA. Medical image matching—a review with classification. IEEE Eng Med Biol. 1993;12:26–39.
63. Viergever MA, Maintz JA, Klein S, Murphy K, Staring M, Pluim JP. A survey of medical image registration—under review. Med Image Anal. 2016;33:140–4.
64. West JB, Fitzpatrick MJ, Wang MY, Dawant BM, Maurer CRJ, Kessler RM, et al. Comparison and evaluation of retrospective intermodality brain image registration techniques. J Comput Assist Tomogr. 1997;21(4):554–66.
65. Fedorov A, Beichel R, Kalpathy-Cramer J, Finet J, Fillion-Robin JC, Pujol S, et al. 3D slicer as an image computing platform for the quantitative imaging network. Magn Reson Imaging. 2012;30:1323–41.
66. Fischl BR. FreeSurfer. Neuroimage. 2012;62:774–81.
67. Jenkinson M, Beckmann CF, Behrens TE, Woolrich MW, Smith SM. Fsl. Neuroimage. 2012;62(2):782–90.
68. Ashburner J. SPM: a history. NeuroImage. 2012;62(2):791–800.
69. Liu L, Mariani SG, De Schlichting E, Grand S, Lefranc M, Signeruret E, et al. Frameless ROSA® robot-assisted lead implantation for deep brain stimulation: technique and accuracy. Oper Neurosurg (Hagerstown, MD). 2020;19:57–64.
70. Cardinale F, Rizzi M, D'Orio P, Casaceli G, Arnulfo G, Narizzano M, et al. A new tool for touch-free patient registration for robot-assisted intracranial surgery: application accuracy from a phantom study and a retrospective surgical series. Neurosurg Focus. 2017;42:E8.
71. Varma T. Use of the NeuroMate stereotactic robot in a frameless mode for functional neurosurgery. Int J Med Robot Comput Assist Surg. 2006;2(April):107–13.

72. Li QH, Zamorano L, Pandya A, Perez R, Gong J, Diaz FG. The application accuracy of the NeuroMate robot—a quantitative comparison with frameless and frame-based surgical localization systems. Comput Aided Surg. 2002;7(2):90–8.
73. Pelizzari CA, Chen GT, Spelbring DR, Weichselbaum RR, Chin-Tu C. Accurate three-dimensional registration of CT, PET, and/or MR images of the brain. J Comput Assist Tomogr. 1989;13(1):20–6.
74. Gonzalez-Martinez JA, Bulacio JC, Thompson S, Gale JT, Smithason S, Najm IM, et al. Technique, results, and complications related to robot-assisted stereoelectroencephalography. Neurosurgery. 2016;78(2):169–80.
75. Machetanz K, Grimm F, Wang S, Bender B, Tatagiba M, Gharabaghi A, et al. Patient-to-robot registration: the fate of robot-assisted stereotaxy. Int J Med Robot Comput Assist Surg. 2021;17(5):e2288.
76. Lemieux L, Lester S, Fish DR. Multimodality imaging and intracranial EEG display for stereotactic surgery planning in epilepsy. Electroencephalogr Clin Neurophysiol. 1992;82:399–407.
77. Cardinale F, Cossu M, Castana L, Casaceli G, Schiariti MP, Miserocchi A, et al. Stereoelectroencephalography: surgical methodology, safety, and stereotactic application accuracy in 500 procedures. Neurosurgery. 2013;72:353–66.
78. Lemieux L, Jagoe R, Fish DR, Kitchen ND, Thomas DG. A patient-to-computed-tomography image registration method based on digitally reconstructed radiographs. Med Phys. 1994;21(11):1749–60.
79. Elder JB, Amar AP, Apuzzo MLJ. Stereotactic and image-guided biopsy. In: Lozano AM, Gildenberg PL, Tasker RR, editors. Textbook of stereotactic and functional neurosurgery. 2nd ed. Berlin: Springer-Verlag; 2009. p. 645–62.
80. Jain D, Sharma MC, Sarkar C, Deb P, Gupta D, Mahapatra A. Correlation of diagnostic yield of stereotactic brain biopsy with number of biopsy bits and site of the lesion. Brain Tumor Pathol. 2006;23:71–5.
81. Dlaka D, Švaco M, Chudy D, Jerbić B, Šekoranja B, Šuligoj F, et al. Brain biopsy performed with the RONNA G3 system: a case study on using a novel robotic navigation device for stereotactic neurosurgery. Int J Med Robot Comput Assist Surg. 2018;14:e1884.
82. Minchev G, Kronreif G, Martínez-Moreno M, Dorfer C, Micko A, Mert A, et al. A novel miniature robotic guidance device for stereotactic neurosurgical interventions: preliminary experience with the iSYS1 robot. J Neurosurg. 2017;126:985–96.
83. Carlson JD, McLeod KE, McLeod PS, Mark J. Stereotactic accuracy and surgical utility of the O-arm in deep brain stimulation surgery. Oper Neurosurg (Hagerstown, MD). 2017;13:96–107.
84. Furlanetti L, Hasegawa H, Oviedova A, Raslan A, Samuel M, Selway R, et al. O-arm stereotactic imaging in deep brain stimulation surgery workflow: a utility and cost-effectiveness analysis. Stereotact Funct Neurosurg. 2021;99(2):93–106.
85. Holewijn RA, Bot M, van den Munckhof P, Schuurman PR. Implementation of intraoperative cone-beam computed tomography (O-arm) for stereotactic imaging during deep brain stimulation procedures. Oper Neurosurg (Hagerstown, MD). 2020;19:E224–9.
86. Holloway KL, Docef A. A quantitative assessment of the accuracy and reliability of O-arm images for deep brain stimulation surgery. Neurosurgery. 2013;72:47–57.
87. Lefranc M, Le Gars D. Robotic implantation of deep brain stimulation leads, assisted by intra-operative, flat-panel CT. Acta Neurochir. 2012;154:2069–74.
88. Smith AP, Bakay RA. Frameless deep brain stimulation using intraoperative O-arm technology. J Neurosurg. 2011;115:301–9.
89. Cardinale F, Moscato A, Colombo PE, Castana L, Cossu M, Torresin A, et al. Intraoperative angiography for intracerebral electrodes planning and implantation: preliminary results with the O-arm system. Abstracts' Volume of the 2nd Meeting of IntraOperative Imaging Society. Istanbul; 2009. p. 13.

90. Cardinale F, Cossu M, Castana L, Schiariti MP, Moscato A, Torresin A, et al. Advances in the surgical technique for stereoelectroencephalography (SEEG) in epilepsy surgery: a retrospective analysis of geometrical accuracy and safety for the implantation of 282 intracerebral electrodes. Acta Neurochir. 2011;153:761.
91. Cardinale F, Miserocchi A, Moscato A, Cossu M, Castana L, Schiariti MP, et al. Talairach methodology in the multimodal imaging and robotics era. In: Scarabin J-M, editor. Stereotaxy and epilepsy surgery. Montrouge: John Libbey Eurotext; 2012. p. 245–72.
92. Arnulfo G, Narizzano M, Cardinale F, Fato MM, Palva JM. Automatic segmentation of deep intracerebral electrodes in computed tomography scans. BMC Bioinformatics. 2015;16:1–12.
93. Desikan RS, Ségonne F, Fischl BR, Quinn BT, Dickerson BC, Blacker D, et al. An automated labeling system for subdividing the human cerebral cortex on MRI scans into gyral based regions of interest. NeuroImage. 2006;31:968–80.
94. Destrieux C, Fischl BR, Dale AM, Halgren E. Automatic parcellation of human cortical gyri and sulci using standard anatomical nomenclature. NeuroImage. 2010;53:1–15.
95. Narizzano M, Arnulfo G, Ricci S, Toselli B, Tisdall MM, Canessa A, et al. SEEG assistant: a 3D slicer extension to support epilepsy surgery. BMC Bioinformatics. 2017;18:1–13.
96. Bourdillon P, Chatillon CÉ, Moles A, Rheims S, Catenoix H, Montavont A, et al. Effective accuracy of StereoElectroEncephaloGraphy (SEEG): robotic tridimensional vs Talairach orthogonal approaches. J Neurosurg. 2019;131:1938–46.
97. Pistol C, Daneasa A, Ciurea J, Rasina A, Barborica A, Oane I, et al. Accuracy and safety of customized stereotactic fixtures for stereoelectroencephalography in pediatric patients. Stereotact Funct Neurosurg. 2021;99(1):17–24.
98. Sharma JD, Seunarine KK, Tahir MZ, Tisdall MM. Accuracy of robot-assisted versus optical frameless navigated stereoelectroencephalography electrode placement in children. J Neurosurg Pediatr. 2019;23:297–302.
99. Lin Z, Wang G, Cheng J, Lin Y, Liu J, Lin J, et al. A robust automated pipeline for localizing SEEG electrode contacts. In: Zeng A, Pan D, Hao T, Zhang D, Shi Y, Song X, editors. Human brain and artificial intelligence. Singapore: Springer Nature; 2019. p. 36–51.
100. Granados A, Vakharia VN, Rodionov R, Schweiger M, Vos SB, O'Keeffe AG, et al. Automatic segmentation of stereoelectroencephalography (SEEG) electrodes post-implantation considering bending. Int J Comput Assist Radiol Surg. 2018;13:935–46.
101. Villalon SM, Paz R, Roehri N, Lagarde S, Pizzo F, Colombet B, et al. EpiTools, a software suite for presurgical brain mapping in epilepsy: intracerebral EEG. J Neurosci Methods. 2018;303:7–15.
102. Li G, Jiang S, Chen C, Brunner P, Wu Z, Schalk G, et al. iEEGview: an open-source multifunction GUI-based Matlab toolbox for localization and visualization of human intracranial electrodes. J Neural Eng. 2019;17:016016.
103. Blenkmann AO, Phillips HN, Princich JP, Rowe JB, Bekinschtein TA, Muravchik CH, et al. iElectrodes: a comprehensive open-source toolbox for depth and subdural grid electrode localization. Front Neuroinform. 2017;11:1–16.
104. Deman P, Bhattacharjee M, Tadel F, Job A-S, Rivière D, Cointepas Y, et al. IntrAnat electrodes: a free database and visualization software for intracranial electroencephalographic data processed for case and group studies. Front Neuroinform. 2018;12:1–11.
105. Higueras-Esteban A, Delgado-Martinez I, Serrano L, Principe A, Perez Enriquez C, Gonzalez Ballester MA, et al. SYLVIUS: a multimodal and multidisciplinary platform for epilepsy surgery. Comput Methods Prog Biomed. 2021;203:106,042.
106. Greene P, Li A, González-Martínez J, Sarma SV. Classification of stereo-EEG contacts in white matter vs. gray matter using recorded activity. Front Neurol. 2021;11:605,696.
107. Arnulfo G, Wang SH, Myrov V, Toselli B, Hirvonen J, Fato MM, et al. Long-range phase synchronization of high-frequency oscillations in human cortex. Nat Commun. 2020;11:5363.
108. Avanzini P, Abdollahi RO, Sartori I, Caruana F, Pelliccia V, Casaceli G, et al. Four-dimensional maps of the human somatosensory system. Proc Natl Acad Sci. 2016;113:1936–43.

109. Balestrini S, Francione S, Mai R, Castana L, Casaceli G, Marino D, et al. Multimodal responses induced by cortical stimulation of the parietal lobe: a stereo-electroencephalography study. Brain. 2015;138:2596–607.
110. Caruana F, Gerbella M, Avanzini P, Gozzo F, Pelliccia V, Mai R, et al. Motor and emotional behaviors elicited by electrical stimulation of the human cingulate cortex. Brain. 2018;141:3035–51.
111. David O, Blauwblomme T, Job A-S, Chabardès S, Hoffmann D, Minotti L, et al. Imaging the seizure onset zone with stereo-electroencephalography. Brain. 2011;134:2898–911.
112. David O, Job A-S, De Palma L, Hoffmann D, Minotti L, Kahane P. Probabilistic functional tractography of the human cortex. NeuroImage. 2013;80:307–17.
113. Ferraro S, Van Ackeren MJ, Mai R, Tassi L, Cardinale F, Nigri A, et al. Stereotactic electroencephalography in humans reveals multisensory signal in early visual and auditory cortices. Cortex. 2020;126:253–64.
114. Mikulan E, Russo S, Parmigiani S, Sarasso S, Zauli FM, Rubino A, et al. Simultaneous human intracerebral stimulation and HD-EEG: ground-truth for source localization methods. Sci Data. 2020;7:127.
115. Rubboli G, Mai R, Meletti S, Francione S, Cardinale F, Tassi L, et al. Negative myoclonus induced by cortical electrical stimulation in epileptic patients. Brain. 2006;129:65–81.
116. Sanz-Leon P, Knock SA, Spiegler A, Jirsa VK. Mathematical framework for large-scale brain network modeling in the virtual brain. NeuroImage. 2015;111:385–430.
117. Lefranc M, Capel C, Pruvot-Occean A-S, Fichten A, Desenclos C, Toussaint P, et al. The impact of the reference imaging modality, registration method and intraoperative flat-panel computed tomography on the accuracy of the ROSA® stereotactic robot. Stereotact Funct Neurosurg. 2014;92(4):242–50.
118. Moran C, Gerard CS, Barua N, Ashida R, Woolley M, Pietrzyk M, et al. Two hundred twenty-six consecutive deep brain stimulation electrodes placed using an "asleep" technique and the neurolmate robot for the treatment of movement disorders. Oper Neurosurg (Hagerstown, MD). 2020;19:530–8.
119. De Benedictis A, Trezza A, Carai A, Genovese E, Procaccini E, Messina R, et al. Robot-assisted procedures in pediatric neurosurgery. Neurosurg Focus. 2017;42(5):E7.
120. Dorfer C, Minchev G, Czech T, Stefanits H, Feucht M, Pataraia E, et al. A novel miniature robotic device for frameless implantation of depth electrodes in refractory epilepsy. J Neurosurg. 2017;126:1622–8.
121. Zheng J, Liu YL, Zhang D, Cui XH, Sang LX, Xie T, et al. Robot-assisted versus stereotactic frame-based stereoelectroencephalography in medically refractory epilepsy. Neurophysiol Clin. 2021;51:111–9.
122. Kim LH, Feng AY, Ho AL, Parker JJ, Kumar KK, Chen KS, et al. Robot-assisted versus manual navigated stereoelectroencephalography in adult medically-refractory epilepsy patients. Epilepsy Res. 2020;159:106253.
123. Rollo PS, Rollo MJ, Zhu P, Woolnough O, Tandon N. Oblique trajectory angles in robotic stereo-electroencephalography. J Neurosurg. 2021;135(1):245–54.
124. Bottan JS, Rubino PA, Lau JC, MacDougall KW, Parrent AG, Burneo JG, et al. Robot-assisted insular depth electrode implantation through oblique trajectories: 3-dimensional anatomical nuances, technique, accuracy, and safety. Oper Neurosurg (Hagerstown, MD). 2020;18(3):278–83.
125. Candela-Cantó S, Aparicio J, López JM, Baños-Carrasco P, Ramírez-Camacho A, Climent A, et al. Frameless robot-assisted stereoelectroencephalography for refractory epilepsy in pediatric patients: accuracy, usefulness, and technical issues. Acta Neurochir. 2018;160:2489–500.
126. Ollivier I, Behr C, Cebula H, Timofeev A, Benmekhbi M, Valenti MP, et al. Efficacy and safety in frameless robot-assisted stereo-electroencephalography (SEEG) for drug-resistant epilepsy. Neurochirurgie. 2017;63(4):286–90.

127. Spyrantis A, Cattani A, Strzelczyk A, Rosenow F, Seifert V, Freiman TM. Robot guided stereoelectroencephalography without computed tomography scan for referencing—analysis of accuracy. Int J Med Robot Comput Assist Surg. 2018;14:e1888.
128. Ho AL, Muftuoglu Y, Pendharkar AV, Sussman ES, Porter BE, Halpern CH, et al. Robot-guided pediatric stereoelectroencephalography: single-institution experience. J Neurosurg Pediatr. 2018;22:489–96.
129. De Momi E, Caborni C, Cardinale F, Castana L, Casaceli G, Cossu M, et al. Automatic trajectory planner for StereoElectroEncephaloGraphy procedures: a retrospective study. IEEE Trans Biomed Eng. 2013;60:986–93.
130. El Hadji S, Moccia S, Scorza D, Rizzi M, Cardinale F, Baselli G, et al. Brain-vascular segmentation for SEEG planning via a 3D fully-convolutional neural network. Proc Annu Int Conf IEEE Eng Med Biol Soc EMBS. 2019:1014–7.
131. Moccia S, De Momi E, El Hadji S, Mattos LS. Blood vessel segmentation algorithms—review of methods, datasets and evaluation metrics. Comput Methods Prog Biomed. 2018;158:71–91.
132. Scorza D, De Momi E, Plaino L, Amoroso G, Arnulfo G, Narizzano M, et al. Retrospective evaluation and SEEG trajectory analysis for interactive multi-trajectory planner assistant. Int J Comput Assist Radiol Surg. 2017;12:1727–38.
133. Vakharia VN, Sparks R, Vos SB, McEvoy AW, Miserocchi A, Ourselin S, et al. The effect of vascular segmentation methods on stereotactic trajectory planning for drug-resistant focal epilepsy: a retrospective cohort study. World Neurosurg X. 2019;4:100,057.
134. Wagstyl K, Adler S, Pimpel B, Chari A, Seunarine K, Lorio S, et al. Planning stereoelectroencephalography using automated lesion detection: retrospective feasibility study. Epilepsia. 2020;61:1406–16.
135. De Momi E, Caborni C, Cardinale F, Casaceli G, Castana L, Cossu M, et al. Multi-trajectories automatic planner for StereoElectroEncephaloGraphy (SEEG). Int J Comput Assist Radiol Surg. 2014;9:1087–97.
136. Sparks R, Zombori G, Rodionov R, Nowell M, Vos SB, Zuluaga MA, et al. Automated multiple trajectory planning algorithm for the placement of stereo-electroencephalography (SEEG) electrodes in epilepsy treatment. Int J Comput Assist Radiol Surg. 2017;12:123–36.
137. Zelmann R, Bériault S, Marinho MM, Mok K, Hall JA, Guizard N, et al. Improving recorded volume in mesial temporal lobe by optimizing stereotactic intracranial electrode implantation planning. Int J Comput Assist Radiol Surg. 2015;10:1599–615.
138. Scorza D, Rizzi M, De Momi E, Cortés C, Bertelsen Á, Cardinale F. Knowledge-based automated planning system for StereoElectroEncephaloGraphy: a center-based scenario. J Biomed Inform. Elsevier Inc. 2020;108:103,460.
139. Vakharia VN, Sparks RE, Granados A, Miserocchi A, McEvoy AW, Ourselin S, et al. Refining planning for stereoelectroencephalography: a prospective validation of spatial priors for computer-assisted planning with application of dynamic learning. Front Neurol. 2020;11:706.
140. Nowell M, Sparks R, Zombori G, Miserocchi A, Rodionov R, Diehl B, et al. Comparison of computer-assisted planning and manual planning for depth electrode implantations in epilepsy. J Neurosurg. 2016;124:1820–8.
141. Scorza D, Moccia S, De Luca G, Plaino L, Cardinale F, Mattos LS, et al. Safe electrode trajectory planning in SEEG via MIP-based vessel segmentation. In: Webster RJ, Fei B, editors. Proc SPIE 10135, med imaging 2017 image-guided proced robot interv model. Orlando: SPIE. Digital Library; 2017. p. 101352C–101352C8.
142. Sparks R, Vakharia VN, Rodionov R, Vos SB, Diehl B, Wehner T, et al. Anatomy-driven multiple trajectory planning (ADMTP) of intracranial electrodes for epilepsy surgery. Int J Comput Assist Radiol Surg. 2017;12:1245–55.
143. Vakharia VN, Sparks R, Rodionov R, Vos SB, Dorfer C, Miller JP, et al. Computer-assisted planning for the insertion of stereoelectroencephalography electrodes for the investigation of drug-resistant focal epilepsy: an external validation study. J Neurosurg. 2019;130:601–10.

144. Bériault S, Al Subaie F, Mok K, Sadikot AF, Pike GB. Automatic trajectory planning of DBS neurosurgery from multi-modal MRI datasets. Med Image Comput Assist Interv. 2011;14:259–66.
145. Bériault S, Al Subaie F, Collins DL, Sadikot AF, Pike GB. A multi-modal approach to computer-assisted deep brain stimulation trajectory planning. Int J Comput Assist Radiol Surg. 2012;7:687–704.
146. Dergachyova O, Zhao Y, Haegelen C, Jannin P, Essert C. Automatic preoperative planning of DBS electrode placement using anatomo-clinical atlases and volume of tissue activated. Int J Comput Assist Radiol Surg Springer International Publishing. 2018;13:1117–28.
147. Essert C, Haegelen C, Lalys F, Abadie A, Jannin P. Automatic computation of electrode trajectories for deep brain stimulation: a hybrid symbolic and numerical approach. Int J Comput Assist Radiol Surg. 2012;7:517–32.
148. Essert C, Fernandez-Vidal S, Capobianco A, Haegelen C, Karachi C, Bardinet E, et al. Statistical study of parameters for deep brain stimulation automatic preoperative planning of electrodes trajectories. Int J Comput Assist Radiol Surg. 2015;10:1973–83.
149. Marcus HJ, Vakharia VN, Sparks R, Rodionov R, Kitchen N, McEvoy AW, et al. Computer-assisted versus manual planning for stereotactic brain biopsy: a retrospective comparative pilot study. Oper Neurosurg. 2020;18:417–22.
150. Segato A, Pieri V, Favaro A, Riva M, Falini A, De Momi E, et al. Automated steerable path planning for deep brain stimulation safeguarding fiber tracts and deep gray matter nuclei. Front Robot AI. 2019;6:1–15.
151. Scorza D, El Hadji S, Cortés C, Bertelsen A, Cardinale F, Baselli G, et al. Surgical planning assistance in keyhole and percutaneous surgery: a systematic review. Med Image Anal. 2021;67:101820.
152. Zanello M, Carron R, Peeters S, Gori P, Roux A, Bloch I, et al. Automated neurosurgical stereotactic planning for intraoperative use: a comprehensive review of the literature and perspectives. Neurosurg Rev. 2021;44:867–88.
153. Benabid AL, Hoffmann D, Lavallée S, Cinquin P, Demongeot J, Le Bas JF, et al. Is there any future for robots in neurosurgery? Adv Tech Stand Neurosurg. 1991;18:3–45.

Part II
Robot Assisted Neurosurgery: Clinical Applications

Chapter 5
Robotics in Functional Neurosurgery

Ryan J. Austerman, Sibi Rajendran, and Amir H. Faraji

Background of Robotic Surgery

Functional neurosurgery has long led the forefront in the use of robotics due to the need for accurate stereotaxy. Deep brain stimulation, epilepsy surgery, and neuro modulatory procedures are among the classic indications. Given the need for extreme precision with target accuracy on the submillimeter scale, the use of robotic technology to minimize human error has become increasingly necessary to advance the field [1]. Ultimately, the goals of using robotics within functional neurosurgery are to improve accuracy and precision to deliver reliable and consistent results by removing random error. While historically these robotic procedures may have been cost-prohibitory, an increasing number of companies designing and implementing successful robotic technology are serving to drive costs down and increased availability. Ideally, this technology could even be implemented in lower or average volume functional neurosurgical centers with minimal expertise or advanced training needed [1].

Stereotactic robots are among the most widely utilized within functional neurosurgery. Among the earliest work includes a study by Kwoh et al. in 1988 where a stereotactic robot (Unimation Puma 200) was interfaced with a CT scanner to conduct brain tumor biopsies under image guidance [2]. The authors highlighted faster procedure time and improved accuracy when the robot was properly calibrated. The control group was a manually adjustable frame without robotic guidance. Similar studies were only in their infancy, given that computed tomography itself only became available in the 1970s [2].

R. J. Austerman · S. Rajendran · A. H. Faraji (✉)
Department of Neurological Surgery, Houston Methodist Hospital, Houston, TX, USA
e-mail: rjausterman@houstonmethodist.org; srajendran2@houstonmethodist.org; ahfaraji@houstonmethodist.org

J. A. González Martínez, F. Cardinale (eds.), *Robotics in Neurosurgery*,
https://doi.org/10.1007/978-3-031-08380-8_5

The most widely used systems currently in the United States (in no particular order) include the ROSA robot (Zimmer Biomet, Warsaw, IN), Neuromate robot (Integrated Surgical Systems, Davis, California), SurgiScope (ISIS Robotics, Saint Martin d'Heres, France), and the Renaissance system (MAZOR Robotics, Caesarea, Israel) [3]. This chapter will place particular emphasis on the ROSA robot, given its widespread availability and adoption within the United States, especially at larger volume academic medical centers performing functional procedures [3].

Techniques for Performing Robotic Surgery and Robot Types

As the ROSA robot is currently the most widely used robot with stereotactic utility, this section will focus on surgical technique using this system as specific to deep brain stimulation with the typical operating room setup shown in Fig. 5.1. The principles herein, however, may be more widely applicable and generalizable.

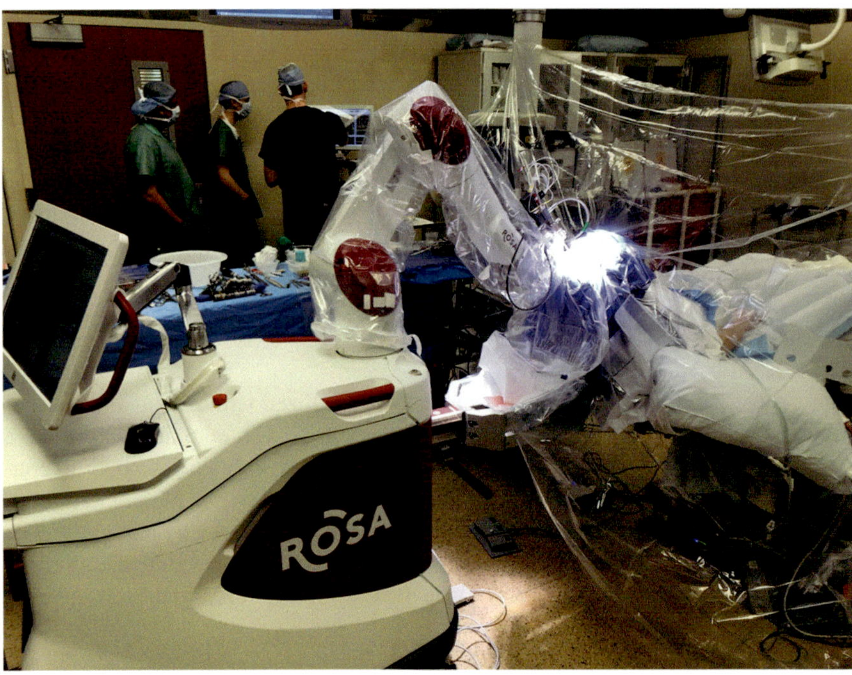

Fig. 5.1 Typical operating setup. The ROSA is positioned in-line with the patient, whose head is elevated to the maximum height possible for attachment of the Leksell frame to the ROSA. A clear operative drape is used to facilitate monitoring of the patient during the "awake" portions of the case. Figure reproduced from Faraji et al. [4]

Planning and Registration

MRI sequences for surgical planning are typically obtained preoperatively. These are merged with volumetric intraoperative CT/O-Arm scan using navigation frame or fiducials for registration. The two primary methods of stereotactic planning are to either [1] use the computer on the robotic system itself or [2] use a laptop provided by the company with pre-installed planning software. The ROSA planning software is based on a specific imaging coordinate system, and in certain cases, a surgeon's preferred third-party software can sometimes be converted into a ROSA-compatible plan. This is rarely necessary for pre-operative planning but becomes relevant when pre-operative anatomical segmentation or tractography or postoperative analysis is warranted.

A plan is created, keeping in mind the usual principles of stereotactic planning with avoidance of vasculature, sulci, and pial and/or ependymal transgressions when possible. Becoming comfortable ahead of time with controlling ROSA's planning software is important as some of the mouse controls and gestures are different than those of common PACS platforms. Besides viewing trajectories in the three usual cardinal planes, the ROSA workstation has a useful view of rotating along the trajectory, giving 360 degrees worth of oblique cuts rotating about the trajectory from entry to target. It also has a typical "probe's eye view" which should be carefully studied. The trajectory length is then set manually according to the indication of surgery.

Three of the most common methods of registration include bone fiducials, laser scanning, and frame pins acting as fiducials. The most common method of registering the ROSA is to use bone fiducials. These are small stainless steel self-tapping screws with a small cup on the other end that accommodates the tip of a ROSA pointer attachment used for stereotactic registration. Placement of the bone fiducials is straight-forward and does not significantly increase operative workflow time. Anywhere from four to six fiducials are placed in the rough shape of a circle centered around the vertex of the head. After shaving and prepping the scalp, fiducials are placed sequentially by [1] making a small stab incision down to skull with a #15 blade, [2] drilling the fiducial into the skull with a hand-held or electric drill, and [3] placing a suture around the fiducial to tamponade any scalp bleeding. After placement, the patient is taken for a volumetric thin-cut CT scan or an analogous portable image is obtained (i.e., with the Medtronic O-Arm). The post-bone-fiducial CT is then merged with the preoperative MRI, and the surgeon can proceed to position the patient. The registration pointer is attached to the robotic arm. Using the robot's foot pedal that unlocks the arm for movement, the tip of the registration probe is carefully brought toward the first fiducial. When the tip is a few centimeters from the fiducial, the robot's movement setting should be changed to "slow," and great care should be taken to remain co-axial with the fiducial to avoid exerting force on it that could displace it from the skull. Once the tip of the probe is inside the cup of the fiducial, the location is recorded on ROSA, and the process is repeated for each fiducial.

A second method of stereotactic registration, with the benefit of being non-invasive and requiring no additional intraoperative CT scan, involves utilization of a laser scanner for surface registration. Although it is still accurate and adequate for certain applications, in the ultra-high precision demanded of DBS, direct bone or frame fiducials are preferred for their increased accuracy.

A third registration technique overcomes some of the inconvenience of bone fiducials while maintaining the same accuracy. Instead of placing fiducials directly into the skull, the centers of each of the four Leksell frame titanium pins are used as a radiographically distinct location on CT or O-Arm scan that can be used in the place of the bone fiducials, as shown in Fig. 5.2. The tip of the registration probe is placed just inside the frame titanium pin's hex key recess which functions in the same manner as the cup of an implanted bone fiducial, as shown in Fig. 5.3.

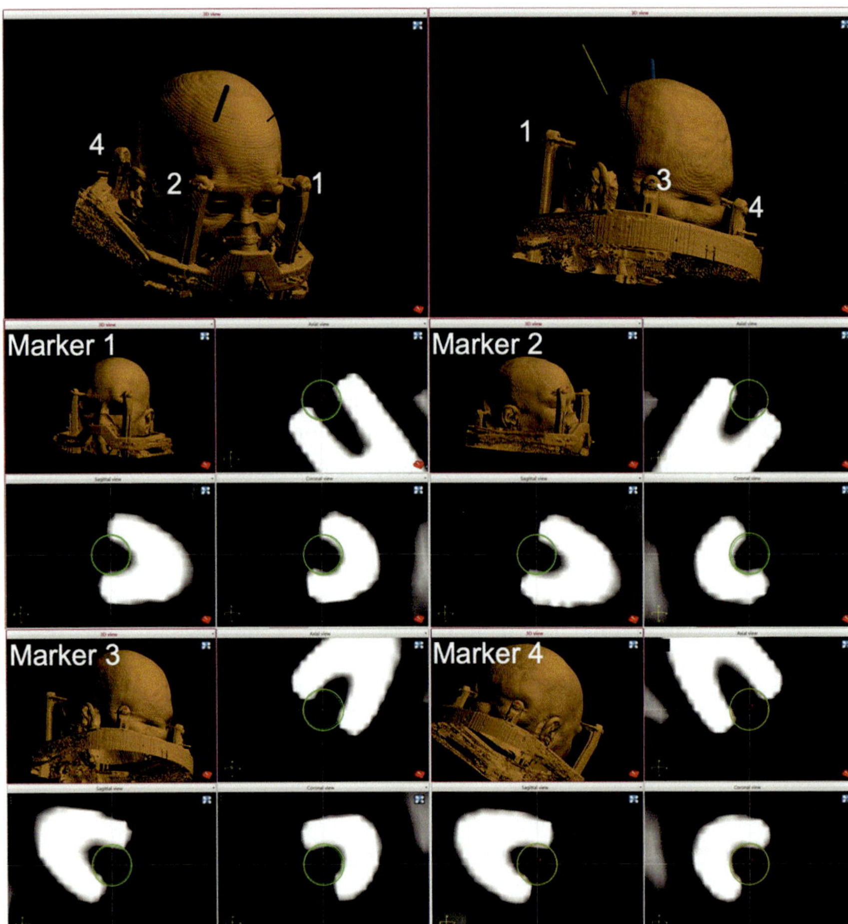

Fig. 5.2 Setting fiducial points on the frame CT. For each of four registration points, the center of the titanium pin head is identified on the CT scan, and these locations are set as "marker" reference points (green circles) in the ROSA software. Figure reproduced from Faraji et al. [4]

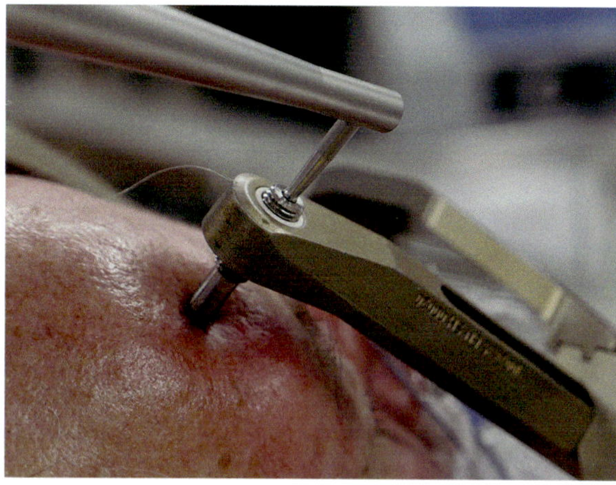

Fig. 5.3 Registration of a frame pin. The ROSA registration tool is shown positioned in the center of the titanium pin opening at the site of the registration marker. The circle corresponding to the registration marker tool has been enhanced in this figure for readability. Figure reproduced from Faraji et al. [4]

A four-point frame (Leksell Stereotactic G-Frame) is placed with the usual technique, but with titanium pins if using them for registration as described above to minimize the scatter artifact on CT scan used for registration. If using bone fiducials, the frame is placed after fiducials have been secured and the registration scan has been completed. After placement of the Leksell frame, or other head fixation device, the patient is placed supine on the operating table in a beach chair position, and the head is secured to the table with the appropriate frame attachment. The neck is typically slightly extended in awake surgery to facilitate airway management. The ROSA is brought toward the patient's head and attached. If using the laser surface registration or Leksell pins as fiducials method, registration can be done at this point [4]. Similarly, the ROSA arm can now be brought to position to visualize entry points and trajectories. Once the position of the patient is satisfactory, two key safety steps must be performed: [1] the robot wheels should be in the locked position and [2] the bed control must be removed or disabled such that it cannot be adjusted while the robot is attached. Bed manipulation with robot attached could have disastrous consequences for both the patient and the robot [4].

Operation

The surgeon can maneuver the arm to the planned entry point and trajectory for a clear visualization of where the incision(s) should be marked. Incision details are not usually impacted by use of the robot and are up to surgeon preference. After prepping the patient and draping, the incision(s) can be opened in the usual fashion. The ROSA arm remains in the "home" position near the base of the unit as the procedure begins. After the incisions have been opened, the arm is brought into the operative field. Of note, personnel must be available during the operation to control the robot settings such as changing trajectories and movement modes. This is often a company representative or equivalent. This may also be done by the surgeon with a sterile drape placed over the robot's touch screen.

The robotic arm can be brought towards the skull to be parallel with the planned trajectory. Depending on surgeon preference and the need for microelectrode recordings (MER) during deep brain stimulation, a burr hole can be placed either with an electric hand drill with a 2.4 mm bit placed directly through the robot's instrument adaptor (i.e., same as sEEG placement), or the entry point can be marked so that it can be opened with a traditional 14 mm perforator in order to accommodate multiple leads for MER. If performing awake surgery, dural opening is avoided until the patient is adequately cooperative with baseline clinical testing done and hemodynamically stability. As with other non-robotic methods of electrode placement, unnecessary CSF egress should be avoided. If no MER is being performed, the dura and pia mater can be opened by placing a biopsy needle or sharp obturator. If MER is being performed, standard cruciate opening of dura and corticectomy is performed. It is important to move the robotic arm out of the way so the surgeon can fully visualize the burr hole and its contents to ensure adequate hemostasis.

Electrode(s) can be placed in usual fashion, with or without MER and/or awake clinical testing being conducted. The final implant placed and secured to the skull with the surgeon's preference of fixation device. One advantage of the robotic workflow is the ability to immediately command the arm to the contralateral side of the head without the need for adjusting any settings, allowing for a smoother workflow and minimizing the opportunity for measurement errors to occur, as shown in Fig. 5.4. The remainder of the procedures involves electrode tunneling and wound closure. Bone fiducials, where applicable, are removed and closed with dissolvable suture.

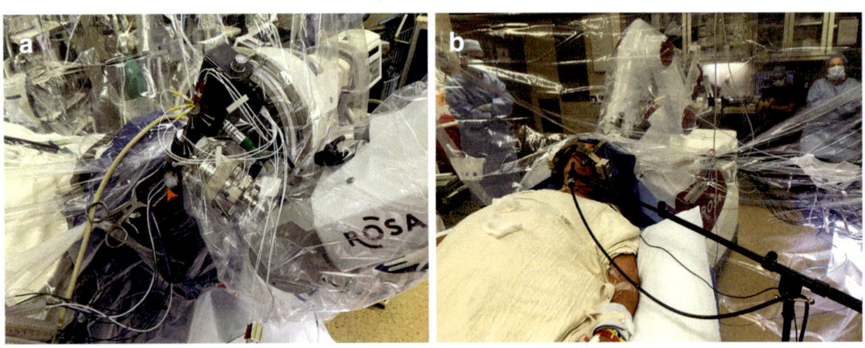

Fig. 5.4 Patient positioning for MER and ECoG. (**a**) ROSA arm in target position, supporting the microdrive and three microelectrodes, with the implantation of two strip electrodes evidenced by their wires protruding from the burr hole (red arrowhead) seen below the ROSA arm. (**b**) Attachment to the ROSA does not preclude the patient from participating comfortably in behavioral research tasks during intracranial recording. Figure reproduced from Faraji et al. [4]

Complication Profile of Robotic Surgery and Literature Review

The overall complication rate of DBS placement with traditional non-robotic techniques is already quite low, and likely not impacted by whether electrodes are placed with a frame or robotic arm. Postop complication rates in a large series of DBS were as follows: asymptomatic intracerebral hemorrhage: 0.5%; asymptomatic intraventricular hemorrhage: 3.4%; symptomatic intracerebral hemorrhage: 1.1%; ischemic infarction: 0.4%; and short-term hemiparesis and/or decreased level of consciousness: 1.7% [5]. A systematic review of long-term hardware complications associated with DBS reported rates of infection: 5.1%; lead migration: 1.6%; lead fracture: 1.5%; IPG malfunction: 1.1% [6]. One area of benefit with robot placement might be accuracy, which may allow for fewer electrode passes and smoother workflow [5].

The ROSA robot has been studied and published on more extensively in its role in sEEG placement. The literature on its use in DBS is small but growing. Neudorfer et al. compared robot-assisted DBS (ROSA) to traditional frame-based DBS in a series of 80 consecutive patients on the basis of "accuracy, precision, reliability, duration of surgery, [effect on] intraoperative imaging quality, safety and maintenance [7]." They observed superior performance of ROSA compared to their existing frame-based workflow. However, it should be cautioned that their existing workflow centered around a Riechert–Mundinger (RM) stereotactic apparatus, and the frame they used with ROSA was a Leksell G-frame, which could confound results [7].

The focus of their study was the robot's impact on accuracy, precision, and reliability. Accuracy, defined by lateral deviations from their initial stereotactic target, was 1.11 ± 0.56 mm with the RM system vs 0.76 ± 0.37 mm with ROSA, $p < 0.001$. Reliability was measured by comparing the frequency of electrodes being off target by more than 2 mm, which did not occur in their ROSA cohort. They also obtained better registration images with CT because metal artifact caused by the RM apparatus was not present when using the ROSA with a Leksell frame. The authors concluded that the observed accuracy, precision, and reliability translated into faster, simpler, and safer procedures.

They also looked at another important factor—duration of surgery—and the impact of robotic-assistance on operative time. Duration of surgery, defined as time from patient in room until final closure (thus accounting for robot setup, planning, etc.) was significantly shorter with ROSA versus the RM apparatus: 325.1 ± 81.6 min versus 394.8 ± 66.6 min, respectively, $p < 0.001$. This equates to more than an hour saved between groups. However, if using the RM apparatus was already a time-consuming workflow, these results might not be as surprising. Furthermore, variation in operative time metrics may be difficult to interpret given differences in staff and infrastructure between different institutions. They attributed the most important sources of saved time to the robot's reliability and accuracy that result in a reduction in lead stimulation testing/recording and need for re-positioning. Furthermore, it is not surprising that changing to a new system of DBS placement—robotic or not—is less efficient, at least initially. Thus, the overall operative time relies less on the technology being used for DBS placement, and more on how consistent and standardized the surgery can be.

Another important point the paper raises is the ease of maintenance on the surgical components other than the robot itself. The size and amount of hardware and instruments that need to be sterilized between cases are less than typical frame-based systems. The Leksell arc is a key determinant of DBS accuracy, yet it must be cleaned and autoclaved after every use. In comparison, all of the targeting with ROSA takes place on the robot which is not sterilized between uses. The only robotic components that must be sterilized between cases are simple instrument holders. This obviates the need for multiple large and expensive frames that must be kept on standby for each case in the event that a replacement is needed for any number of reasons.

Notably, but not surprisingly, the authors found a significant reduction in operative time in the first half of their patient series compared to the second half. Improvements in workflow efficiency and outcome are a common finding in several papers on the subject, which will be described below.

In a similar paper also comparing ROSA to an institutions existing workflow, Paff et al. compared the performance of ROSA to that of a CRW frame workflow [8]. However, the authors focused more on clinical outcomes than intraoperative performance. Patients implanted via ROSA or CRW frame had equivalent levodopa equivalent daily doses (LEDD) and mean motor scores when measured at 6, 12, and 24 months postoperatively [8].

The authors reported an increased complication rate in the ROSA group versus the CRW group. However, the significance of this is unclear for a few reasons. First, their overall complication rate is higher than expected both in the CRW and ROSA patient groups. Their sample consisted of 33 CRW patients and 27 ROSA patients, and the difference between complication rate did not achieve statistical significance. They reported 11% wound and hardware infectious complications with ROSA versus 6% in the CRW group. Similarly, their rates of observed cognitive, psychiatric, and motor side effects were higher than average in both groups. It is also important to reiterate that this is a small sample size consisting of retrospective and nonrandomized data.

In contrast to Neudorfer et al's improvement in operative time with the robot, these authors instead experienced an increase in time (447.9 ± 48.4 min with ROSA vs 375.6 ± 69.2 min with CRW frame, $p = 0.00275$). However, this group was comparing ROSA to a simpler frame-based system (CRW) than the RM system used by Neudorfer et al. Nonetheless, the contrasting findings highlight the fact that use of surgical robots in general may have an upfront time investment in setting them up that is sometimes later paid off by improved efficiency and accuracy. If patients experience better results, an increase in operative time may be justified.

Because no retrospective data on their frame-based accuracy was available, this was only analyzed for the robotic group. They compared the accuracy of left and right-sided leads via 3-dimensional vector error and found 1.36 ± 0.83 mm and

1.81±0.78 mm, respectively, not statistically significant. It is important to note that accuracies are measured differently between publications, with some only evaluating error in 2-dimensions via lateral or radial deviations, and others (such as this one) evaluating error with the third dimension of electrode depth. Error in electrode depth is generally not caused by issues with the robot, and instead results from errors in measurement or surgical technique. Also, when MER is performed, the final electrode depth is perhaps variable compared to the initial target. Three-dimensional errors will therefore be higher than those calculated for only two dimensions.

Faraji et al. published their experience using ROSA on a series of patients undergoing DBS lead placement in the ventrointermediate nucleus (Vim), subthalamic nucleus (STN), or globus pallidus interna (GPi)[4]. They measured the radial error (two dimensional, as described above) of implanted leads and found it to be similar to that of typical frame-based implantation techniques. However, they observed an improvement in accuracy when comparing the second half of their patient series to the first half. This highlights the importance of the learning curve that exists for all new devices (Overall error 1.14 ± 0.11 mm, error in first ten patients 1.46 ± 0.19 mm, error in the second ten patients 0.86 ± 0.09 mm, $p = 0.006$) [4]. Similarly, Liu et al. performed a rigorous analysis for electrode placement accuracy with ROSA, without comparing to another workflow. In this large series of 119 patients undergoing implantation of 192 leads, all were placed with submillimeter accuracy using ROSA [9]. This group used the traditional bone fiducial technique for registration, and used MER similar to Faraji et al. This study focused on the accuracy of ROSA (and different imaging modalities to assess lead placement) and did not include data on patient outcomes or complications [9].

Due to the established accuracy of ROSA—often better than many previous institutional workflows—some have questioned whether MER or awake surgery is even necessary for DBS placement. Is the robot's accuracy a substitute for the data provided by awake testing or MER, especially in an era of advancements in anatomic segmentation and DBS target imaging? This is an even more pertinent question with the advent of directional and segmented DBS leads for electric field contouring.

Jin et al. compared their ROSA DBS implantation patients on the basis of asleep versus awake lead placement [10]. In their large retrospective cohort of 153 DBS patients implanted with a total of 306 electrodes, they compared operative time, complications, outcome assessments, and programming settings. All patients were registered with bone fiducials and implanted with assistance of MER. The only significant difference between the two groups was that operative time, measured from skin incision to closure, was expectedly longer in the awake group versus those under general anesthesia. Surgery took 1.09 ± 0.46 h in the general anesthesia group and 1.54 ± 0.57 h in the awake group, $p < 0.0001$. There was a slight decrease in the length of the MER portion of the case in the asleep versus awake group (12.03 ± 1.77 min vs 12.89 ± 2.73 min, $p = 0.0338$), but this was not clinically significant. When comparing several DBS programming settings between different implantation groups, there was one significant finding of "amplitude stimulation for neuromodulation" being less in the general anesthesia versus local anesthesia groups (2.33 ± 0.62 V general anesthesia, 2.77 ± 0.70 V local anesthesia, $p = 0.0018$). This finding remained significant even after Bonferroni correction of alpha for their list of pairwise comparisons. There was no significant difference in electrode placement accuracy (0.71 ± 0.25 mm in the general anesthesia group and 0.76 ± 0.23 mm in the awake group, $p = 0.3031$). The reduction in operative time with equivalent target accuracy and complication rates contributes to the case for asleep DBS in PD. Given that the primary motivator of awake surgery is the ability to perform macrostimulation and test for side effects, will refinements in electrode technology such as directional targeting further reduce the need for it [8]?

A study from Lefranc et al. in 2017 similarly compared DBS patients implanted via ROSA between asleep and awake surgery to evaluate whether the accuracy of the robot was equivalent to awake surgery with clinical testing [11]. They looked at a total of 23 patients who underwent bilateral STN DBS for PD. They found no significant differences in required stimulation voltages or other device parameters. Both groups had similar improvement in their PD symptoms in the short term as well as 1 year after surgery. Operative time was significantly lower in the GA group than the awake group, (375 versus 442 min, $p = 0.00032$), partially due to time saved by not clinically testing. Both groups had similar complication rates. They looked at a total of 23 patients who underwent bilateral STN DBS for PD. They found no significant differences in required stimulation voltages or other device parameters. Both groups had similar improvement in their PD symptoms in the short term as well as 1 year after surgery. Operative time was significantly lower in the GA group than the awake group, (375 versus 442, $p = 0.00032$), partially due to time saved by not clinically testing. Both groups had similar complication rates [11].

While the majority of robotic DBS placement workflows and publications focus on the ROSA, a few other systems have been used and described. The Mazor Renaissance was initially developed for spinal applications and cleared by the FDA for intracranial surgery in 2012 [12]. Ho et al. described their experience with this system that consists of a small skull-mounted tower and instrument holder to guide electrode entry and targeting [13]. They compared their outcomes using the Mazor Renaissance to their prior workflow using the Medtronic Nexframe system and had positive results. They observed a significantly shorter operative time when using the Mazor robot over the Nexframe system (281 versus 325 min, $p = 0.013$). Like so many other papers, there is a trend of decreasing operative time with experience, especially when comparing the first and second halves of their cohort: 302.6 versus 256.5 min, $p = 0.0398$). With the Mazor robot, they required fewer electrode passes than with the Nexframe (1.05 versus 1.45, $p = 0.0007$). Both groups had similar complication rates.

Another robotic system for DBS placement is the Renshaw Neuromate, which has also been used in stereotactic neurosurgical procedures. One of the early papers describing robot-assisted DBS implantation was with a Neuromate, published in 2004 by Varma et al., in a series of DBS for PD, tremor, and cervical dystonia [14]. The robot at the time was registered with a complex ultrasonic system and microphone array to localize the arm in three-dimensional space. Even with technology dating back to 2003 and early methods of stereotactic registration, they still achieved a mean error of 1.7 mm.

Other publications have described various institutions' experiences with updated versions of the Renshaw Neuromate. Candela et al. described their experience with the device in a prospective cohort of children undergoing DBS placement for movement disorders after developing a center for this specific patient population [15]. Their implanted electrode error was 1.24 mm. The only significant complication in their series of six patients was that their first implanted electrode was displaced medially by 4 mm, which impaired the ability to stimulate with some of the contacts [15].

Another publication on the Neuromate by von Langsdorff, Paqun, and Fontaine assessed its accuracy in a series of 17 consecutive patient implanted with a total of 30 electrodes and found mean accuracy of 0.86 ± 0.32 mm [16]. They did not analyze other variables such as operative time or complications.

Pointers for Complication Avoidance or Workflow Improvement

As several of the papers discussed above have demonstrated, experience with the robot system is critical. Increased comfort with it results in significant improvements in both operative time and accuracy.

Mastery of the bone or frame fiducial registration process is essential. Specifically, understanding the behavior of the arm when bringing the registration tip into the cup of the fiducial. There is a slight tendency for it to slowly "bob" up and down by a millimeter every half second or so. Timing when you remove your foot from the pedal just as the "down bob" of the motion occurs results in the best possible accuracy. Finesse with this step of the operation can lead to near-zero RMS errors and better accuracy. The RMS is also limited by the resolution of the registration imaging—therefore a fine-cut CT scan is preferred if accuracy is desired.

Maintain as much of your prior workflow when transitioning to using ROSA to temper the learning curve as much as possible. For example, Faraji et al. use the standard Leksell distance to center of 190 mm when using ROSA. By always keeping the electrode driver starting distance—10 mm regardless of whether MER is used, with reduction in the z-axis error is reduced. A standardized workflow limits the opportunity for the introduction of error.

Do not forget to unplug the operative bed and make everyone in the operating room aware that it cannot be adjusted after attaching ROSA. This is a critical safety point.

If using ROSA with an attached Alpha Omega microdrive, note that the arm is imbalanced due to the added weight. Thus, confirm that the arm is not unlocked when electrode guide tubes are in the brain.

Follow stereotactic best practices such as always confirming proper length measurements. Do not assume the robot has any "intelligence" regarding this step (or any step at all for the matter).

Working with the same set of operating room and ancillary staff is vital, as the learning curve on equipment assembly the order by which steps are executed is steep.

Check patient comfort regarding their neck position multiple times, as it cannot be changed after registration of ROSA.

References

1. Vazhayil V, et al. An overview of robotics in functional neurosurgery. Indian J Neurosurg. 2019;08:006–10.
2. Kwoh YS, Hou J, Jonckheere EA, Hayati S. A robot with improved absolute positioning accuracy for CT guided stereotactic brain surgery. IEEE T Bio-med Eng. 1988;35:153–60.
3. Faria C, et al. Review of robotic technology for stereotactic neurosurgery. IEEE Rev Biomed Eng. 2015;8:125–37.
4. Faraji AH, Kokkinos V, Sweat JC, Crammond DJ, Richardson RM. Robotic-assisted stereotaxy for deep brain stimulation lead implantation in awake patients. Oper Neurosurg. 2020;19:444–52.
5. Fenoy AJ, Simpson RK. Risks of common complications in deep brain stimulation surgery: management and avoidance: clinical article. J Neurosurg. 2014;120:132–9.
6. Jitkritsadakul O, et al. Systematic review of hardware-related complications of deep brain stimulation: do new indications pose an increased risk? Brain Stimul. 2017;10:967–76.
7. Neudorfer C, Hunsche S, Hellmich M, Majdoub FE, Maarouf M. Comparative study of robot-assisted versus conventional frame-based deep brain stimulation stereotactic neurosurgery. Stereot Funct Neuros. 2018;96:327–34.
8. Paff M, et al. Two-year clinical outcomes associated with robotic-assisted subthalamic lead implantation in patients with Parkinson's disease. J Robotic Surg. 2020;14:559–65.
9. Liu L, et al. Frameless ROSA® robot-assisted lead implantation for deep brain stimulation: technique and accuracy. Oper Neurosurg. 2019;19:57–64.
10. Jin H, et al. A comparative study of asleep and awake deep brain stimulation robot-assisted surgery for Parkinson's disease. Npj Park Dis. 2020;6:27.
11. Lefranc M, et al. Asleep robot-assisted surgery for the implantation of subthalamic electrodes provides the same clinical improvement and therapeutic window as awake surgery. World Neurosurg. 2017;106:602–8.
12. 510(k) Premarket notification for Mazor renaissance system with brain application. https://www.accessdata.fda.gov/scripts/cdrh/cfdocs/cfpmn/pmn.cfm?ID=K120812. Accessed 5 July 2021.
13. Ho AL, et al. Frameless robot-assisted deep brain stimulation surgery: an initial experience. Oper Neurosurg. 2019;17:424–31.
14. Varma TRK, et al. Use of the NeuroMate stereotactic robot in a frameless mode for movement disorder surgery. Stereot Funct Neuros. 2004;80:132–5.
15. Candela S, et al. Frameless robot-assisted pallidal deep brain stimulation surgery in pediatric patients with movement disorders: precision and short-term clinical results. J Neurosurg Pediatrics. 2018;22:416–25.
16. von Langsdorff D, Paquis P, Fontaine D. In vivo measurement of the frame-based application accuracy of the Neuromate neurosurgical robot. J Neurosurg. 2015;122:191–4.

Chapter 6
Robotics in Epilepsy Surgery

Hussam Abou-Al-Shaar, Arka N. Mallela, Danielle Corson, James Sweat, and Jorge Alvaro González Martínez

Introduction

The practice of epilepsy surgery has significantly changed in the last decade although fundamentals and core concepts have remained largely unchanged. With recent radiological and computational innovations, modern techniques, including the use of robotic devices, are increasingly utilized in many surgical fields. In this sense, epilepsy surgery is not an exception [1–17]. At present, assistant robotic devices have been mainly applied for stereotactic localization and placement of recording electrodes or different types of probes that require precise placement, as in stereoelectroencephalography (SEEG), deep brain stimulation (DBS), responsive nerve stimulators (RNS), and laser interstitial thermal therapy (LITT) procedures. The application of robotic devices has reshaped the practice of epilepsy surgery, bringing relevant advantages in relation to the more standard stereotactic frame-based methods. Namely, robots have the potential to increase the accuracy and the capability of performing numerous insertion trajectories without the need for time-consuming coordinate adjustments. These technical aspects can potentially translate to relevant clinical advantages, creating reproducible surgical results and a more acceptable margin of error in the implantations, reducing peri-operative complications and overall operative time [2, 5, 9, 17].

H. Abou-Al-Shaar · A. N. Mallela · D. Corson · J. Sweat · J. A. González Martínez (✉)
Department of Neurological Surgery and Epilepsy Center, University of Pittsburgh Medical Center, Pittsburgh, PA, USA
e-mail: aboualshaarh@upmc.edu; mallelaan@upmc.edu; wagnerdm@upmc.edu; sweatj@upmc.edu; gonzalezjo@upmc.edu

J. A. González Martínez, F. Cardinale (eds.), *Robotics in Neurosurgery*,
https://doi.org/10.1007/978-3-031-08380-8_6

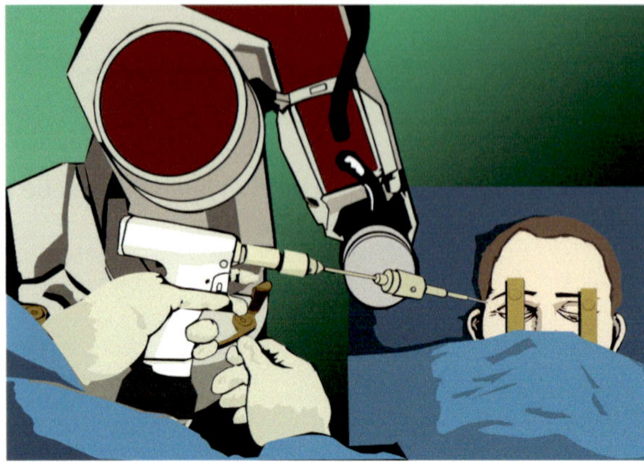

Fig. 6.1 Artist representation of Robotic SEEG demonstrating the robotic device incorporated into the epilepsy surgery armamentarium

One of the most widespread applications of robotics in epilepsy surgery is the stereotactic placement of depth electrodes through the SEEG method (Fig. 6.1) [18]. Briefly, the SEEG is a presurgical invasive monitoring method that allows precise intracortical recordings in multiple non-contiguous lobes, within the three-dimension stereotaxic space, following a highly formulated hypotheses of implantation that seeks to understand the spatiotemporal organization of the epileptiform activity. In many centers, mostly outside Europe, the method represents a shift in the diagnostic and treatment paradigms as compared to the practice of invasive monitoring through the subdural implantation technique. Among other advantages, the avoidance of large craniotomies and their related complications are clear benefits of SEEG procedures [5, 11, 17, 19–31].

The SEEG stereotaxic method and related stereotactic technique were originally developed and described by Jean Talairach and Jean Bancaud. In the initial implantations by Tailarach and Bancaud, and still utilized in some surgical centers, stereotactic frames and the double grid system, in association with teleangiography, were used as the main instruments for precisely implanting the depth electrodes [32–37]. Despite its long-reported clinical successful application, we could speculate that the technical complexity regarding the placement of SEEG depth electrodes using conventional stereotactic frames might have contributed to the limited and late widespread clinical application in centers outside France and Italy. The multiple steps procedures, the need for multiple coordinate adjustments and verifications, and the complexity of imaging fusion are examples of how technical challenges associated with the placement of depth electrodes might have delayed the more general application of this method. The availability of modern robotic devices, with multiples advantages related to versatility, practicality, and precision, was an important driving force in the utilization of the SEEG method in centers outside Europe. Over the past decade, there has been an exponential increase in robotic SEEG procedures in the United States and this may be related, among other factors, to the availability of robotic devices [18].

Robotic SEEG

SEEG Planning

It is important to note that the basic stereotaxic principles related to conventional (non-robotic) and robotic implantations are similar. The development of the SEEG robotic implantation plan demands a clear formulation of the specific anatomo-electro-functional hypotheses to be tested [38–42]. Similar to conventional SEEG, the hypotheses are typically generated during multidisciplinary patient management conferences (PMCs) based on the results of various non-invasive evaluations that include semiology, scalp EEG, imaging, neuropsychology, and other types of non-invasive information. In general sense, SEEG depth electrode placements are designed to sample the anatomic lesion (if identified), potential structure(s) related to the ictal onset, and possible pathway(s) of early and late propagation of epileptiform activity. The entry, intermediate points of interest, and targets are reached using commercially available depth electrodes in various lengths and variable number of contacts, depending on the specific brain region of interest to be explored. Depth electrodes are inserted using orthogonal/semiorthogonal or oblique/semi-oblique orientations, allowing intracranial recording from lateral, intermediate, and/or deep cortical and subcortical structures in a three-dimensional (3D) arrangement, thus accounting for the dynamic, spatiotemporal organization of the epileptic discharges (Fig. 6.2). It is fundamentally important to separate the SEEG method (a stereotaxic method of seizure localization) from techniques related to the implantation of depth electrodes (a stereotactic technique: frame-based, frameless-based, robotic or conventional).

The protocol and procedures related to SEEG robotic implantation will vary from center to center, but the fundamental principles of explorations and interpretation of SEEG recordings should remain similar, regardless of the applied technique. Specifically, at our center, the discussions related to the hypotheses of implantation and the potential location of electrodes are carried out during multidisciplinary patient management conferences, which take place days or weeks before the implantation. The conclusions of the discussions are documented in the patient's medical record, including the hypotheses of implantation and the possible location of electrodes. The electrodes are then represented in the Talairach stereotactic space as a common stereotactic coordinate system, allowing the precise translation of the original implantation map to the robot stereotactic software (Fig. 6.2). Volumetric preoperative magnetic resonance images (T1, contrasted with Gadolinium contrast, e.g., Multihance®—0.1 mmol/kg) are obtained the day before surgery, DICOM format images are digitally transferred to robot's native planning software, and 3D volumetric reconstructions are generated (axial, coronal, and sagittal) and reformatted based on the topographic location of the anterior commissure (AC)-posterior commissure (PC) line. Trajectories are created to maximize sampling from

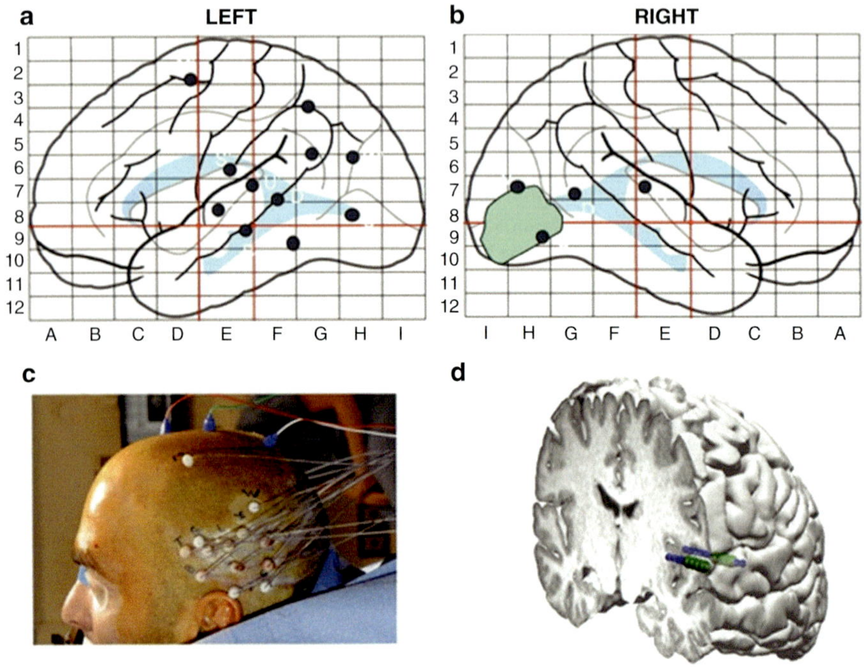

Fig. 6.2 SEEG planning and anatomical representation in Robotic SEEG. (**a**) and (**b**) illustrate the SEEG planning before the implantation. In this patient, we demonstrate the plan for bilateral SEEG implantation in temporal-occipital regions. The green area in the (**b**) panel represents a possible lesion observed on preoperative MRI. (**c**) illustrates the intraoperative aspect of robotic SEEG implantation. (**d**) depicts the three-dimensional representation of electrodes (blue) in the superior temporal gyrus on the left hemisphere. The green circles represent the areas where ictal recordings demonstrated the onset on the epileptiform activity

superficial and deep cortical and subcortical areas within the pre-selected zones of interest. The trajectories are oriented orthogonally (or semi-orthogonally) in the majority of cases to facilitate the anatomo-electrophysiological correlation during the extra-operative recording phase and to avoid possible trajectory shifts due to excessive angled entry points. All trajectories are evaluated for safety and target accuracy in their individual reconstructed planes (axial, sagittal, and coronal), and any trajectory that appears to compromise vascular structures is adjusted appropriately without affecting sampling from the areas of interest (Fig. 6.3). A set working distance of 200 mm from the drilling platform to the target is initially utilized for each trajectory as starting point, later adjusted in order to maximally reduce the working distance and consequently increase the implantation accuracy. The overall implantation schemas are analyzed using the 3D cranial reconstruction capabilities, and external trajectory positions are examined for any entry sites that would be prohibitively close (less than 1.5 cm distance) at the skin level.

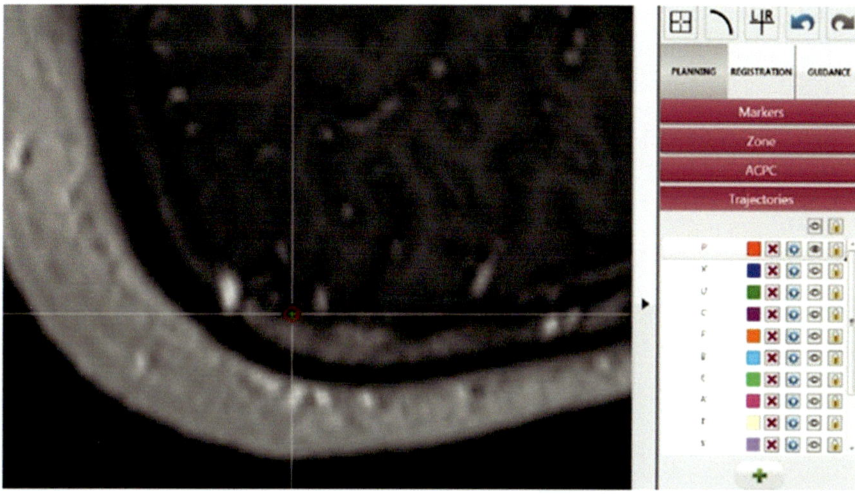

Fig. 6.3 Aspect of robotic SEEG planning using the robotic device native software. The picture illustrates that the entry point is in the preoperative contrasted MRI. Note the absence of vascular structures at the entry point location

The Surgical Implantation

The following description is related to the implantation technique applied to ROSA robotic system (Zimmer Biomet). Initially, patients undergo general anesthesia. For each patient, the head is placed into a three-point fixation head holder. The robot is then positioned such that the working distance (distance between the base of the robotic arm and the midpoint of the cranium) is fixed and approximately 70 cm. The robot is locked into position, and the head holder device is secured to the robot. No additional position adjustments are made to the operating table or to the robot during the implantation procedure. The operating table bed control is disconnected to prevent inadvertent movements of the patient. After positioning and securing the patient to the robot, image registration takes place. For SEEG procedures, we apply semi-automatic laser based facial recognition or fiducial-based registration (Fig. 6.4). Accuracy of the registration process is then confirmed by correlating additional independently chosen surface landmarks with the registered MRI. If calculated error is higher than 2 mm, the registration process is repeated, until an optimal registration accuracy is reached.

After prepping, draping, and trajectory confirmation, the arm movement is initiated using a foot pedal. A 2 mm diameter handheld drill is introduced through the platform and used to create a small opening in the skin and then skull, enough to support the guiding bolt. The dura is opened with an insulated dura perforator and monopolar cautery at low settings. Guiding bolts are screwed into the skull firmly,

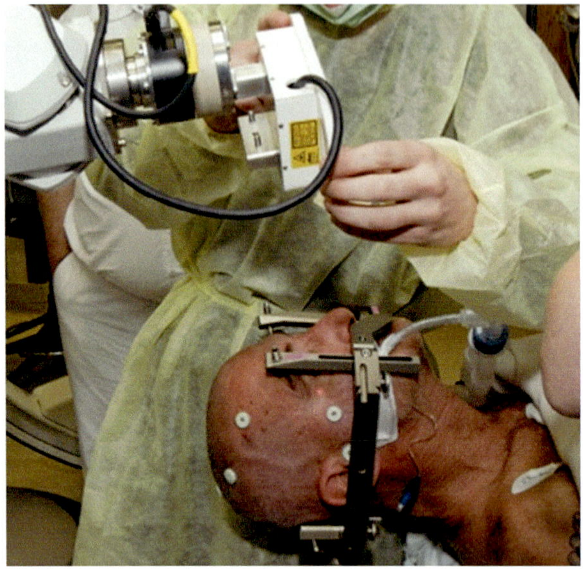

Fig. 6.4 Robotic laser registration in SEEG procedure

and the distance from drilling platform to the retaining bolt is measured. This process is repeated for each trajectory. A small stylet (2 mm in diameter) is then set to the previously recorded electrode distance. The stylet is passed gently into the parenchyma, guided by the implantation bolt, followed immediately by the insertion of the pre-measured electrode.

After implantation of all electrodes, the patient is removed from the fixation device. Fluoroscopy is then utilized in the AP plane to confirm the general accuracy of implanted electrode trajectories. A postimplantation volumetric computed tomography (CT) scan of the brain without contrast, with 1 mm cuts, is obtained for each patient. Following SEEG implantation, patients are subjected to clinical monitoring and electrographic recording of all seizure events at the epilepsy monitoring unit [43].

Results of SEEG Robotic Implantations

In a recent report, the authors analyzed a large series of patients with medically refractory focal epilepsy who underwent robotic stereotactic placement of depth electrodes for extraoperative brain monitoring using the SEEG technique [43]. The analyzed data included demographic and seizure semiology, number and location of implanted SEEG electrodes, time of planning, time of procedure, location of the epileptogenic zone, type of surgical resection, application accuracy, and procedure-related complications. Postoperative seizure outcome was measured using the Engel classification [44]. In total, one hundred patients with refractory focal epilepsy underwent 101 robotic-assisted SEEG procedures. All procedures were completed without cancellations due to hardware or software malfunctioning. The time for planning was 30 min in average (ranging from 15 to 60 min). The average operative time was 130 min (range from 45 to 160 min). Analyses of the robot-assisted SEEG recordings resulted in hypothetical localization of the epileptogenic zone in 97 patients (97%). Sixty-eight patients underwent surgical resection guided by robot-assisted SEEG evaluations, corresponding to 70.1% of the patients with localizable seizures.

In vivo application accuracy, tested in 500 consecutive trajectories, demonstrated the mean entry point error of 1.38 mm (±0.8 mm) and the mean target point error of 2.31 mm (±0.9 mm). Despite the tendency of higher target point errors when compared to entry point errors, statistical analyses failed to demonstrate a statistically significant difference. Regarding the occurrence of adverse events, the authors reported a total of 4 patients (4%) with surgical complications related to intracranial bleeding (2 subdural hematomas and 2 intraparenchymal hematomas). All events of intracranial bleeding were related to the entry point of frontal and parietal located electrodes. Of the 4 patients with intracranial hematomas, 3 patients were asymptomatic with small volume bleeds (<2 cm^3) located in non-eloquent cortical areas. These were considered minor complications, and no surgical intervention or changes in the standard treatment course or hospital stay were necessary. The major complication rate of the reported series was 1%. Given the total number of implanted electrodes (n = 1245), the risk of major hemorrhagic complication per electrodes was 0.08%. Regarding seizure outcome reported in the series, the mean follow-up after robotic SEEG-guided resection was 18 months (ranging from 6 to 30 months). From the group of patients who underwent resective surgery (68 patients), 45 (66.2%) had class I seizure-free outcome postoperatively at last follow-up and 11 (16.2%) had rare disabling seizures after surgery (Class II). Seven patients (10.3%) had worthwhile improvement in seizures (Class III), and 5 patients (7.3%) had no worthwhile improvement in seizures (Class IV). The authors concluded that the results using the reported robotic method parallel previous reports regarding the utility and safety of the traditional SEEG method in the treatment of patients with medically refractory and difficult to localize seizures. This demonstrates that the robotic SEEG method is a reliable, safe, simplified, and time-efficient alternative to the more conventional methods of SEEG implantation. Various studies have also reported similar results and conclusions demonstrating that robotic-assisted stereotactic procedures are safe, accurate, efficient, and comparable to frame-based devices [11, 14, 25, 32, 43, 45].

Reports describing and analyzing comparisons between robotic versus conventional depth electrodes implantations are sparse and a controversial topic. Authors advocating robotic implantation have described its possible superiority to frameless non-robotic systems, but a "head-to-head" comparison is still missing. Eljamel and colleagues [46] have used a robotic device to insert depth electrodes for intraoperative epileptic focus, achieving an average registration accuracy of 1.4 mm compared to 2.6 mm with an image-guided surgery system. Among several factors, the rigid and stable platform for skull drilling provided by robotic devices may have contributed to the difference in accuracy between these two techniques.

Beyond the SEEG method and technique, there are multiple reports of robotics applications in other areas of epilepsy and functional neurosurgery. In particular, there has been novel and innovative use of these technologies in ablative procedures such as MR-guided laser interstitial thermal therapy (MRgLITT or LITT) or radiofrequency ablations, in neuromodulation procedures such as responsive neurostimulation (RNS), and in deep brain stimulation (DBS). We detail the further robotic application in the field of epilepsy surgery in the subsequent sections.

Robotic Ablative Procedures

Stereotactic ablative procedures require the accurate placement of an ablative probe (for laser or radiofrequency procedures) into a specific target previously defined in stereotactic space, often determined by prior SEEG exploration or by MRI visible lesions that are thought to be the epileptogenic zone. As such, robots have two immediate roles: first, for the accurate stereotactic placement of the ablative device, and second, the steerable control of the inserted ablative probe. Previous authors have successfully demonstrated the ablation of epileptogenic periventricular nodular heterotopias in patients with medically resistant epilepsy [47]. After appropriate preoperative imaging, the authors utilized the ROSA® system to accurately guide the placement of the laser catheter (Visualase, Medtronic, Dublin, Ireland) in conjunction with intraoperative MRI. In this report, there were no complications following the ablation. In a similar method, other authors utilized the ROSA® system to guide the placement of a radiofrequency ablation catheter in 5 patients (ages 6 months to 13 years) with hypothalamic hamartomas and consequent gelastic seizures [48]. Four of five patients had grade I seizure outcome, and there were no permanent complications.

Robotic Placement of Responsive Neurostimulation Electrodes

Responsive neurostimulation (RNS) (NeuroPace Inc., Mountain View, CA) is an alternative to ablative therapies for medically refractory focal epilepsy. RNS can detect epileptiform patterns and delivers electrical stimulation along two stereotactically implanted electrodes to terminate seizures. As with other epilepsy implantation procedures, accurate placement of the electrodes is paramount. As such, robotic stereotaxy is a powerful surgical adjunct for RNS implantation (Fig. 6.5). McGovern and colleagues [9] demonstrated robotic implantation of RNS electrodes in 12

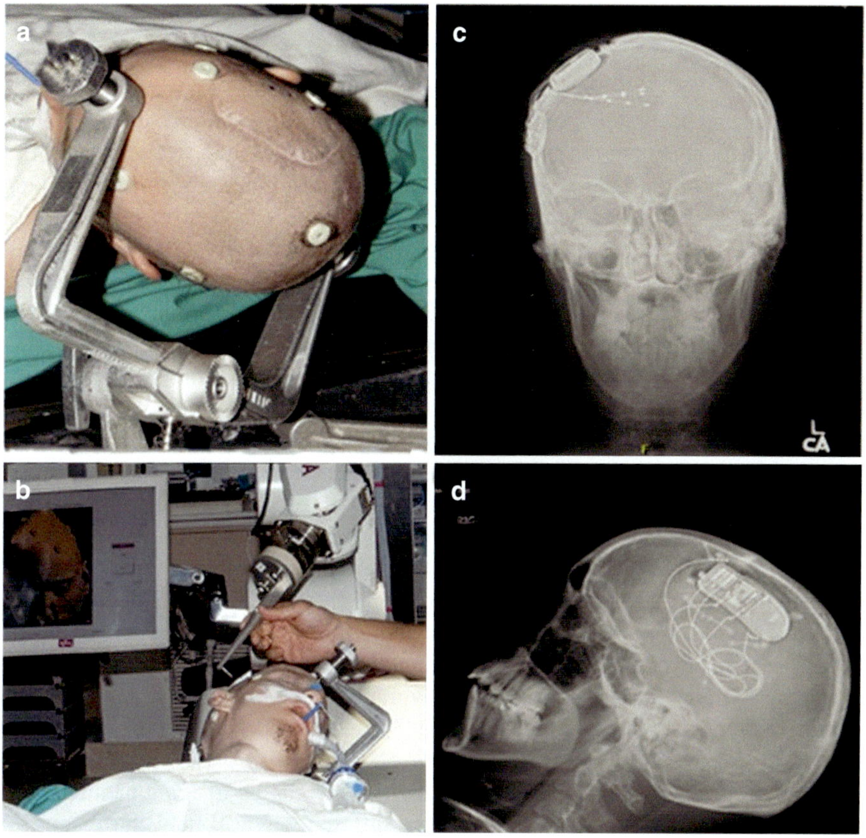

Fig. 6.5 Robotic implantation of response neuro stimulation device. (**a**) Head position using Mayfield head holder. (**b**) Robotic registration using scalp fiducials. Panels (**c**) and (**d**) showing AP and lateral postimplantation RNS device X-rays using the robotic technique

patients, with an overall seizure reduction rate of approximately 40% at 2 years. Notably, 10 of the 12 patients had implantation in temporal lobe structures, with the other two in orbitofrontal cortex and premotor cortex. Similarly, Chan et al. demonstrated successful robotic implantation of RNS in eight patients with mesial temporal lobe epilepsy. Four patients had one-year follow-up, of which one had a grade I outcome and 2 had grade II outcomes. Finally, Tran and colleagues have recently reported ROSA-based RNS implantation in 16 patients. At 1-year follow-up of 8 patients, there was an average of 90% seizure reduction [49]. There is demonstrably increasing usage of robotic stereotaxy in RNS, but further studies will be required to understand the benefits in terms of electrode accuracy, operative efficiency, and seizure freedom.

Conclusions

Stereotactic robots can precisely guide the placement of electrodes and laser probes in 3D space and accurately perform multiple stereotactic trajectories using a frameless setup with adequate precision and in a short period of time. These capabilities avoid the need for multiple, time-consuming frame coordinate adjustments, making the procedures less susceptible for human errors and consequently complications. These advantages suggest that surgical robots are an ideal platform for the placement of SEEG electrodes. Other reports related to DBS, RNS, and LITT procedures using robotic capabilities have been described, highlighting the feasibility and similar advantages in comparison with the SEEG robotic [9, 50, 51].

Concerning safety, the SEEG robotic technique has been demonstrated to be a safe technique, with major morbidity rate of 1% compatible with other SEEG series that applied more conventional stereotactic guidance techniques. Most of the published series reported a morbidity rate ranging from 0 to 5.6% [1, 17, 23, 43]. Spire and colleagues [52] described their experience with robotic implantation of depth electrodes in four patients concurrently undergoing craniotomy and placement of subdural monitoring electrodes for the evaluation of intractable epilepsy with one complication after subdural grid placement but no complication related to depth electrode implantation. By obtaining compatible results with our larger series, the authors also believed that the SEEG system allows the safe and accurate placement of depth electrodes in an efficient manner while obviating the need of reposition the patient or removing the stereotactic frame. The main disadvantage of robotic surgery is its initial cost.

Technological developments in imaging guidance, digital imaging methods, and the more widely use of robotized devices in different medical fields have contributed to the recent and progressive systematic application of robotic surgery in neurosurgery. This statement is specifically relevant in epilepsy surgery and particularly relevant for the SEEG method. The intrinsic features of the SEEG method and technique, with its absolute necessity for high accuracy in multiple trajectories, provide the ideal clinical scenario for the routine application of robotics. The robotic technique is demonstrated to be safe, accurate, and efficient in anatomically defining the epileptogenic zone, proving its feasibility, minimal invasiveness, and reliability, without compromising efficiency. Although further studies are needed, the initial promising results are encouraging and possibly predictive of the further widespread application of this technology in the field of epilepsy surgery as well as in other neurosurgery subspecialties in the near future.

Acknowledgement *Disclosure of Funding:* none.

References

1. Sutherland GR, Maddahi Y, Gan LS, Lama S, Zareinia K. Robotics in the neurosurgical treatment of glioma. Surg Neurol Int. 2015;6(Suppl 1):S1–8. https://doi.org/10.4103/2152-7806.151321.
2. Ballantyne GH, Marescaux JGP. Primer of robotic & telerobotic surgery. Lippincott Williams & Wilkins; 2004.
3. Fomenko A, Serletis D. Robotic stereotaxy in cranial neurosurgery: a qualitative systematic review. Neurosurgery. 2018;83(4):642–50. https://doi.org/10.1093/neuros/nyx576.
4. Scorza D, De Momi E, Plaino L, et al. Retrospective evaluation and SEEG trajectory analysis for interactive multi-trajectory planner assistant. Int J Comput Assist Radiol Surg. 2017;12(10):1727–38. https://doi.org/10.1007/s11548-017-1641-2.
5. Cardinale F, Rizzi M. Stereotactic accuracy must be as high as possible in stereoelectroencephalography procedures. J Robot Surg. 2017;11(4):485–6. https://doi.org/10.1007/s11701-017-0723-z.
6. De Benedictis A, Trezza A, Carai A, et al. Robot-assisted procedures in pediatric neurosurgery. Neurosurg Focus. 2017;42(5):E7. https://doi.org/10.3171/2017.2.FOCUS16579.
7. Vakharia VN, Sparks R, O'Keeffe AG, et al. Accuracy of intracranial electrode placement for stereoencephalography: a systematic review and meta-analysis. Epilepsia. 2017;58(6):921–32. https://doi.org/10.1111/epi.13713.
8. Abel TJ, Varela Osorio R, Amorim-Leite R, et al. Frameless robot-assisted stereoelectroencephalography in children: technical aspects and comparison with Talairach frame technique. J Neurosurg Pediatr. 2018;22(1):37–46. https://doi.org/10.3171/2018.1.PEDS17435.
9. McGovern RA, Alomar S, Bingaman WE, Gonzalez-Martinez J. Robot-assisted responsive neurostimulator system placement in medically intractable epilepsy: instrumentation and technique. Oper Neurosurg (Hagerstown, Md). 2019;16(4):455–64. https://doi.org/10.1093/ons/opy112.
10. De Momi E, Caborni C, Cardinale F, et al. Automatic trajectory planner for StereoElectroEncephaloGraphy procedures: a retrospective study. IEEE Trans Biomed Eng. 2013;60(4):986–93. https://doi.org/10.1109/TBME.2012.2231681.
11. Cardinale F, Cossu M, Castana L, et al. Stereoelectroencephalography: surgical methodology, safety, and stereotactic application accuracy in 500 procedures. Neurosurgery. 2013;72(3):353–66.; discussion 366. https://doi.org/10.1227/NEU.0b013e31827d1161.
12. Meng F, Ding H, Wang G. A stereotaxic image-guided surgical robotic system for depth electrode insertion. Annu Int Conf IEEE Eng Med Biol Soc IEEE Eng Med Biol Soc Annu Int Conf. 2014;2014:6167–70. https://doi.org/10.1109/EMBC.2014.6945037.
13. Enatsu R, Bulacio J, Najm I, et al. Combining stereo-electroencephalography and subdural electrodes in the diagnosis and treatment of medically intractable epilepsy. J Clin Neurosci Off J Neurosurg Soc Australas. 2014;21(8):1441–5. https://doi.org/10.1016/j.jocn.2013.12.014.
14. Arnulfo G, Narizzano M, Cardinale F, Fato MM, Palva JM. Automatic segmentation of deep intracerebral electrodes in computed tomography scans. BMC Bioinformatics. 2015;16:99. https://doi.org/10.1186/s12859-015-0511-6.
15. von Langsdorff D, Paquis P, Fontaine D. In vivo measurement of the frame-based application accuracy of the Neuromate neurosurgical robot. J Neurosurg. 2015;122(1):191–4. https://doi.org/10.3171/2014.9.JNS14256.
16. Golby A, editor. Image-guided neurosurgery. Elsevier Academic Press; 2015.
17. Cardinale F, Casaceli G, Raneri F, Miller J, Lo RG. Implantation of Stereoelectroencephalography electrodes: a systematic review. J Clin Neurophysiol Off Publ Am Electroencephalogr Soc. 2016;33(6):490–502. https://doi.org/10.1097/WNP.0000000000000249.

18. Abou-Al-Shaar H, Brock AA, Kundu B, Englot DJ, Rolston JD. Increased nationwide use of stereoencephalography for intracranial epilepsy electroencephalography recordings. J Clin Neurosci Off J Neurosurg Soc Australas. 2018;53:132–4. https://doi.org/10.1016/j.jocn.2018.04.064.
19. Gonzalez-Martinez J, Mullin J, Vadera S, et al. Stereotactic placement of depth electrodes in medically intractable epilepsy. J Neurosurg. 2014;120(3):639–44. https://doi.org/10.3171/2013.11.JNS13635.
20. Cossu M, Fuschillo D, Cardinale F, et al. Stereo-EEG-guided radio-frequency thermocoagulations of epileptogenic grey-matter nodular heterotopy. J Neurol Neurosurg Psychiatry. 2014;85(6):611–7. https://doi.org/10.1136/jnnp-2013-305514.
21. McGovern RA, Ratneswaren T, Smith EH, et al. Investigating the function of deep cortical and subcortical structures using stereotactic electroencephalography: lessons from the anterior cingulate cortex. J Vis Exp. 2015;(98) https://doi.org/10.3791/52773.
22. Cardinale F, Cossu M. SEEG has the lowest rate of complications. J Neurosurg. 2015;122(2):475–7. https://doi.org/10.3171/2014.7.JNS141680.
23. Mullin JP, Smithason S, Gonzalez-Martinez J. Stereo-Electro-Encephalo-Graphy (SEEG) with robotic assistance in the presurgical evaluation of medical refractory epilepsy: a technical note. J Vis Exp. 2016;(112) https://doi.org/10.3791/53206.
24. Bartolomei F, Lagarde S, Wendling F, et al. Defining epileptogenic networks: contribution of SEEG and signal analysis. Epilepsia. 2017;58(7):1131–47. https://doi.org/10.1111/epi.13791.
25. Bancaud J, Angelergues R, Bernouilli C, et al. Functional stereotaxic exploration (SEEG) of epilepsy. Electroencephalogr Clin Neurophysiol. 1970;28(1):85–6.
26. Talairach J, Bancaud J, Bonis A, et al. Surgical therapy for frontal epilepsies. Adv Neurol. 1992;57:707–32.
27. Gonzalez-Martinez J, Lachhwani D. Stereoelectroencephalography in children with cortical dysplasia: technique and results. Child's Nerv Syst ChNS Off J Int Soc Pediatr Neurosurg. 2014;30(11):1853–7. https://doi.org/10.1007/s00381-014-2499-z.
28. Gonzalez-Martinez J, Bulacio J, Alexopoulos A, Jehi L, Bingaman W, Najm I. Stereoelectroencephalography in the "difficult to localize" refractory focal epilepsy: early experience from a north American epilepsy center. Epilepsia. 2013;54(2):323–30. https://doi.org/10.1111/j.1528-1167.2012.03672.x.
29. Gonzalez-Martinez J, Najm IM. Indications and selection criteria for invasive monitoring in children with cortical dysplasia. Child's Nerv Syst ChNS Off J Int Soc Pediatr Neurosurg. 2014;30(11):1823–9. https://doi.org/10.1007/s00381-014-2497-1.
30. Serletis D, Bulacio J, Bingaman W, Najm I, González-Martínez J. The stereotactic approach for mapping epileptic networks: a prospective study of 200 patients. J Neurosurg. 2014;121(5):1239–46. https://doi.org/10.3171/2014.7.JNS132306.
31. Vadera S, Burgess R, Gonzalez-Martinez J. Concomitant use of stereoelectroencephalography (SEEG) and magnetoencephalographic (MEG) in the surgical treatment of refractory focal epilepsy. Clin Neurol Neurosurg. 2014;122:9–11. https://doi.org/10.1016/j.clineuro.2014.04.002.
32. Talairach J, De Aljuriaguerra J, David M. A stereotaxic study of the deep encephalic structures in man; technic; physiopathologic and therapeutic significance. Presse Med. 1952;60(28):605–9.
33. Talairach J. Stereotaxic radiologic explorations. Rev Neurol (Paris). 1954;90(5):556–84.
34. Talairach J, TOURNOUX P. Apparatus for hypophysial stereotaxis by nasal approach. Neurochirurgie. 1955;1(1):127–31.
35. Talairach J, TOURNOUX P. Stereotaxic localization of central gray nuclei. Neurochirurgia (Stuttg). 1958;1(1):88–93. https://doi.org/10.1055/s-0028-1095515.
36. Talairach J, David M TP. L'exploration Chirurgicale Stéréotaxique de Lobe Temportal Dans l'épilepsie Temporale. libraires de l'Academie de medecine; 1958.
37. Talairach J, Bancaud J, Bonis A, Szikla G, Tournoux P. Functional stereotaxic exploration of epilepsy. Confin Neurol. 1962;22:328–31. https://doi.org/10.1159/000104378.

38. Bancaud J, Bonis A, Talairach J, Tournoux P, Szikla G, Saw V. The value of stereotaxic functional exploration in the localization of expansive lesions. Rev Obstet Ginecol Venez. 1961;105:219–20.
39. Talairach J, Bancaud J, Bonis A, Tournoux P, Szikla G, Morel P. Functional stereotaxic investigations in epilepsy. Methodological remarks concerning a case. Rev Neurol (Paris). 1961;105:119–30.
40. Bancaud J, Talairach J. Epilepsy of the supplementary motor area: a particularly difficult diagnosis in children. Rev Neuropsychiatr Infant. 1965;13(6):483–99.
41. Bancaud J, Talairach J. Functional organization of the supplementary motor area. Data obtained by stereo-E.E.G. Neurochirurgie. 1967;13(3):343–56.
42. J T. Atlas d'anatomie Stéréotaxique Du Télencéphale, Études Anatomo-Radiologiques. Masson et Cie. 1967;
43. González-Martínez J, Bulacio J, Thompson S, et al. Technique, results, and complications related to robot-assisted stereoelectroencephalography. Neurosurgery. 2016;78(2):169–80. https://doi.org/10.1227/NEU.0000000000001034.
44. Engel J. Surgical treatment of the epilepsies. Lippincott Williams & Wilkins; 1993.
45. Yaffe R, Burns S, Gale J, et al. Brain state evolution during seizure and under anesthesia: a network-based analysis of stereotaxic EEG activity in drug-resistant epilepsy patients. Annu Int Conf IEEE Eng Med Biol Soc IEEE Eng Med Biol Soc Annu Int Conf. 2012;2012:5158–61. https://doi.org/10.1109/EMBC.2012.6347155.
46. Eljamel MS. Robotic application in epilepsy surgery. Int J Med Robot. 2006;2(3):233–7. https://doi.org/10.1002/rcs.97.
47. Gonzalez-Martinez J, Vadera S, Mullin J, et al. Robot-assisted stereotactic laser ablation in medically intractable epilepsy: operative technique. Neurosurgery. 2014;10(Suppl 2):163–7. https://doi.org/10.1227/NEU.0000000000000286.
48. Tandon V, Chandra PS, Doddamani RS, et al. Stereotactic radiofrequency thermocoagulation of hypothalamic hamartoma using robotic guidance (ROSA) coregistered with O-arm guidance-preliminary technical note. World Neurosurg. 2018;112:267–74. https://doi.org/10.1016/j.wneu.2018.01.193.
49. Tran DK, Paff M, Mnatsakanyan L, et al. A novel robotic-assisted technique to implant the responsive neurostimulation system. Oper Neurosurg (Hagerstown, Md). 2020;18(6):728–35. https://doi.org/10.1093/ons/opz226.
50. McGovern RA, Knight EP, Gupta A, et al. Robot-assisted stereoelectroencephalography in children. J Neurosurg Pediatr. 2018;23(3):288–96. https://doi.org/10.3171/2018.7.PEDS18305.
51. RossL,NaduvilAM,BulacioJC,NajmIM,Gonzalez-MartinezJA.Stereoelectroencephalography-guided laser ablations in patients with neocortical pharmacoresistant focal epilepsy: concept and operative technique. Oper Neurosurg (Hagerstown, Md). 2018;15(6):656–63. https://doi.org/10.1093/ons/opy022.
52. Spire WJ, Jobst BC, Thadani VM, Williamson PD, Darcey TM, Roberts DW. Robotic image-guided depth electrode implantation in the evaluation of medically intractable epilepsy. Neurosurg Focus. 2008;25(3):E19. https://doi.org/10.3171/FOC/2008/25/9/E19.

Chapter 7
Robotic SEEG-Guided Radiofrequency Thermal Ablation

Marc Guénot and Massimo Cossu

History and Principles of SEEG-Guided Radiofrequency Thermocoagulation

Stereoelectroencephalography (SEEG) is required in many patients suffering from pharmacoresistant focal epilepsy to define the optimal cortical resection. It consists of stereotactic implantation of depth electrodes in the brain, in order to identify the exact location(s) of the epileptogenic area(s), as well as the pathways of discharge propagation. Nowadays, the indirect targeting provided by the use of the Talairach's atlas [1, 2] has been mostly replaced, thanks to MRI imaging, by a direct targeting.

The idea to use stereotactically implanted electrodes to perform lesions by means of radiofrequency waves is not a new idea, and a first paper reporting an effect on epilepsy was published in 1965 [3]. Initially, treatment of epilepsy was not the main purpose of this procedure, which aimed at healing unmanageable behavioral disorders by selective amygdalotomy [4]. Several lesioning techniques have been proposed, but the use of radiofrequency heating remains the most popular due to its intrinsic advantages. From the 70s to the 90s, stereotactic lesioning as a surgical treatment of focal epilepsy was largely developed. The rate of improvement in terms of seizure frequency was reported to vary from 50 to 85%. However, this literature displayed results which are difficult to interpret given the surgical techniques and outcome assessment used. Notably, presurgical assessment was less rigid,

M. Guénot (✉)
Department of Functional Neurosurgery, P. Wertheimer Hospital, Hospices Civils de Lyon, University of Lyon, Lyon, France
e-mail: marc.guenot@chu-lyon.fr

M. Cossu
"Claudio Munari" Center for Epilepsy Surgery, Azienda Socio-Sanitaria Territoriale Grande Ospedale Metropolitano Niguarda, Milano, Italy
e-mail: massimo.cossu@ospedaleniguarda.it

J. A. González Martínez, F. Cardinale (eds.), *Robotics in Neurosurgery*,
https://doi.org/10.1007/978-3-031-08380-8_7

verification of site and size of lesion is difficult, and follow-up data are poor. In 1999, Parrent & Blume carried out a single study to assess the safety and efficacy of stereotactic ablation of the amygdala and hippocampus for the treatment of medial temporal lobe epilepsy [5]. They concluded that extensive amygdalo-hippocampal ablation improved seizure outcome compared with more limited ablation, but that results were not as good as with temporal lobectomies in a comparable patient group.

Due to the rather disappointing results of stereotactic lesioning for epilepsy, this technique, while popular in the 60s and 70s, was largely abandoned at the end of the last century.

As all the results previously quoted were obtained following unique focal stereotactic lesions based mainly on non-invasive investigations (which did not allow accurate delineation of the ictal onset zone), an evolution of this procedure has been represented since about 15 years now taking benefit of the SEEG technique [6]. This improves its efficiency by creating lesions not targeted a priori on a selected structure but aiming at a total or partial destruction of the epileptogenic zone, as tailored in each individual patient by the SEEG exploration [7]. This technique named **SEEG-guided RF-thermocoagulation** (SEEG-guided RF-TC, or thermo-SEEG) provides a solution to some limits of stereotactic procedures previously described and offers multiple advantages supported by several lines of evidences:

(a) The per-operative bleeding risk is low as the electrodes are already in place, for recording purposes (this procedure does not require passage of electrodes through brain beyond the passages required by diagnostic SEEG electrodes).
(b) Performing lesions on electrodes which are also used for diagnostic recordings allows a quality of target selection that is not possible to obtain with a stereotactic procedure using a planning based on non-invasive data.
(c) The numerous available targets due to the high number of implanted electrodes allow proceeding to numerous RF-thermocoagulations with a possibility to create confluent lesions using contiguous targets (Fig. 7.1).
(d) Electrical stimulations are systematically performed during the video-SEEG recording sessions to mimic the possible side effects of a lesion. Consequently, there is no need for supplementary stimulation during the procedure, a plus for the patient.
(e) RF-thermocoagulation provides well-circumscribed lesions with impedance monitoring.
(f) Anesthesia is not required and patient can be monitored by a neurologist during the procedure.
(g) Performing RF-thermocoagulation has no impact on the feasibility and on the operative risks of a further conventional surgery, if needed.
(h) These lesions are well tolerated by the patient.

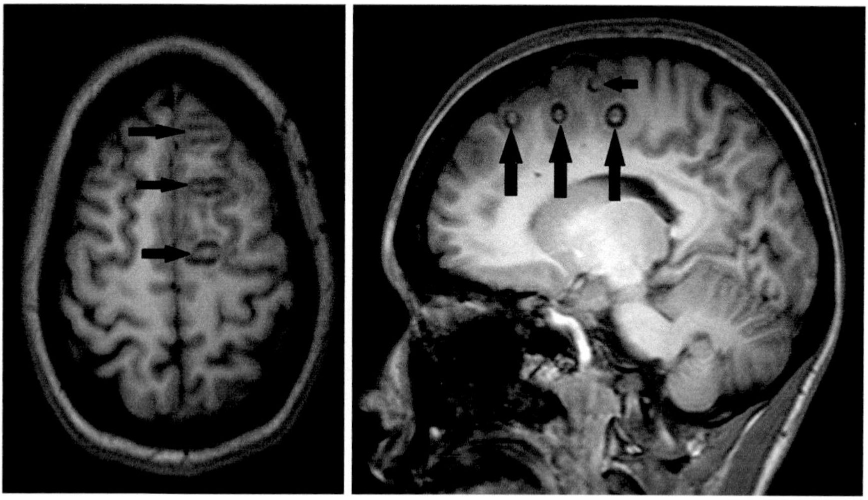

Fig. 7.1 MRI scan displaying multiple post SEEG-guided RF-TC lesions (arrows) using contiguous targets along the electrodes

Modus Operandi

SEEG-guided RF-TC consists of RF-TC delivered between two contiguous contacts of the same electrode located in every selected target [8]. The production of an RF thermal lesion is initiated by the propagation of the RF current between the two contacts, thus creating an electric field. Oscillatory movements of tissue ions within this electric field result in tissue heating, with thermal necrosis occurring when temperatures increase between 50° and 100 ° C. Cell death is the result of protein coagulation and irreversible damage to key cytosolic and mitochondrial enzymes, and to nucleic acid–histone protein complexes [9, 10].

Reported coagulation parameters, useful to increase the local temperature to 78°–82 ° C, slightly differ from center to center, mainly depending on the RF generator employed [11, 12]. However, there is evidence that increasing (progressively and with a constant linear velocity) the voltage of the delivered current until these parameters spontaneously collapse (usually in a few seconds) provides larger lesions than using fixed parameters [13]. On average, the volume of a single RF lesion produced between two adjacent contacts ranges from 85 to 100 mm^3 [12, 13]. When multiple RF-TC are carried out on a same electrode track, this results in confluent lesions (Fig. 7.2). Recent studies have reported the possibility to apply RF also between contacts situated on distinct adjacent electrodes (cross-bonding RF-TC), provided that the distance between the selected contacts is less than 7 mm [14]. In those instances, placing a dense array of electrodes in the presumed epileptogenic area or lesion may facilitate the shaping of the coagulation volume according to

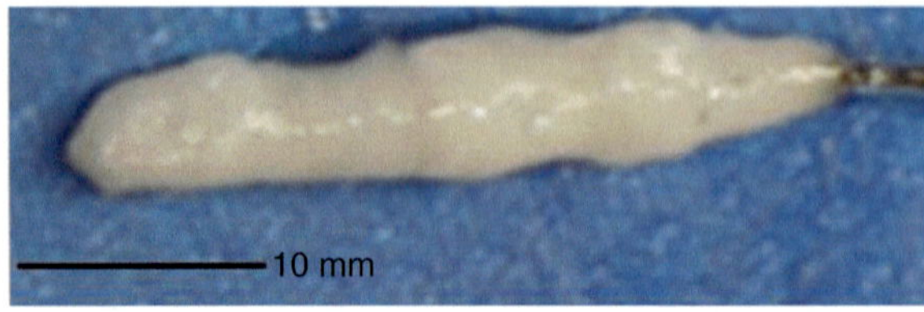

Fig. 7.2 Visual aspect of multiple RF-TC performed in egg-white on adjacent contacts of a SEEG electrode

specific requirements, as reported in the treatment of hypothalamic hamartomas [15] and hippocampal sclerosis-related epilepsy [16].

During the RF-TC procedure, patients undergo a real time clinical evaluation by a neurologist. A control of SEEG activity is performed immediately after RF-TC. Ablation of the electrodes is performed at the end of the procedure (except for patients in whom further recording is required to assess the effect of RF-TC on seizures) and patients are discharged after 24 h of clinical follow-up in the epilepsy department. In selected cases submitted to extensive coagulation, oral steroids may be prescribed for preventing excessive perilesional edema.

Indications and Results: Review

Indications

All the patients must previously benefit from a comprehensive presurgical non-invasive investigation, which consists of long-term scalp video-EEG monitoring, neuropsychological testing, high resolution 1.5 T or 3 T Magnetic Resonance Imaging (MRI), and metabolic imaging (18Fluorodeoxyglucose Positron Emission Tomography (PET) scan). Some patients also undergo ictal Single Photon Emission Computerized Tomography (SPECT) and magnetic source imaging of interictal paroxysmal activity using magneto-encephalography (MEG). Typically, long-term intracranial EEG monitoring using phase II invasive SEEG exploration is performed in patients for whom data obtained from phase I non-invasive investigations are not congruent enough to propose direct surgery. Patients are informed of the aims and risks of SEEG recordings and of RF-TC.

Patients are considered eligible for RF-TC when SEEG findings indicate that (i) all or the major part of the epileptogenic zone is accessible to RF-TC (procedure aiming at avoiding a feasible surgery); (ii) when the epileptic network, although unilateral, is widely distributed or include eloquent or deep and inaccessible areas (palliative therapeutic option when surgery is not feasible) [17].

Furthermore, SEEG-guided RF-TC is indicated whenever it may represent a curative option and is therefore employed as a first-line treatment, as in selected cases of epilepsy associated with periventricular nodular heterotopia [18, 19] (Fig. 7.3), hypothalamic hamartomas [15], hippocampal sclerosis [16], and focal

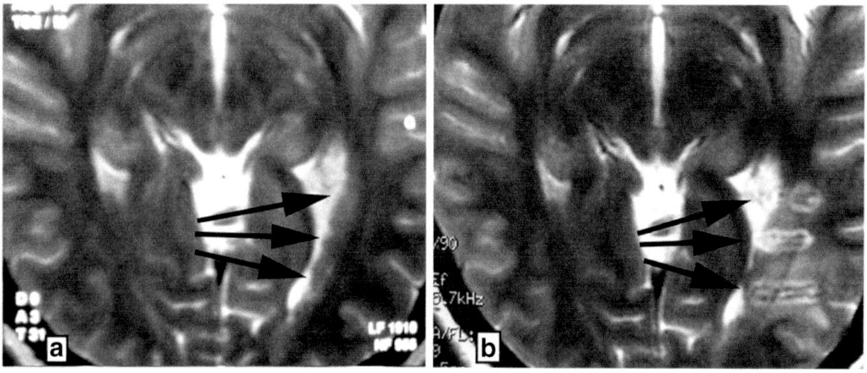

Fig. 7.3 MRI scans displaying a left posterior periventricular heterotopia (arrow) before (**a**) and after (**b**) SEEG-guided RF-TC

cortical dysplasia [20]. In similar cases, SEEG is used as a diagnostic and therapeutic tool, and electrodes are typically arranged a priori for maximizing the coverage of the presumed epileptogenic lesion(s) or structures [11] in order to both evaluate their contribution to seizure generation and to include as much as possible of epileptogenic tissue within the coagulation volume.

Finally, SEEG-guided RF-TC may be a useful prognostic tool in cases amenable to surgical resections according to SEEG findings: indeed, it has been postulated that even a partial or transient response to RF-TC (i.e., absence or decreased frequency/intensity of seizures) may herald a favorable seizure outcome after resection. It has been reported that the outcome at 2 months after SEEG-guided RFTC is a predictive factor of success for patients who finally undergo conventional epilepsy surgery [21].

Selection of Targets for RF-TC

Targets are chosen in cortical sites showing either a low amplitude fast pattern or spike-wave discharges at the onset of the seizures, in intralesional location, and/or in contacts where electrical stimulation induces habitual seizures [12, 22]. Interictal paroxysmal activities are not usually considered for planning thermo-coagulation sites, with the exception of focal cortical dysplasias type II, where interictal spikes are recognized as biomarkers of these lesions [23].

Safety Profile of RF-TC

Before RF-TC, a functional mapping is systematically performed using low- and high-frequency electrical stimulations, for disclosing cortical and subcortical structures involved in essential neurological functions. Sites where stimulation induces, for instance, motor responses, or language disorders are excluded from the coagulation plan prepared by the neurophysiologist. Furthermore, selection of contacts lying in close proximity (usually <2 mm) to vascular structures must be carefully evaluated for the risk of hemorrhagic or ischemic injury.

Concerning the safety, a few transient side effects have been reported, including seizures or local fleeting pain during RF delivery and development of transient local brain swelling around the coagulated region [24], whereas unexpected severe permanent neurological morbidity is very rare [21]. As a whole, the rate of neurological deficits still present 1 year after the procedure ranges from 0 to 4% across series, averaging 2.5% of treated cases [25]. This occurs mainly if RF-TC is performed within highly eloquent areas [12, 25], when postoperative morbidity is generally expected according to functional mapping, and it may be anticipated and discussed with the patients. With the reported rates of permanent deficits and of transient side effects, SEEG-guided RF-TC can be considered as the safest procedure for surgical treatment of drug-resistant focal epilepsy.

Seizure Outcome

Available data indicate that seizure freedom after SEEG-guided RF-TC is achieved by 23% of cases, whereas a favorable response (>50% reduction of seizure frequency) is observed in more than half of patients [25]. Although a significant subset of responders at 1 year of follow-up have been shown to maintain their status for the following 2–10 years [21], maintenance over time of achieved benefits (seizure freedom, decreased frequency, or intensity of seizures) is an issue still waiting for full elucidation. This aspect has relevant implications on timing of eventual resective surgery and, more importantly, on management of antiepileptic medications, especially in patients rendered seizure free after RF-TC.

The best results are observed in epilepsies associated with cortical developmental malformations, particularly focal cortical dysplasias and heterotopias [19, 20]. Promising results have been reported in hypothalamic hamartomas [15] and in hippocampal sclerosis-related epilepsy [16], while the effect of RF-TC is less favorable in non-lesional epilepsy cases [25]. The benefit-risk ratio of the SEEG-guided RF-TC procedure proves to be particularly favorable for patients in whom surgery is not feasible or risky.

Refinements Provided by Robotic SEEG Implantation

Accuracy of stereotactic techniques is essential to maximize both efficacy and safety of SEEG evaluations for two main reasons. First, the cortical regions included in the exploration plan must be sampled with the greatest possible accuracy, as suboptimal targeting may result in misinterpretation of collected data and errors in the identification of the epileptogenic zone. Second, electrode implantation must follow avascular trajectories, since damage to arteries or veins, especially at the cortical entry point, may have severe neurological consequences secondary to intracranial hemorrhage.

The SEEG methodology, introduced in the last century at Saint Anne Hospital, Paris, France [1, 2], has been constantly updated over time, but its baseline stereotactic features have been so far maintained unchanged. Along with modern neuroimaging, the advent of robot-assisted technologies has strongly influenced the evolution of SEEG implantation technique [26]: the main yields include reduction of surgical time, gain in targeting accuracy, enhanced safety profile, increased amount and quality of collected data [27–30].

In addition, the implementation of structural and functional multimodal imaging in the pre-implantation workflow has proven essential for image-guided planning and control of robot-assisted procedures.

The contribution of robot assistance to the improved accuracy of implants has increased the indications for SEEG-guided RF-TC when the procedure is specifically performed for curative purposes. For instance, in periventricular nodular heterotopias, nodules are frequently located at the level of the ventricular trigone, with the optic radiations running in close proximity to the lesion. Robotized electrode placement allows extremely precise targeting of the nodules, thus enabling effective RF-ablation of the nodules without injury to the subjacent white matter (Fig. 7.4).

The same applies to focal small-sized, bottom-of-the-sulcus focal cortical dysplasias type II, whose coagulation requires absolute precision of targeting due to their small size (Fig. 7.5) and to their location, as in the rolandic area, where they are frequently contiguous to the cortico-spinal and thalamocortical tracts.

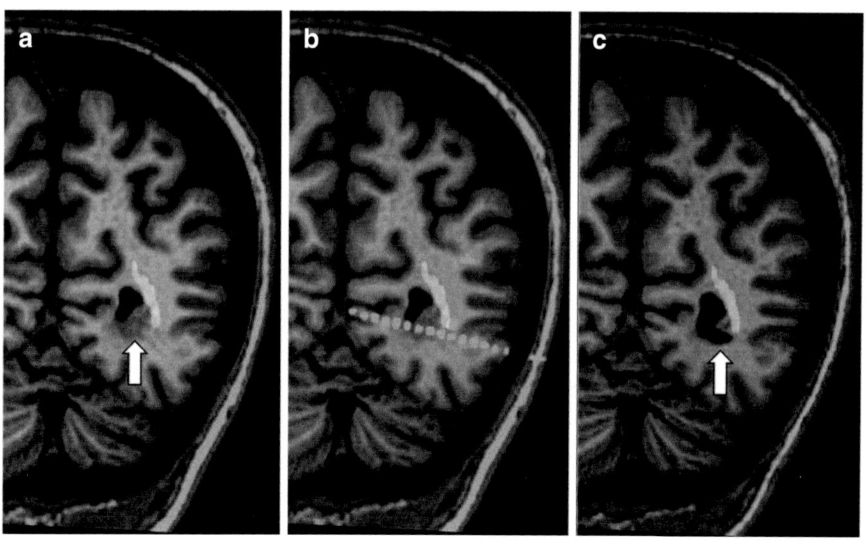

Fig. 7.4 T1-weighted MR scan of a periventricular nodular heterotopy (arrow) of the left occipital horn, displaying the optic radiation obtained from DTI-based fiber-tracking (**a**). In (**b**) the SEEG electrode placed with robotic assistance within the nodule and brushing the inferior border of the optic radiation is shown. The nodule has been coagulated (arrow) sparing the optic radiation (**c**)

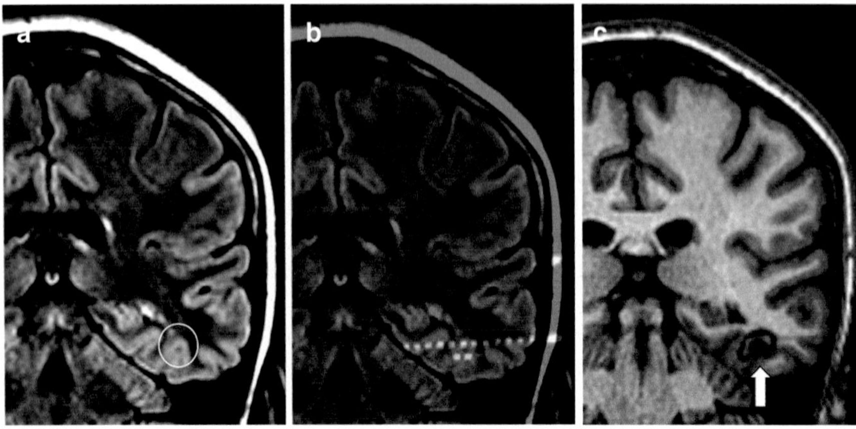

Fig. 7.5 This subtle bottom-of-sulcus focal cortical dysplasia of the left temporal basal cortex (**a**, open circle) was targeted by two electrodes placed under robot assistance (**b**). After SEEG monitoring, multiple confluent RF-TCs resulted in complete ablation of the lesion (**c**) and sustained seizure freedom

The introduction of robot devices for SEEG implants has also made possible optimal sampling of the insular cortex, which, although frequently implicated in peri-sylvian epilepsies, was considered poorly accessible to electrodes placed with less recent traditional techniques, due to the dense screen of vascular structures covering this area. Besides improving the safety of the typical trans-opercular orthogonal trajectories, the robotic arm allows targeting the insula through oblique trans-frontal and trans-parietal trajectories. Thanks to these multiple approaches, an intense coverage of the insula cortex may be achieved, and potentially curative RF-TC may be carried out in this region. In selected patients, favorable seizure outcome in insular epilepsy has been obtained by RF-TC, avoiding the risks of conventional open surgery in this highly critical region [31] (Fig. 7.6).

Conclusions, Perspectives

SEEG-guided RF-TC is a safe technique, being efficient in many selected cases. More than two third of patients show a short-term improvement and approximately half of them are responders at 1 year follow-up, with a not negligible subset of patients maintaining this status.

Complications are minor, rare, and reversible in many cases. No long-term side effects, particularly on cognitive function, are observed. Thus, it is possible to treat targets located very near to cortical areas with high functional value (language or primary visual zone) or poorly accessible to conventional surgical procedure (insular cortex). The use of SEEG electrodes for performing multiple RF-thermolesions also appears to provide a unique opportunity to have large access to the

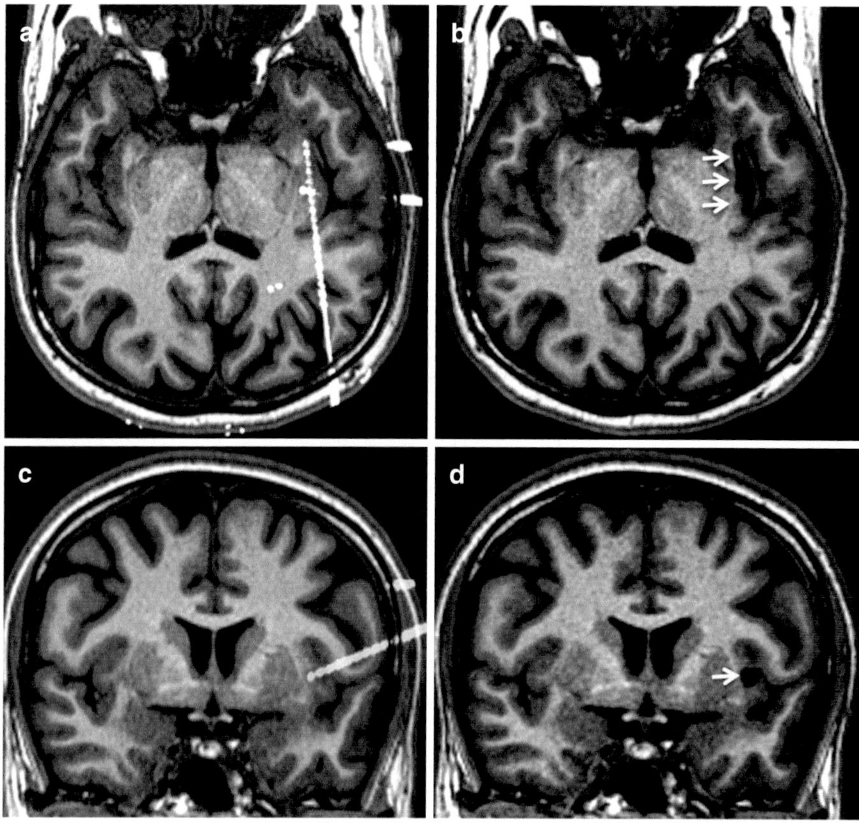

Fig. 7.6 Left boxes illustrate a robot-assisted SEEG implant with accurate targeting of the insular cortex through multiple trajectories (**a**, **c**). On the right, same slices showing post-coagulation (arrows) MR scans (**b**, **d**)

epileptogenic network. In some specific situations, SEEG-guided RF-TC represents an effective, first-line treatment alternative to high-risk conventional surgery.

The benefit-risk ratio of the thermo-SEEG procedure proves particularly favorable for the patients in whom surgery is not feasible or risky. In these cases, thermo-SEEG proves to be a safe therapeutic option, the results of which compare favorably to those of other palliative therapeutic procedures such as vagus nerve stimulation, multiple subpial transection, callosotomy, or deep intracerebral stimulations.

The rather recent advent of robot-assisted technologies, through reduction of surgical time, major gain in targeting accuracy, enhanced safety profile, and increased amount of collected data, does strongly contribute to significant improvements of the SEEG-guided RF-thermocoagulation efficiency. It allows, in the daily practice, to increase its indications, especially when the procedure is specifically performed for curative purposes related to lesions located very close to highly functional areas, or when the insular cortex is involved.

References

1. Talairach J, David M, Tournoux P. Atlas d'Anatomie Stereotaxique. Paris: Masson and Cie Editeurs; 1957.
2. Bancaud J, Talairach J, Bonis A, Schaub C, Szikla G, Morel P, et al. La stereo-electro-encephalographie dans l'epilepsie. Paris: Masson; 1965.
3. Schwab RS, Sweet WH, Mark VH, Kjellberg RN, Ervin FR. Treatment of intractable temporal lobe epilepsy by stereotactic amygdala lesions. Trans Am Neurol Assoc. 1965;90:12–9.
4. Narabayashi H, Nagao T, Saito Y, Yoshida M, Nagahata M. Stereotaxic amygdalotomy for behavior disorders. Arch Neurol. 1963;9:11–26.
5. Parrent AG, Blume WT. Stereotactic amygdalohippocampotomy for the treatment of medial temporal lobe epilepsy. Epilepsia. 1999;40:1408–16.
6. Guénot M, Isnard J, Ryvlin P, Fischer C, Mauguière F, Sindou M. SEEG-guided RF thermocoagulation of epileptic foci: feasibility, safety, and preliminary results. Epilepsia. 2004;45:1368–74.
7. Guenot M, Isnard J. Multiple SEEG-guided RF-thermolesions of epileptogenic foci. Neurochirurgie. 2008;54:441–7.
8. Isnard J, Taussig D, Bartolomei F, Bourdillon P, Catenoix H, Chassoux F, et al. French guidelines on stereoelectroencephalography (SEEG). Clin Neurophysiol. 2018;48:5–13.
9. Goldberg SN. Radiofrequency tumor ablation: principles and techniques. Eur J Ultrasound. 2001;13:129–47.
10. Cosman ER Jr, Cosman ER Sr. Electric and thermal field effects in tissue around radiofrequency electrodes. Pain Med. 2005;6:405–24.
11. Guénot M, Isnard J, Catenoix H, Mauguière F, Sindou M. SEEG-guided RF-thermocoagulation of epileptic foci: a therapeutic alternative for drug-resistant non-operable partial epilepsies. Adv Tech Stand Neurosurg. 2011;36:61–78.
12. Cossu M, Fuschillo D, Casaceli G, Pelliccia V, Castana L, Mai R, et al. Stereoelectroencephalography-guided radiofrequency thermocoagulation in the epileptogenic zone: a retrospective study on 89 cases. J Neurosurg. 2015;123:1358–67.
13. Bourdillon P, Isnard J, Catenoix H, Montavont A, Rheims S, Ryvlin P, Ostrowsky-Coste K, Mauguière F, Guénot M. SEEG-guided radiofrequency thermocoagulation (SEEG RF-TC): from in vitro and in vivo data to technical guidelines. World Neurosurg. 2016;94:73–7.
14. Wang D, Wei P, Shan Y, Ren L, Wang Y, Zhao G. Optimized stereoelectroencephalography-guided radiofrequency thermocoagulation in the treatment of patients with focal epilepsy. Ann Transl Med. 2020;8:15.
15. Wei PH, An Y, Fan XT, Wang YH, Yang YF, Ren LK, et al. Stereoelectroencephalography-guided radiofrequency Thermocoagulation for hypothalamic hamartomas: preliminary evidence. World Neurosurg. 2018;114:e1073–8.
16. Fan X, Shan Y, Lu C, An Y, Wang Y, Du J, et al. Optimized SEEG-guided radiofrequency thermocoagulation for mesial temporal lobe epilepsy with hippocampal sclerosis. Seizure. 2019;71:304–11.
17. Catenoix H, Mauguière F, Guénot M, Ryvlin P, Bissery A, Sindou M, et al. SEEG-guided thermocoagulations: a palliative treatment of nonoperable partial epilepsies. Neurology. 2008;71:1719–26.
18. Cossu M, Fuschillo D, Cardinale F, Castana L, Francione S, Nobili L, et al. Stereo-EEG-guided radio-frequency thermocoagulations of epileptogenic grey-matter nodular heterotopy. J Neurol Neurosurg Psychiatry. 2014;85:611–7.
19. Mirandola L, Mai RF, Francione S, Pelliccia V, Gozzo F, Sartori I, et al. Stereo-EEG: diagnostic and therapeutic tool for periventricular nodular heterotopia epilepsies. Epilepsia. 2017;58:1962–71.
20. Catenoix H, Mauguière F, Montavont A, Ryvlin P, Guénot M, Isnard J. Seizures outcome after stereoelectroencephalography-guided thermocoagulations in malformations of cortical development poorly accessible to surgical resection. Neurosurgery. 2015;77:9–14.

21. Bourdillon P, Isnard J, Catenoix H, Montavont A, Rheims S, Ryvlin P, et al. Stereoelectroencephalography-guided radiofrequency thermocoagulation (SEEG-guided RF-TC) in drug-resistant focal epilepsy: results from a 10-year experience. Epilepsia. 2017;58:85–93.
22. Bourdillon P, Rheims S, Catenoix H, Montavont A, Ostrowsky-Coste K, Isnard J, et al. Surgical techniques: stereoelectroencephalography-guided radiofrequency-thermocoagulation (SEEG-guided RF-TC). Seizure. 2020;77:64–8.
23. Chassoux F, Devaux B, Landré E, Turak B, Nataf F, Varlet P, et al. Stereoelectroencephalography in focal cortical dysplasia: a 3D approach to delineating the dysplastic cortex. Brain. 2000;123:1733–51.
24. Cossu M, Cardinale F, Casaceli G, Castana L, Consales A, D'Orio P, et al. Stereo-EEG–guided radiofrequency thermocoagulations. Epilepsia. 2017;58(Suppl. 1):66–72.
25. Bourdillon P, Cucherat M, Isnard J, Ostrowsky-Coste K, Catenoix H, Guénot M, et al. Stereo-electroencephalography-guided radiofrequency thermocoagulation in patients with focal epilepsy: a systematic review and meta-analysis. Epilepsia. 2018;59:2296–304.
26. Cardinale F, Cossu M, Castana L, Casaceli G, Schiariti MP, Miserocchi A, et al. Stereoelectroencephalography: surgical methodology, safety, and stereotactic application accuracy in 500 procedures. Neurosurgery. 2013;72:353–66.
27. Cardinale F, Rizzi M, D'Orio P, Casaceli G, Arnulfo G, Narizzano M, et al. A new tool for touch-free patient registration for robot-assisted intracranial surgery: application accuracy from a phantom study and a retrospective surgical series. Neurosurg Focus. 2017;42(5):E8.
28. Mullin JP, Shriver M, Alomar S, Najm I, Bulacio J, Chauvel P, et al. Is SEEG safe? A systematic review and meta-analysis of stereo-electroencephalography-related complications. Epilepsia. 2016;57:386–401.
29. Vakharia VN, Sparks R, O'Keeffe AG, Rodionov R, Miserocchi A, McEvoy A, et al. Accuracy of intracranial electrode placement for stereoencephalography: a systematic review and meta-analysis. Epilepsia. 2017;58:921–32.
30. Bourdillon P, Châtillon CE, Moles A, Rheims S, Catenoix H, Montavont A, Ostrowsky-Coste K, Boulogne S, Isnard J, Guénot M. Effective accuracy of stereoelectroencephalography: robotic 3D versus Talairach orthogonal approaches. J Neurosurg. 2018;131:1–9.
31. Mullatti N, Landre E, Mellerio C, Oliveira AJ, Laurent A, Turak B, et al. Stereotactic thermocoagulation for insular epilepsy: lessons from successes and failures. Epilepsia. 2019;60:1565–79.

Chapter 8
Robotics in Laser Ablation Procedures

Yusuke S. Hori, Jorge Alvaro González Martínez, and Gene H. Barnett

Introduction

Laser interstitial thermal therapy (LITT) is a relatively new stereotactic and minimally invasive procedure for treating various intracranial conditions [1, 2]. The concept of this treatment is laser thermal ablation that resulting in hyperthermia and tissue necrosis. An initial application of this technique for brain tumor was reported in 1983 using an experimental tumor model [3].

Early on, this technique had several limitations including the lack of real-time monitoring to predict the extent of ablation. The development of magnetic resonance thermography (MRT) has enabled intraoperative real-time guidance of the thermal delivery and monitoring of the temperature changes in the tissue [4], thus leading to practical use of LITT in the clinical setting.

An early report of LITT for brain tumor patients was reported by Sugiyama et al. in 1990 [5]. Since then, an increasing number of the studies have demonstrated the

Y. S. Hori
Rose Ella Burkhardt Brain Tumor and Neuro-Oncology Center, Department of Neurological Surgery, Neurological Institute, Cleveland Clinic, Cleveland, OH, USA
e-mail: horiy@ccf.org

J. A. González Martínez
Department of Neurological Surgery and Epilepsy Center, University of Pittsburgh Medical Center, Pittsburgh, PA, USA
e-mail: gonzalezjo@upmc.edu

G. H. Barnett (✉)
Rose Ella Burkhardt Brain Tumor and Neuro-Oncology Center, Department of Neurological Surgery, Neurological Institute, Cleveland Clinic, Cleveland, OH, USA

Cleveland Clinic Lerner College of Medicine of Case Western Reserve University, Cleveland, OH, USA
e-mail: BARNETG@ccf.org

J. A. González Martínez, F. Cardinale (eds.), *Robotics in Neurosurgery*, https://doi.org/10.1007/978-3-031-08380-8_8

efficacy and safety of LITT in several intracranial conditions. To date, glioblastoma and brain metastasis are the most reported brain tumors [1]. Previous reports including multicenter studies have shown the positive effect of LITT on progression-free survival of glioblastoma patients [6, 7]. Several studies have also reported the results of local control of brain metastases in patients treated with LITT, especially for those with recurrent tumor [8, 9]. de Franca SA et al. conducted a meta-analysis to compare the post-treatment outcome of LITT with stereotactic radiosurgery (SRS) and showed that LITT significantly reduced the absolute risk of post-treatment adverse effects when compared with SRS. Nonetheless, there is still a lack of prospective and larger studies comparing these therapies [10]. The efficacy of LITT for radiation necrosis has also been reported [11–13]. Recent studies have shown comparable results between LITT and craniotomy, and the possible superiority of LITT compared with bevacizumab when treating radiation necrosis [14, 15].

Regarding patient selection, the efficacy of LITT has been reported for both newly diagnosed and recurrent brain tumor patients [16–19]. Importantly, even in the elderly population, LITT has shown its feasibility with shorter hospital length of stay and low mortality rates postoperatively [20]. A common location of the tumor is deep-seated lesions not-easily accessible by traditional surgical treatments [21]. With respect to the lesion size, tumors less than 3 cm are those most effectively treated. Kamath et al. have indicated that tumor greater than 3 cm in diameter conveys a higher rate of complications [22].

As a future application of LITT with other treatment modalities, Vega et al. have recently reported the potential hybrid therapy of LITT and SRS in spinal metastatic tumor [23]. Several reports have also proposed a combination therapy with LITT and surgical resection of brain tumor to overcome the limitations in size and post-procedural edema [24, 25]. An appropriate combination of LITT and other therapies and the possible indications have to be further explored in the upcoming decade.

Neuro-Oncological Applications

Technically, the initial step of the procedure is often to conduct stereotactic biopsy to confirm a diagnosis, followed by insertion of the laser probe (Figs. 8.1 and 8.2). This may be accomplished by using a stereotactic frame or neuro-navigation system. For the NeuroBlate System (Monteris Medical, Plymouth, MN), typically an anchoring bolt is then secured in a twist drill hole, a robotic probe driver secured to it, then the laser probe itself threaded through the driver and into the brain. The tumor margin and the location of the laser probe are confirmed using intraoperative magnetic resonance imaging (MRI) (Figs. 8.3 and 8.4). The probe driver allows the rotation and depth of the probe to be robotically controlled from the MRI control room. Rotation is important when a "side firing" laser probe is used. A superficial region of the tumor is ablated first to minimize the intraoperative seeding of tumor cells from probe retraction, and then deeper areas are treated. Temperature changes in the lesion are monitored during the procedure using MRT (Figs. 8.5 and 8.6) and

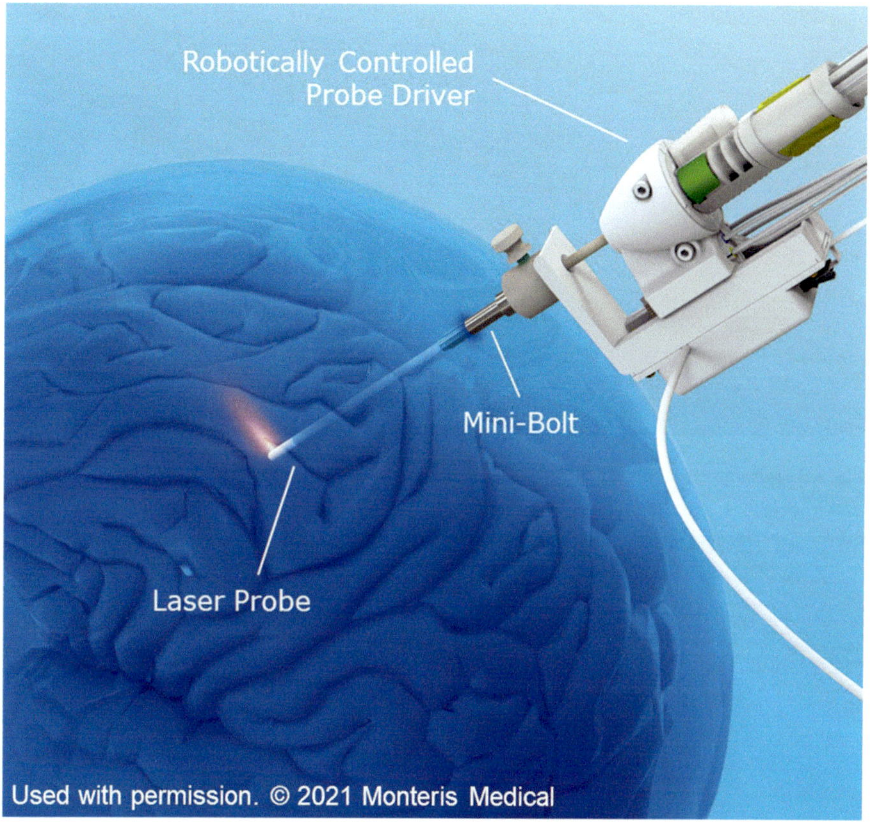

Fig. 8.1 Illustration of laser probe in LITT procedure. Used with permission. © 2021 Monteris Medical

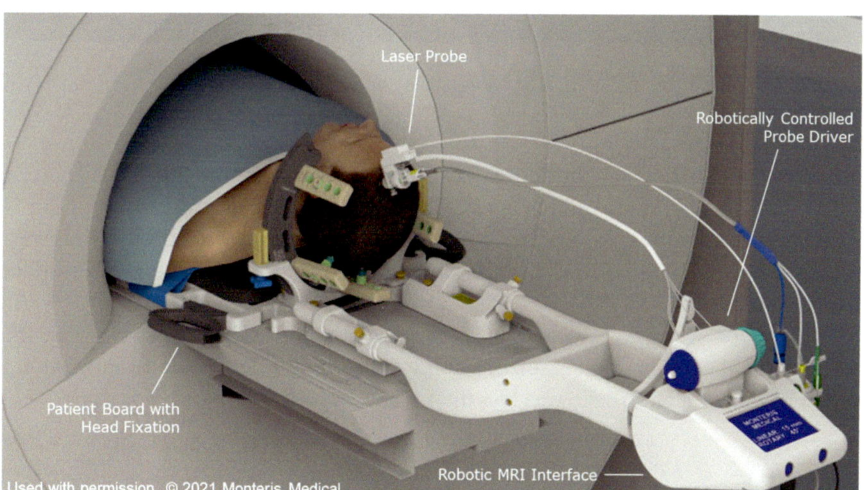

Fig. 8.2 Illustration of entire system used during LITT procedure. Used with permission. © 2021 Monteris Medical

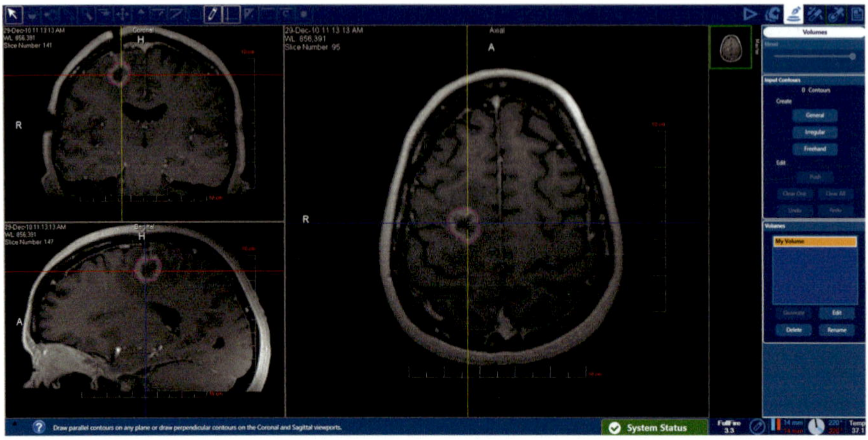

Fig. 8.3 Intraoperative use of MRI to define tumor contour (pink line)

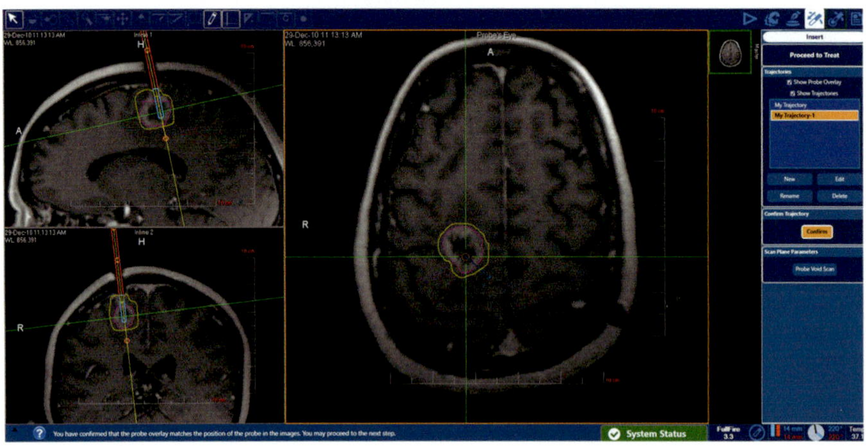

Fig. 8.4 The location of the laser probe confirmed by intraoperative MRI (near vertical pair of red and blue lines)

predicted thermal damage threshold lines are generated every several seconds. After confirming that an entire tumor was included in the ablation area, the probe is removed, along with its associated hardware, and a simple wound closure is performed. A postoperative MRI scan is obtained the next day, and typical hospital length of stay is 1–3 days.

A previous systemic review of postoperative complications has shown that the most frequent complication is seizure, followed by motor deficits and wound infection. The rate of hemorrhage was less than 1% [17]. In summary, LIIT is a relatively

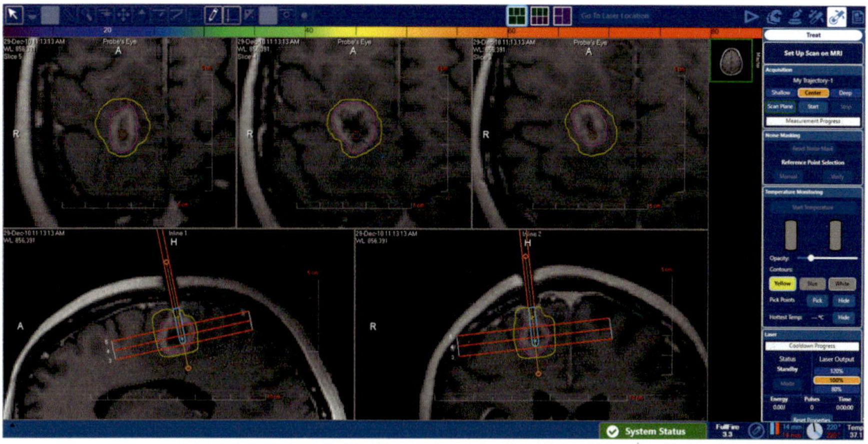

Fig. 8.5 Intraoperative real-time monitoring of tissue temperature changes yellow line indicating heating area (thermal equivalent of 43 °C for 2 min) outside of which tissue is expected to recover

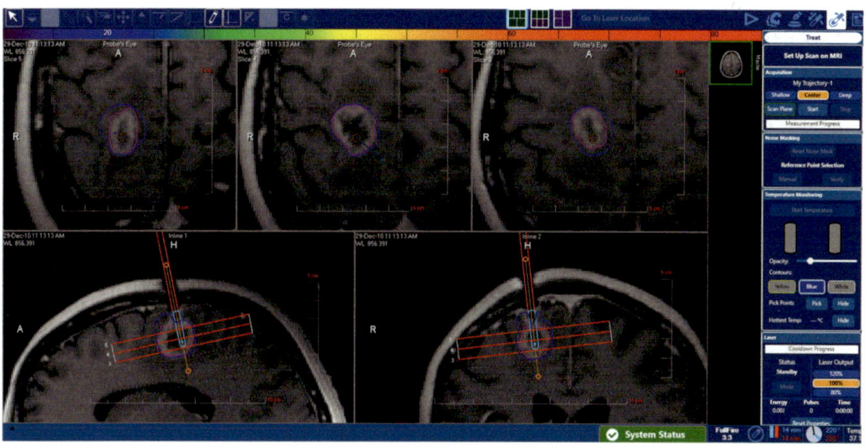

Fig. 8.6 Intraoperative real-time monitoring of tissue temperature changes region within blue line resulting in a necrotic area (thermal equivalent of 43 °C for 10 min or greater)

new, minimally invasive surgical modality with applications for some intracranial and spinal tumors. Patient selection is important, and the technique is particularly suited to small, deep-seated tumors. Common candidate lesions include newly diagnosed or recurrent high-grade gliomas and post-SRS failures of recurrent tumor or radiation necrosis. The procedures are typically tolerated well with low complication rates, short hospital stay and results comparable to or exceeding those of conventional surgery.

Epilepsy Applications

Robotic assistant devices for the placement of laser catheters are also applied in epilepsy procedures. Like the oncological applications, the robotic devices are used here to promote a precise and safe implantation of laser probes into predefined targets and/or trajectories.

The application of robotic devices is utilized in temporal and extra-temporal epilepsies, in lesional or non-lesional scenarios. In mesial temporal lobe epilepsies, robots can be applied to guide the placement of laser probes in the mesial temporal lobe structures such as the hippocampus, parahippocampus, and amygdala. Similar to other frame or frameless methods of implantation, stereotactic robots promote a precise positioning of laser catheters with great practicality and precision, despite been a frameless system. Arguably, this is the main advantage of applying robots in laser applications for epilepsy. In non-lesional epilepsy cases, where oftentimes the SEEG method is applied for better definition and localization of the epileptogenic zone (EZ), the robotic application is used in both procedures: first when planning and inserting the stereoelectroencephalography (SEEG) depth electrodes, and second when selecting the SEEG trajectory that best fit the location of the EZ and, subsequently, the final placement of the laser probe.

The application of robotic implanted laser catheters for medically refractory epilepsy is vast and diverse. The treatment of epileptogenic lesions such as tubers (in tuberous sclerosis) and mesial temporal sclerosis (via selective laser amygdalohippocampectomy), MRI identified focal cortical dysplasias, hamartomas, and post-stroke epilepsy have all been described in the literature. The advantages associated with laser ablative procedures are attributed to the small surgical access, the precision in the anatomical location of the generated lesions and their dimensions, and the relative short ablation time associated with each treatment. All these features can potentially translate into a safer, cost-effective, and more efficient treatment option for patients with medically intractable focal epilepsy caused by a specific MRI-visible etiology or in non-lesional mesial temporal lobe epilepsy. The application of the SEEG technique in combination of the laser method with the purpose of disrupting specific epileptic networks in patients with non-lesional and extra-temporal medically refractory epilepsy is a novel method that still lacks validation in efficacy and safety. Perhaps the main disadvantage of laser ablative procedures for epilepsy is the lack of electrophysiological feedback during the surgical intervention.

Robotic Ablative procedures: Similar to the oncological described procedures (Figs. 8.7, 8.8, 8.9), stereotactic ablative procedures require the accurate placement of an ablative device (laser or radiofrequency) to a target defined in stereotactic space, often one determined by prior SEEG investigation. As such, robots have two immediate roles—first, the accurate stereotactic placement of the ablative device, and second, the control and insertion of the ablative device. Gonzalez-Martinez and colleagues have successfully demonstrated, for the first time, ablation of an epileptogenic periventricular nodular heterotopia in 19-year-old female with medically

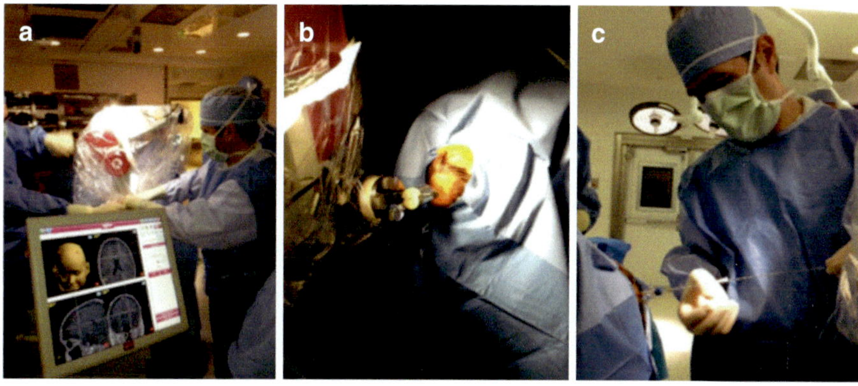

Fig. 8.7 Intraoperative photographs showing (**a** and **b**) robot guiding trajectory; (**c**) laser applicator through guiding bolt

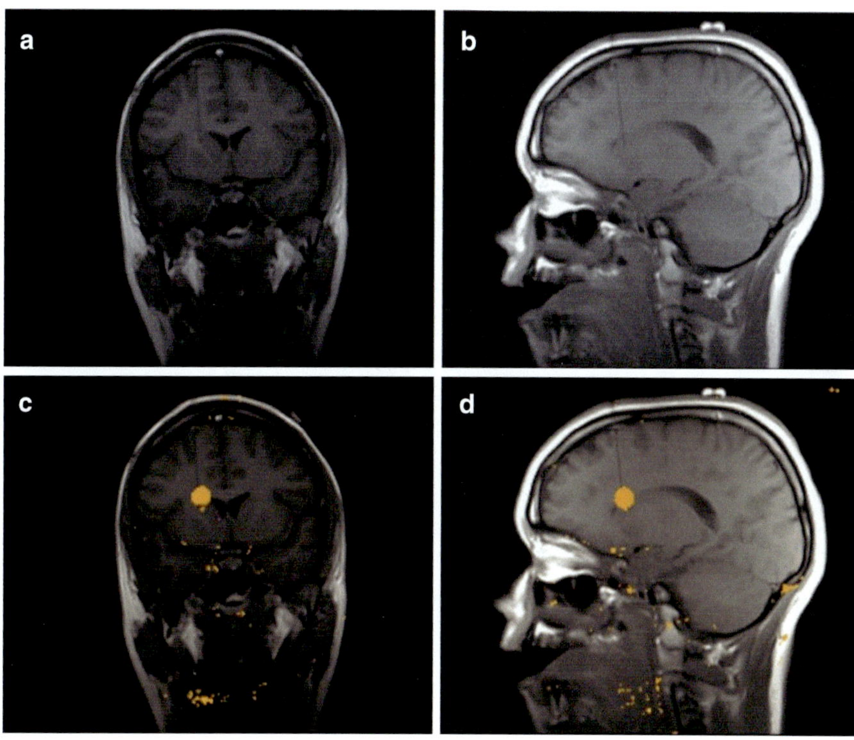

Fig. 8.8 (**a** and **b**) Intraoperative T1 non-contrast coronal and sagittal views; (**c** and **d**) defining the lesion contour; (**e** and **f**) intraoperative real-time monitoring of tissue temperature changes

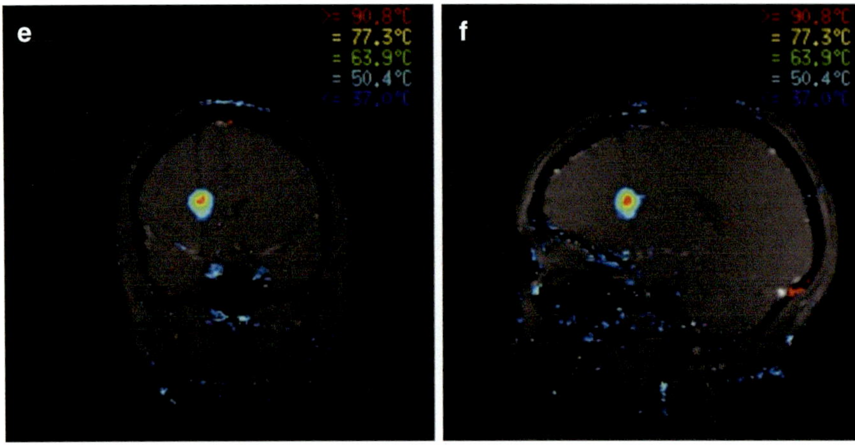

Fig. 8.8 (continued)

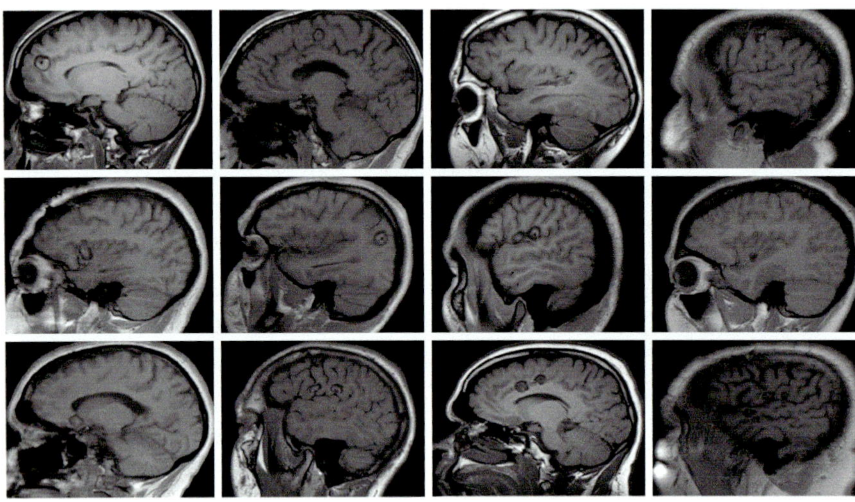

Fig. 8.9 T1 sagittal MRIs depicting the postoperative aspect of robotic SEEG guided laser ablation procedures in medically refractory epileptic patients

resistant epilepsy [26]. After appropriate preoperative imaging, the authors utilized the ROSA® system to accurately guide the placement of the laser catheter (Visualase, Medtronic, Dublin, Ireland) in conjunction with intraoperative MRI. There were no complications following ablation. In a similar method, Tandon and colleagues utilized the ROSA® system to guide the placement of a radiofrequency ablation catheter in 5 patients (ages 6 months to 13 years) with hypothalamic hamartomas and consequent gelastic seizures [27]. Four of five patients had grade I seizure outcome, and there were no permanent complications.

Summary: Laser Interstitial Thermal Therapy is emerging as an important surgical tool for the management of some cranial and spinal tumors, as well as some cases of lesional as well as non-lesional epilepsy. Robotics can be used to direct the laser probe to the target, and to manipulate the depth and rotation of the laser probe intracranially.

References

1. Missios S, Bekelis K, Barnett GH. Renaissance of laser interstitial thermal ablation. Neurosurg Focus. 2015;38(3):E13.
2. Diaz R, Ivan ME, Hanft S, Vanni S, Manzano G, Jagid J, Komotar RJ. Laser interstitial thermal therapy: lighting the way to a new treatment option in neurosurgery. Neurosurgery. 2016;79(Suppl 1):S3–7.
3. Bown SG. Phototherapy in tumors. World J Surg. 1983;7(6):700–9.
4. De Poorter J. Noninvasive MRI thermometry with the proton resonance frequency method: study of susceptibility effects. Magn Reson Med. 1995;34(3):359–67.
5. Sugiyama K, Sakai T, Fujishima I, Ryu H, Uemura K, Yokoyama T. Stereotactic ijnterstitial laser-hyperthermia using Nd-YAG laser. Stereotact Funct Neurosurg. 1990;54–55:501–5.
6. Mohammadi AM, Hawasli AH, Rodriguez A, Schroeder JL, Laxton AW, Elson P, Tatter SB, Barnett GH, Leuthardt EC. The role of laser interstitial thermal therapy in enhancing progression-free survival of difficult-to-access high-grade gliomas: a multicenter study. Cancer Med. 2014;3(4):971–9.
7. Kamath AA, Friedman DD, Akbari SHA, Kim AH, Tao Y, Luo J, Leuthardt EC. Glioblastoma treated with magnetic resonance imaging-guided laser interstitial thermal therapy: safety, efficacy, and outcomes. Neurosurgery. 2019;84(4):836–43.
8. Beechar VB, Prabhu SS, Bastos D, Weinberg JS, Stafford RJ, Fuentes D, Hess KR, Rao G. Volumetric response of progressing post-SRS lesions treated with laser interstitial thermal therapy. J Neuro-Oncol. 2018;137(1):57–65.
9. Bastos DCA, Rao G, Oliva ICG, Loree JM, Fuentes DT, Stafford RJ, Beechar VB, Weinberg JS, Shah K, Kumar VA, Prabhu SS. Predictors of local control of brain metastasis treated with laser interstitial thermal therapy. Neurosurgery. 2020;87(1):112–22.
10. de Franca SA, Tavares WM, Salinet ASM, Teixeira MJ, Paiva WS. Laser interstitial thermal therapy as an adjunct therapy in brain tumors: a meta-analysis and comparison with stereotactic radiotherapy. Surg Neurol Int. 2020;11:360.
11. Rammo R, Asmaro K, Schultz L, Scarpace L, Siddiqui S, Walbert T, Kalkanis S, Lee I. The safety of magnetic resonance imaging-guided laser interstitial thermal therapy for cerebral radiation necrosis. J Neuro-Oncol. 2018;138(3):609–17.
12. Ahluwalia M, Barnett GH, Deng D, Tatter SB, Laxton AW, Mohammadi AM, Leuthardt E, Chamoun R, Judy K, Asher A, Essig M, Dietrich J, Chiang VL. Laser ablation after stereotactic radiosurgery: a multicenter prospective study in patients with metastatic brain tumors and radiation necrosis. J Neurosurg. 2018;130(3):804–11.
13. Luther E, McCarthy D, Shah A, Semonche A, Borowy V, Burks J, Eichberg DG, Komotar R, Ivan M. Radical laser interstitial thermal therapy ablation volumes increase progression-free survival in biopsy-proven radiation necrosis. World Neurosurg. 2020;136:e646–59.
14. Hong CS, Deng D, Vera A, Chiang VL. Laser-interstitial thermal therapy compared to craniotomy for treatment of radiation necrosis or recurrent tumor in brain metastases failing radiosurgery. J Neuro-Oncol. 2019;142(2):309–17.
15. Sujijantarat N, Hong CS, Owusu KA, Elsamadicy AA, Antonios JP, Koo AB, Baehring JM, Chiang VL. Laser interstitial thermal therapy (LITT) vs. bevacizumab for radiation necrosis in previously irradiated brain metastases. J Neuro-Oncol. 2020;148(3):641–9.

16. Viozzi I, Guberinic A, Overduin CG, Rovers MM, Ter Laan M. Laser interstitial thermal therapy in patients with newly diagnosed glioblastoma: a systematic review. J Clin Med. 2021;10(2):355.
17. Montemurro N, Anania Y, Cagnazzo F, Perrini P. Survival outcomes in patients with recurrent glioblastoma treated with laser interstitial thermal therapy (LITT): a systematic review. Clin Neurol Neurosurg. 2020;195:105942.
18. Thomas JG, Rao G, Kew Y, Prabhu SS. Laser interstitial thermal therapy for newly diagnosed and recurrent glioblastoma. Neurosurg Focus. 2016;41(4):E12.
19. Sloan AE, Ahluwalia MS, Valerio-Pascua J, Manjila S, Torchia MG, Jones SE, Sunshine JL, Phillips M, Griswold MA, Clampitt M, Brewer C, Jochum J, McGraw MV, Diorio D, Ditz G, Barnett GH. Results of the NeuroBlate system first-in-humans phase I clinical trial for recurrent glioblastoma: clinical article. J Neurosurg. 2013;118(6):1202–19.
20. Ginalis EE, Danish SF. Magnetic resonance-guided laser interstitial thermal therapy for brain tumors in geriatric patients. Neurosurg Focus. 2020;49(4):E12.
21. Shah AH, Burks JD, Buttrick SS, Debs L, Ivan ME, Komotar RJ. Laser interstitial thermal therapy as a primary treatment for deep inaccessible gliomas. Neurosurgery. 2019;84(3):768–77.
22. Kamath AA, Friedman DD, Hacker CD, Smyth MD, Limbrick DD Jr, Kim AH, Hawasli AH, Leuthardt EC. MRI-guided interstitial laser ablation for intracranial lesions: a large single-institution experience of 133 cases. Stereotact Funct Neurosurg. 2017;95(6):417–28.
23. Vega RA, Ghia AJ, Tatsui CE. Percutaneous hybrid therapy for spinal metastatic disease: laser interstitial thermal therapy and spinal stereotactic radiosurgery. Neurosurg Clin N Am. 2020;31(2):211–9.
24. Wright J, Chugh J, Wright CH, Alonso F, Hdeib A, Gittleman H, Barnholtz-Sloan J, Sloan AE. Laser interstitial thermal therapy followed by minimal-access transsulcal resection for the treatment of large and difficult to access brain tumors. Neurosurg Focus. 2016;41(4):E14.
25. Pisipati S, Smith KA, Shah K, Ebersole K, Chamoun RB, Camarata PJ. Intracerebral laser interstitial thermal therapy followed by tumor resection to minimize cerebral edema. Neurosurg Focus. 2016;41(4):E13.
26. Gonzalez-Martinez J, Vadera S, Mullin J, Enatsu R, Alexopoulos AV, Patwardhan R, Bingaman W, Najm I. Robot-assisted stereotactic laser ablation in medically intractable epilepsy: operative technique. Neurosurgery. 2014;10(Suppl 2):167–72.
27. Tandon V, Chandra PS, Doddamani RS, Subianto H, Bajaj J, Garg A, Tripathi M. Stereotactic radiofrequency Thermocoagulation of hypothalamic hamartoma using robotic guidance (ROSA) Coregistered with O-arm guidance-preliminary technical note. World Neurosurg. 2018;112:267–74.

Chapter 9
Nuances of Robotics Applied in Children

Aswin Chari, Hani J. Marcus, and Martin M. Tisdall

Introduction

Within the range of operations carried out by paediatric neurosurgeons, a subset is ideally suited to robotic assistance. Many of the conditions treated are congenital or developmental abnormalities that distort the 'normal' anatomy, increasing reliance on careful evaluation and planning based on pre-operative imaging.

The smaller scale of the paediatric brain and spine demands increased precision. In infants, minimally invasive approaches have the added advantage of reducing blood loss and the need for transfusion.

The evidence base for robot-assisted paediatric neurosurgery is relatively sparse, and the majority of robot-assisted neurosurgical procedures are developed in adults before being extended to children. The numbers of cases in paediatric neurosurgery are smaller which makes developing an independent evidence base difficult. Therefore, the general approach for the majority is to use the procedures as developed and evidenced in adults but modified to the specific needs of children.

The first use of robotics in paediatric neurosurgery was approximately 20 years ago, with reports of robot-assisted endoscopy in 16- and 18-year-old patients [1, 2].

A. Chari (✉) · M. M. Tisdall
Department of Neurosurgery, Great Ormond Street Hospital, London, UK

Developmental Neurosciences, Great Ormond Street Institute of Child Health, University College London, London, UK
e-mail: aswin.chari.18@ucl.ac.uk; martin.tisdall@gosh.nhs.uk

H. J. Marcus
Victor Horsley Department of Neurosurgery, National Hospital for Neurology and Neurosurgery, London, UK

Wellcome EPSRC Centre for Interventional and Surgical Sciences, University College London, London, UK
e-mail: h.marcus@ucl.ac.uk

J. A. González Martínez, F. Cardinale (eds.), *Robotics in Neurosurgery*,
https://doi.org/10.1007/978-3-031-08380-8_9

Since then, robotic assistance has been used for a wide variety of procedures in paediatric neurosurgery and, for some operations such as stereoelectroencephalography (SEEG) and the biopsy or ablation of deep lesions, has become the standard of care. In this chapter, we discuss general and procedure-specific considerations for adapting robot-assisted procedures to paediatric neurosurgery. Where available, we also present the evidence for the safety and efficacy of their use.

General Considerations

Head Immobilisation

Head immobilisation is one of the key considerations in paediatric cranial neurosurgery. Traditional pin-based head immobilisation devices that are routinely used in adults should be used with caution in children (especially those under 3 years) due to thin cranial vault bone which may even have areas deficient of bone. Electromagnetic neuronavigation systems have provided an alternative to rigid immobilisation for a number of procedures including image-guided ventricular catheter placement and biopsy. However, the vast majority of robotic systems still require rigid head immobilisation.

Therefore, in their current form, cranial robot-assisted procedures may only be possible in children who are suitable for skull pin immobilisation, with a minimum age of approximately 1 year of age [3]. Rigid immobilisation devices such as the MAYFIELD® and DORO® systems have been modified for paediatric use by increasing the support under the head, increasing the number of pins and using specifically designed paediatric pins. These modified systems are compatible with frameless robotic workflows but must be used with caution [4]; although the DORO® system does not specify a minimum age of use, the MAYFIELD® system clearly states minimum age of 5 years. The placement of the pins must be carefully considered to avoid areas of thin or deficient skull and may require assessment on a preoperative CT scan. In addition, pins can be modified (for example, with the modified rubber stopper technique) to reduce the risk of skull fracture and skin complications; such innovations require careful evaluation prior to widespread adoption as they fall outside of the devices' stated indications for use [5, 6].

Frame-based systems such as the Leksell® system also do not have a minimum age on the indications for use but the forces on the pins must be adjusted carefully to balance between ensuring reliable fixation and the risks of skull fracture or plunging. In our practice, we have developed a number of nuances to frame application in children (specifically for SEEG) outlined in Fig. 9.1. These include ensuring that the frame is placed orthogonal to the head and skull base with the base just below nose and external auditory meatus; if it is too high, it impedes the insertion of low temporal electrodes and, if it is too low, it precludes safe fixation of the frame to the robot due to impingement on the shoulders.

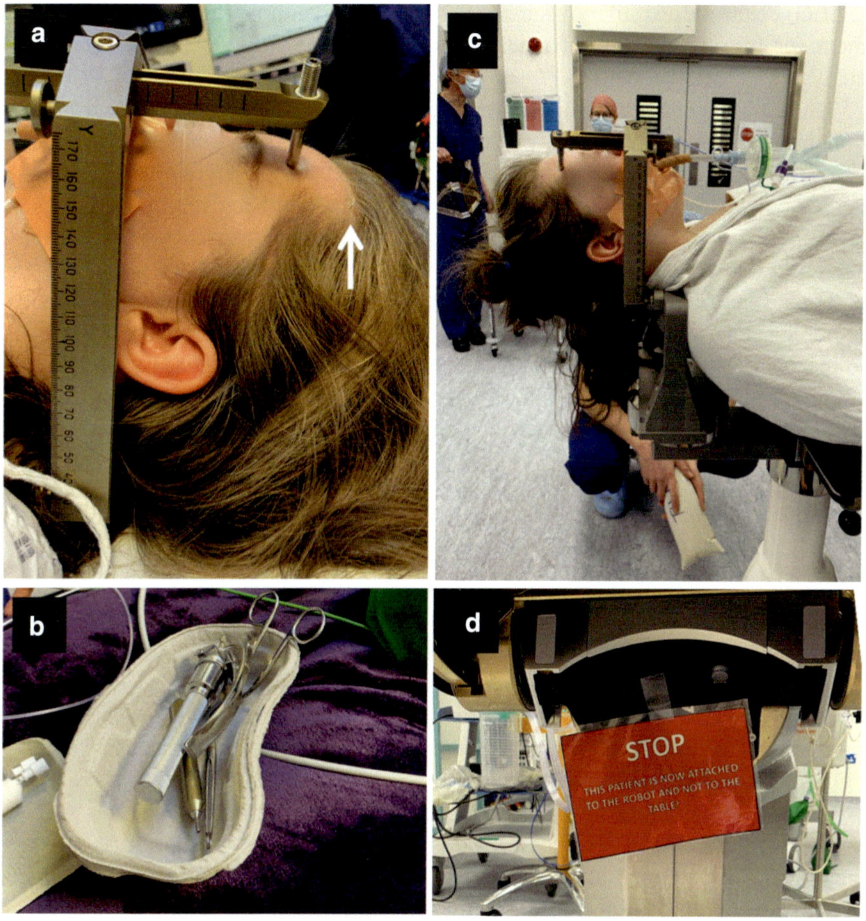

Fig. 9.1 Application of a frame for SEEG. (**a**) Final frame position including the staple (arrow) that acts to validate registration accuracy. (**b**) Ensuring safe transfer to the CT scanner with the screwdriver that facilitates rapid access to the mouth in the event of an airway emergency. (**c**) Optimal positioning allows access to the temporal base for low temporal electrodes whilst ensuring the shoulders remain away from the frame attachment. (**d**) Ensuring safety at the operating table by disconnecting the operating table remote. This sign warns people in the operating room not to move the operating table. The remote is disconnected and stored in a predefined location for ease of access in the event of an emergency

Image Registration

A key consideration of whether to choose a frame-based or frameless workflow is registration accuracy. Frameless workflows can use fiducial (bone-anchored or skin) or surface-based registrations, both of which have been shown to be both safe and accurate. In the paediatric literature, median entry point and target point localisation errors of approximately 1 and 1.5 mm have been shown with frameless registration and 0.7 and 1.1 mm with frame-based registration for stereoelectroencephalography

(SEEG) electrodes; similar differences of 0.5 mm target point localisation improvement for frame-based over frameless systems have also been shown in a meta-analysis and meta-regression [7–9].

The differences are small, and frame-based registration is associated with additional steps of requiring frame application and image acquisition with the frame in situ. However, this must be considered in the context of the alternatives. Even with contemporary equipment, skin fiducials or surface-based registrations show poor levels of accuracy (errors in the region of 2.5 and 5.3 mm, respectively) [10]. Bone-anchored fiducials, whilst possible under local anaesthesia in adults, require a general anaesthetic in children; in this case, as a frame is more accurate, we currently prefer a frame-based workflow. A regular part of our workflow to ensure accuracy is to place a skin staple near the forehead prior to acquisition of the CT scan with the frame. This provides a validation of registration accuracy as we plan a trajectory to the outer tip of the staple prior to beginning the procedure (Fig. 9.1c).

Safety in Moving the Patient

For frame-based and some frameless procedures (for example, MRI-guided laser interstitial thermal therapy (LiTT)), there is a requirement to move between the anaesthetic room, operating table, and the scanner (which may be located within the operating theatre or independently in the radiology department). Although not unique to paediatrics, this is more often performed under general anaesthesia in children and safety during these transfers must be carefully considered. From this perspective, simulation is an important part of introducing new procedures such as robotic surgery [11]. At our centre, we ensure that a member of the surgical team stays with the patient at all times, with a screw driver in case an anaesthetic emergency requires urgent removal of the frame (Fig. 9.1d).

In the operating theatre, once the frame is secured to the robot, the head is fixed to the robot and not associated with the table. This poses a risk that moving the table could lead to the body moving with the head being fixed in position to the robot. Therefore, as a safety measure, once adequately positioned, the operating table remote is disconnected and stored in a predetermined location to ensure that the table doesn't get moved inadvertently (Fig. 9.1d).

Procedure-Specific Considerations

Stereoelectroencephalography (SEEG)

The need for high levels of accuracy across multiple trajectories makes SEEG ideal for robot-assisted procedures. There is increasing evidence for its safety and efficacy in children [12–15]. In terms of adaptations in children, there are a number of key issues to consider.

The first is whether SEEG is even technically possible as a method of intracranial evaluation. Children with epilepsy often have learning difficulties and challenging behaviour and this can lead to issues with compliance with SEEG; although rare, we have encountered instances of children pulling out one (or all) electrodes during the monitoring period; tolerability is therefore something we consider seriously. In addition, in young children, the skull may be too thin to allow securing of the anchor bolts and we therefore do not perform SEEG in those <3 years old. However, there are reports of successful implantation in children <3 years old using a frameless immobilisation workflow [4].

The second major consideration is the range of aetiologies undergoing SEEG in children. Extratemporal aetiologies are more common than in adults, including some with deeper locations such as insular epilepsies and periventricular nodular heterotopias. Therefore, it makes sense to consider whether the chosen electrodes can also deliver thermocoagulation, which can be performed safely in children and which we use as a prognostic test [16].

Once the decision to undertake SEEG has been made, the acquisition of adequate pre-operative imaging is crucial to safe trajectory planning. At our centre, we acquire 3D T1 MPRAGE, FLAIR and gadolinium-enhanced T1 MRI sequences as a minimum at 3 T and dual energy CT angiography (DECTA) most commonly under general anaesthesia; this requires additional planning and anaesthetic risks but ensures high quality images are obtained (Fig. 9.2). Although digital subtraction angiography (DSA) has been shown to be safe in children at select high volume centres [17] and is commonly used in adults prior to SEEG [18], we believe the vessel delineation from gadolinium-enhanced T1 MRI and DECTA are sufficient and mitigate against even the small risks of stroke and access vessel complications of DSA. Novel MRI sequences such as a gadolinium-enhanced T1 spoiled gradient recalled echo sequence have been shown to be even more sensitive to vasculature than traditional gadolinium-enhanced T1 MRI, and these can be acquired without radiation exposure.

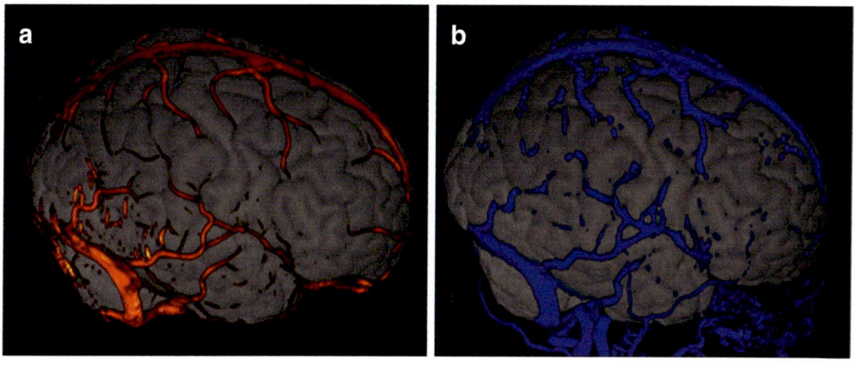

Fig. 9.2 Pre-operative planning for SEEG showing vessel delineation using (**a**) gadolinium-enhanced T1 and (**b**) DECTA

The operation itself, once adequately planned, becomes relatively straightforward. Our approach is to cycle through all the trajectories (prior to formal prepping and draping) with the laser pointer attached to the robotic arm. This ensures that all the trajectories can be reached, and the entry points can be marked. If there are occipital electrodes, prone positioning may be necessary. In such cases, one must be vigilant to select the correct orientation on the robotic software prior to starting.

Biopsies

Robot-assisted biopsies are indicated for deeper lesions involving the subcortical structures and brainstem. As the role of biopsy in diffuse midline H3K27M-mutant glioma (formerly diffuse intrinsic pontine glioma) is firmly established [19–21], this is the most common indication for robot-assisted biopsy in the paediatric population. There are a number of technical nuances to consider around both the choice of biopsy location and trajectory.

Biopsy location can be guided by thorough radiological evaluation of all available MRI sequences. This includes arterial spin labelling to identify areas of increased metabolic turnover (high cerebral blood flow and perfusion) in order to maximise the yield, which can approach 90–100% [21–23].

Biopsy trajectory for diffuse midline H3K27M-mutant glioma includes both trans-cerebellar and transcortical approaches. At our institution, we tend to favour a trans-cerebellar peduncle approach over the transcortical approach for the majority of cases [22]. In order to facilitate this, the frame application needs to be optimised (Fig. 9.3). In order to gain access to the posterior fossa, the head needs to be flexed and therefore, the frame is applied with an AP tilt so cervical spine flexion is produced once the frame is fixed in a vertical orientation. The posts of the Leksell® frame may impede access and therefore, we routinely remove the post on the side of the biopsy. This should be performed before the localisation CT scan is done as removal of the post can cause the frame to move slightly.

MRI-Guided Laser Interstitial Thermal Therapy (LiTT) for Epilepsy

MRI-guided LiTT has opened the possibilities of treating deep-seated drug resistant epilepsies, in particular hypothalamic hamartoma and insular lesions which are both more common in children (Fig. 9.4) [24]. As they are both deep-seated lesions and, in the case of the insula, with dense vasculature, LiTT catheter placement using robotic assistance is warranted to increase accuracy. Whilst most lesions may be addressed through a single trajectory that optimises the ablated volume, multiple trajectories must sometimes be used [25]. LiTT has become almost the standard of

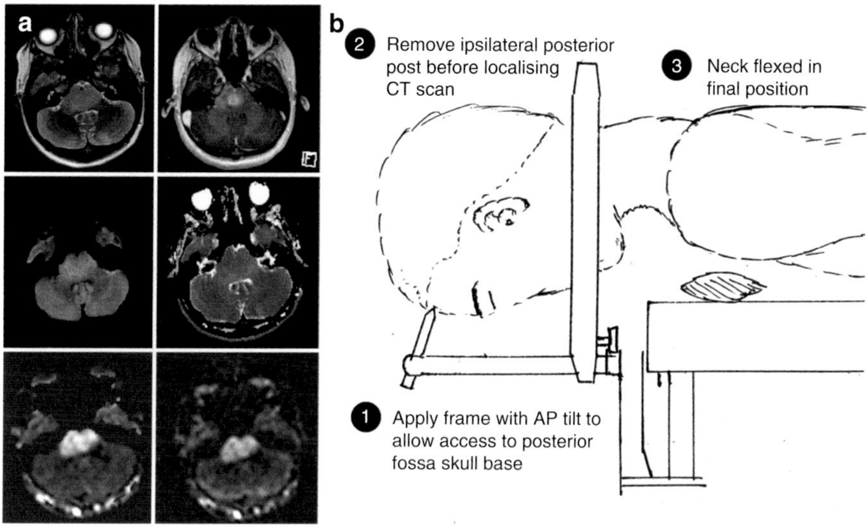

Fig. 9.3 Optimisation measures for frame-based trans-cerebellar biopsy of brainstem lesions. (**a**) Example of the contribution of arterial spin labelling sequences to the choice of biopsy site in a 13-year-old with presumed diffuse midline glioma in the pons. Top row shows T2 and gadolinium-enhanced T1, middle row shows diffusion weighted imaging and apparent diffusion coefficient maps, bottom row shows relative cerebral blood flow and perfusion imaging maps from arterial spin labelling. Given these findings, a location on the right side adjacent to the middle cerebral peduncle was chosen for biopsy which confirmed WHO Grade IV midline glioma, H3K27M mutant. (**b**) Optimisation of the operation including placement of the frame at a tilt to allow it to be flat once the head is flexed, removal of the post before localisation of the CT scan for a trans-cerebellar biopsy of a brainstem tumour

care for hypothalamic hamartoma although long-term seizure freedom and permanent or transient complications are not yet well reported [26]. Insular LiTT catheters have predominantly been placed following parasagittal trajectories that facilitate coverage of the putative seizure onset zone (usually aligned to one of the insular gyri) and safe access without having to traverse the vasculature of the operculo-insular fissure [27].

In terms of future directions, it remains to be definitively established, for the less accessible insular dysplasias, whether LiTT is non-inferior to open resective surgery [28] and whether there is any role for LiTT for lesions that are equally accessible via open resective surgery.

LiTT is also an option for other disconnective procedures such as corpus callosotomy and hemispherotomy in children [29, 30]. Although the current evidence is only in the form of case reports and small case series for these indications, the proof-of-principle that disconnections can be achieved exists from diffusion imaging validation studies that also use computer-assisted planning to optimally plan the trajectories [31].

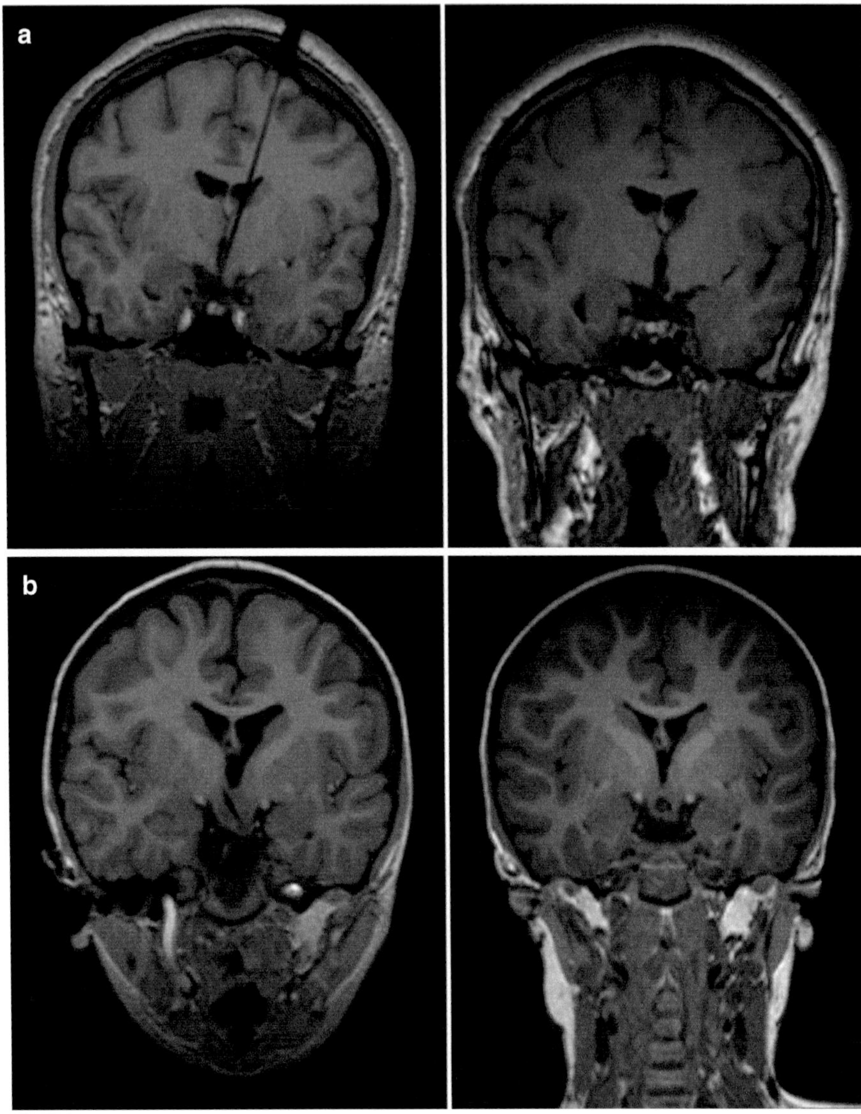

Fig. 9.4 Intra-operative (left) and post-operative (right) images of epileptogenic lesions treated by LiTT. (**a**, **b**) Hypothalamic hamartoma. (**c**) Posterior insular epilepsy

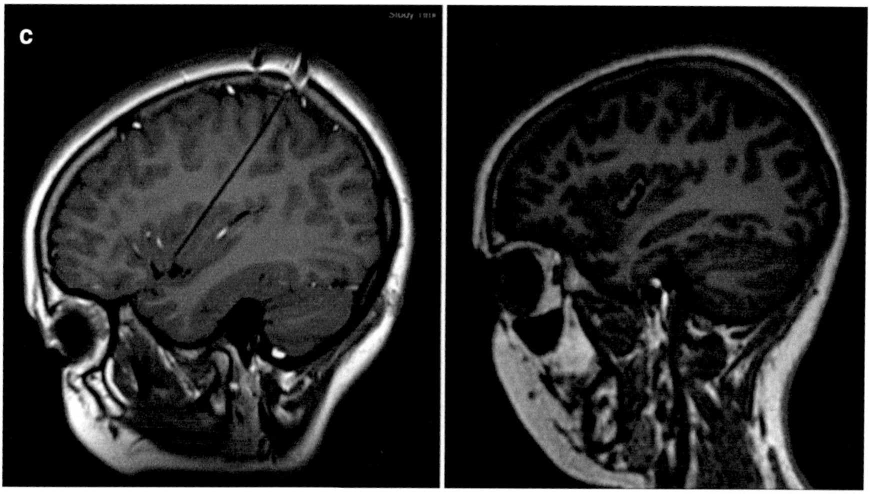

Fig. 9.4 (continued)

Deep Brain Stimulation or Lesioning

The remit of indications for deep brain stimulation or lesioning is more limited in the paediatric population but includes movement disorders (especially dystonia), epilepsy and psychiatric disorders. Robotic assistance has been successfully used for the accurate placement of electrodes in a handful of cases [8, 32]. Apart from accuracy considerations, there are few specific nuances to paediatric robot-assisted DBS electrode implantation. The main nuances to paediatric DBS surround the placement of the implantable pulse generators in alternative locations to reduce the incidence of infection and technical issues surrounding recharging, which is beyond the scope of the robot-assisted component of the procedure [33].

Endoscopic Procedures

Conceptually, endoscopic procedures (as opposed to stereotactic procedures) require some tissue manipulation. Alongside the precision provided by accurate trajectory planning, there is scope for improving performance through integrating haptic feedback and robot-assisted movement of the endoscopic instruments to provide increased degrees of freedom [34]. Whilst the instruments are not in widespread use, robotic systems integrating haptic feedback have been used for the more routine endoscopic procedures (third ventriculostomy, septostomy, cyst fenestration) as well as disconnection of hypothalamic hamartoma. [8, 35] Robotic assistance can be particularly useful in pathology where there is non-dilated or morphologically abnormal ventricular anatomy, although, it may be helpful to start with the more straightforward cases (third ventriculostomy with large ventricles) during the learning period.

Robotic guidance has also been for endoscope-assisted hemispherotomy using a para-endoscopic hybrid technique through a small interhemispheric transcallosal approach [36]. This technique uses a 10 mm endoscope that allows an extended field-of-view and has been shown to have equivalent outcomes to an open hemispherotomy technique with reduced blood loss and post-operative length of stay [36].

Convection-Enhanced Drug Delivery

Robot-assisted implantation of convection-enhanced drug delivery (CED) catheters has been purported to have immense potential for conditions such as Parkinson's disease, Alzheimer's disease and glioma although a recent randomised controlled trial in Parkinson's disease did not show efficacy [37, 38]. In the paediatric sphere, the main interest has been in CED for diffuse midline H3K27M-mutant glioma. Results of CED using therapeutic agents for diffuse midline H3K27M-mutant glioma have so far only been published from animal studies. Although there are ongoing clinical trials in humans, it is unknown whether robot-assisted techniques are being utilised for catheter implantation in these patients [39, 40].

Spinal Surgery

Paediatric spinal surgery, with the emphasis on scoliosis surgery, lends itself ideally to robot-assisted pedicle screw placement; the sagittal and rotational curvatures distort normal anatomy, and the smaller pedicles necessitate high levels of accuracy. Experience of these robotic systems that can be used with either intra-operative fluoroscopy registered to pre-operative CT scans or intra-operative CT scans shows high levels of accuracy (successful screw placement in 98.7%) [41, 42]. CT scan protocols have been optimised to reduce radiation exposure by up to 90% and found not to compromise registration accuracy [43]. In an initial experience of 40 cases, Gonzalez et al. report only 4 cases with technical system problems, all of which were resolved following troubleshooting [41].

Endovascular Neurosurgery

The first-in-human use of a neuroendovascular robot has just been reported, with authors purporting increased procedural and technical accuracy and reduced radiation exposure, all of which would be extremely beneficial in the paediatric population. With the growing indications for neuroendovascular intervention including intraarterial chemotherapy for retinoblastoma, there is potential for the robot-assisted approach to be particularly beneficial in children [44].

Foetal Neurosurgery

As the indications for foetal surgery expand beyond myelomeningocele to include other conditions such as hydrocephalus and encephaloceles [45, 46], there is scope for robotic integration into this expanding field of neurosurgery. This is particularly attractive for foetoscopic techniques and, indeed, early innovators created ovine models of robot-assisted foetoscopic techniques almost 20 years ago, although, as far as the authors are aware, these have yet to be translated [47].

Concluding Remarks

The potential benefits of robot-assisted neurosurgery in children are myriad, including increased safety and accuracy and reductions in blood loss and radiation exposure. As evidence slowly accumulates, we will undoubtedly see increased uptake and it remains to be seen whether the results in high volume specialised centres can be reproduced more widely. The nuances covered in this chapter may be important in ensuring high levels of safety and accuracy in paediatric robot-assisted procedures.

References

1. Zimmermann M, Krishnan R, Raabe A, Seifert V. Robot-assisted navigated neuroendoscopy. Neurosurgery. 2002;51(6):1446–51; discussion 1451-1452.
2. Vougioukas VI, Hubbe U, Hochmuth A, Gellrich NC, van Velthoven V. Perspectives and limitations of image-guided neurosurgery in pediatric patients. Childs Nerv Syst. 2003;19(12):783–91.
3. Berry C, Sandberg DI, Hoh DJ, Krieger MD, McComb JG. Use of cranial fixation pins in pediatric neurosurgery. Neurosurgery. 2008;62(4):913–8; discussion 918–919.
4. Alexander H, Fayed I, Oluigbo CO. Rigid cranial fixation for robot-assisted stereoelectroencephalography in toddlers: technical considerations. Oper Neurosurg (Hagerstown). 2020;18(6):614–20.

5. LoPresti MA, Nguyen J, Lam SK. Pinning in pediatric neurosurgery: the modified rubber stopper technique. J Neurosurg Pediatrics. 2020;1(aop):1–6.
6. Chari A, Tisdall MM, Marcus HJ. Letter to the editor. Systematic and safe approaches to innovation in pediatric pinning. J Neurosurg Pediatrics. 2020;26(5):601–2.
7. Sharma JD, Seunarine KK, Tahir MZ, Tisdall MM. Accuracy of robot-assisted versus optical frameless navigated stereoelectroencephalography electrode placement in children. J Neurosurg Pediatr. 2019;23(3):297–302.
8. Benedictis AD, Trezza A, Carai A, Genovese E, Procaccini E, Messina R, et al. Robot-assisted procedures in pediatric neurosurgery. Neurosurg Focus. 2017;42(5):E7.
9. Philipp LR, Matias CM, Thalheimer S, Mehta SH, Sharan A, Wu C. Robot-assisted Stereotaxy reduces target error: a meta-analysis and meta-regression of 6056 trajectories. Neurosurgery. 2021;88(2):222–33.
10. Mongen MA, Willems PWA. Current accuracy of surface matching compared to adhesive markers in patient-to-image registration. Acta Neurochir. 2019;161(5):865–70.
11. Candela-Cantó S, Alamar M, Aláez C, Muchart J, Forero C, de la Gala C, et al. Highly realistic simulation for robot-assisted hypothalamic hamartoma real-time MRI-guided laser interstitial thermal therapy (LITT). Childs Nerv Syst. 2020;36(6):1131–42.
12. Taussig D, Chipaux M, Lebas A, Fohlen M, Bulteau C, Ternier J, et al. Stereo-electroencephalography (SEEG) in 65 children: an effective and safe diagnostic method for pre-surgical diagnosis, independent of age. Epileptic Disord. 2014;16(3):280–95.
13. McGovern RA, Knight EP, Gupta A, Moosa ANV, Wyllie E, Bingaman WE, et al. Robot-assisted stereoelectroencephalography in children. J Neurosurg Pediatr. 2018;23(3):288–96.
14. Ho AL, Feng AY, Kim LH, Pendharkar AV, Sussman ES, Halpern CH, et al. Stereoelectroencephalography in children: a review. Neurosurg Focus. 2018;45(3):E7.
15. Sacino MF, Huang SS, Schreiber J, Gaillard WD, Oluigbo CO. Is the use of stereotactic electroencephalography safe and effective in children? A meta-analysis of the use of stereotactic electroencephalography in comparison to subdural grids for invasive epilepsy monitoring in pediatric subjects. Neurosurgery. 2019;84(6):1190–200.
16. Chipaux M, Taussig D, Dorfmuller G, Dorison N, Tisdall MM, Boyd SG, et al. SEEG-guided radiofrequency thermocoagulation of epileptic foci in the paediatric population: feasibility, safety and efficacy. Seizure. 2019;70:63–70.
17. Lin N, Smith ER, Scott RM, Orbach DB. Safety of neuroangiography and embolization in children: complication analysis of 697 consecutive procedures in 394 patients. J Neurosurg Pediatr. 2015;16(4):432–8.
18. Vakharia VN, Sparks R, Vos SB, McEvoy AW, Miserocchi A, Ourselin S, et al. The effect of vascular segmentation methods on stereotactic trajectory planning for drug-resistant focal epilepsy: a retrospective cohort study. World Neurosurg X. 2019;4:100057.
19. Fonseca A, Afzal S, Bowes L, Crooks B, Larouche V, Jabado N, et al. Pontine gliomas a 10-year population-based study: a report from the Canadian Paediatric Brain Tumour Consortium (CPBTC). J Neuro-Oncol. 2020;149(1):45–54.
20. Vitanza NA, Monje M. Diffuse intrinsic pontine glioma: from diagnosis to next-generation clinical trials. Curr Treat Options Neurol. 2019;21(8):37.
21. Hamisch C, Kickingereder P, Fischer M, Simon T, Ruge MI. Update on the diagnostic value and safety of stereotactic biopsy for pediatric brainstem tumors: a systematic review and meta-analysis of 735 cases. J Neurosurg Pediatr. 2017;20(3):261–8.
22. Dawes W, Marcus HJ, Tisdall M, Aquilina K. Robot-assisted stereotactic brainstem biopsy in children: prospective cohort study. J Robot Surg. 2019;13(4):575–9.
23. Gupta M, Chan TM, Santiago-Dieppa DR, Yekula A, Sanchez CE, Elster JD, et al. Robot-assisted stereotactic biopsy of pediatric brainstem and thalamic lesions. J Neurosurg Pediatr. 2020;27:317–24.
24. Hoppe C, Helmstaedter C. Laser interstitial thermotherapy (LiTT) in pediatric epilepsy surgery. Seizure. 2020;77:69–75.

25. Gireesh ED, Lee K, Skinner H, Seo J, Chen P-C, Westerveld M, et al. Intracranial EEG and laser interstitial thermal therapy in MRI-negative insular and/or cingulate epilepsy: case series. J Neurosurg. 2020;135:751–9.
26. Bourdillon P, Ferrand-Sorbet S, Apra C, Chipaux M, Raffo E, Rosenberg S, et al. Surgical treatment of hypothalamic hamartomas. Neurosurg Rev. 2021;44:753–62.
27. Alexander H, Cobourn K, Fayed I, Oluigbo CO. Magnetic resonance-guided laser interstitial thermal therapy for the treatment of nonlesional insular epilepsy in pediatric patients: technical considerations. Pediatr Neurosurg. 2020;55(3):155–62.
28. Hale AT, Sen S, Haider AS, Perkins FF, Clarke DF, Lee MR, et al. Open resection versus laser interstitial thermal therapy for the treatment of pediatric insular epilepsy. Neurosurgery. 2019;85(4):E730–6.
29. Chua MMJ, Bushlin I, Stredny CM, Madsen JR, Patel AA, Stone S. Magnetic resonance imaging-guided laser-induced thermal therapy for functional hemispherotomy in a child with refractory epilepsy and multiple medical comorbidities. J Neurosurg Pediatr. 2020;27:30–5.
30. Caruso JP, Janjua MB, Dolce A, Price AV. Retrospective analysis of open surgical versus laser interstitial thermal therapy callosotomy in pediatric patients with refractory epilepsy. J Neurosurg Pediatr. 2021;27:420–8.
31. Vakharia VN, Sparks RE, Vos SB, Bezchlibnyk Y, Mehta AD, Willie JT, et al. Computer-assisted planning for minimally invasive anterior two-thirds laser corpus callosotomy: a feasibility study with probabilistic tractography validation. Neuroimage Clin. 2020;25:102174.
32. Candela S, Vanegas MI, Darling A, Ortigoza-Escobar JD, Alamar M, Muchart J, et al. Frameless robot-assisted pallidal deep brain stimulation surgery in pediatric patients with movement disorders: precision and short-term clinical results. J Neurosurg Pediatr. 2018;22(4):416–25.
33. Kaminska M, Perides S, Lumsden DE, Nakou V, Selway R, Ashkan K, et al. Complications of deep brain stimulation (DBS) for dystonia in children—the challenges and 10 year experience in a large paediatric cohort. Eur J Paediatr Neurol. 2017;21(1):168–75.
34. Francis P, Eastwood KW, Bodani V, Looi T, Drake JM. Design, modelling and teleoperation of a 2 mm diameter compliant instrument for the da Vinci platform. Ann Biomed Eng. 2018;46(10):1437–49.
35. Calisto A, Dorfmüller G, Fohlen M, Bulteau C, Conti A, Delalande O. Endoscopic disconnection of hypothalamic hamartomas: safety and feasibility of robot-assisted, thulium laser-based procedures. J Neurosurg Pediatr. 2014;14(6):563–72.
36. Chandra PS, Subianto H, Bajaj J, Girishan S, Doddamani R, Ramanujam B, et al. Endoscope-assisted (with robotic guidance and using a hybrid technique) interhemispheric transcallosal hemispherotomy: a comparative study with open hemispherotomy to evaluate efficacy, complications, and outcome. J Neurosurg Pediatr. 2018;23(2):187–97.
37. Barua NU, Gill SS, Love S. Convection-enhanced drug delivery to the brain: therapeutic potential and neuropathological considerations. Brain Pathol. 2014;24(2):117–27.
38. Whone A, Luz M, Boca M, Woolley M, Mooney L, Dharia S, et al. Randomized trial of intermittent intraputamenal glial cell line-derived neurotrophic factor in Parkinson's disease. Brain. 2019;142(3):512–25.
39. Singleton WGB, Bienemann AS, Woolley M, Johnson D, Lewis O, Wyatt MJ, et al. The distribution, clearance, and brainstem toxicity of panobinostat administered by convection-enhanced delivery. J Neurosurg Pediatr. 2018;22(3):288–96.
40. PhD SM MD. An open label single arm phase I/II study of MTX110 delivered by convection-enhanced delivery (CED) in patients with diffuse intrinsic pontine glioma (DIPG) previously treated with external beam radiation therapy. clinicaltrials.gov; 2021 Jan. Report No.: NCT03566199. Available from: https://clinicaltrials.gov/ct2/show/NCT03566199
41. Gonzalez D, Ghessese S, Cook D, Hedequist D. Initial intraoperative experience with robotic-assisted pedicle screw placement with stealth navigation in pediatric spine deformity: an evaluation of the first 40 cases. J Robotic Surg. 2021;15:687–93.

42. Shaw KA, Murphy JS, Devito DP. Accuracy of robot-assisted pedicle screw insertion in adolescent idiopathic scoliosis: is triggered electromyographic pedicle screw stimulation necessary? J Spine Surg. 2018;4(2):187–94.
43. Sensakovic WF, O'Dell MC, Agha A, Woo R, Varich L. CT radiation dose reduction in robot-assisted pediatric spinal surgery. Spine (Phila Pa 1976). 2017;42(7):E417–24.
44. Al Saiegh F, Chalouhi N, Sweid A, Mazza J, Mouchtouris N, Khanna O, et al. Intra-arterial chemotherapy for retinoblastoma via the transradial route: technique, feasibility, and case series. Clin Neurol Neurosurg. 2020;194:105824.
45. Cavalheiro S, Silva da Costa MD, Nicácio JM, Dastoli PA, Capraro Suriano I, Barbosa MM, et al. Fetal surgery for occipital encephalocele. J Neurosurg Pediatr. 2020;26:605–12.
46. Cavalheiro S, da Costa MDS, Mendonça JN, Dastoli PA, Suriano IC, Barbosa MM, et al. Antenatal management of fetal neurosurgical diseases. Childs Nerv Syst. 2017;33(7):1125–41.
47. Aaronson OS, Tulipan NB, Cywes R, Sundell HW, Davis GH, Bruner JP, et al. Robot-assisted endoscopic intrauterine myelomeningocele repair: a feasibility study. Pediatr Neurosurg. 2002;36(2):85–9.

Chapter 10
Robot-Assisted Endoscopy

Alessandro De Benedictis, Carlotta Ginevra Nucci, Camilla Rossi-Espagnet, Andrea Carai, and Carlo Efisio Marras

Introduction

Over the last 30 years, the use of medical robots has rapidly expanded from the industrial sector to many surgical fields, such as soft-tissue, urological, orthopedic, general, and cardiac surgeries. Neurosurgeons were also involved in developing robotic technology, with the aim of improving feasibility and quality of treatment of different diseases, including tumors, epilepsy, disturbances of cerebrospinal fluid (CSF) circulation, movement disorders, and psychiatric diseases [1, 2].

In this context, growing experience showed that robotic assistances offer several advantages in comparison with traditional approaches, in terms of safety, versatility, repeatability, precision, visuo-manual coordination, and feedback. This is especially true when considering the pediatric neurosurgical field, which is often characterized by challenging aspects, including small size and deeply located targets, their relationships with critical neurovascular structures, frequent finding of malformation variants, and impossibility of using the stereotactic frame [1, 3].

Neuroendoscopy is a well-established and diffuse technique, allowing several possible applications by minimally invasive approaches, such as treatment of obstructive hydrocephalus and intracranial cysts, resection, or biopsy of tumors and

A. De Benedictis · C. G. Nucci · A. Carai · C. E. Marras (✉)
Neurosurgery Unit, Department of Neurosciences, Bambino Gesù Children's Hospital, IRCCS, Rome, Italy
e-mail: alessandro.debenedictis@opbg.net; carlotta.nucci@opbg.net; andrea.carai@opbg.net; carloefisio.marras@opbg.net

C. Rossi-Espagnet
Neuroradiology Unit, Imaging Department of Radiology, Bambino Gesù Children's Hospital, IRCCS, Rome, Italy

Neuroradiology Unit, NESMOS Department, Sapienza University, Rome, Italy
e-mail: mcamilla.rossi@opbg.net

J. A. González Martínez, F. Cardinale (eds.), *Robotics in Neurosurgery*, https://doi.org/10.1007/978-3-031-08380-8_10

malformations. Moreover, endoscopy is routinely used in children, not only because of the high incidence of hydrocephalus-related diseases, but also for the frequent finding of an altered ventricular anatomy, due to morphological variants or pathological distortions [4].

The combined use of standard stereotactic methods and robotic technology for endoscopy approaches was first described by Benabid et al. in 1992. The author stated that *"positioning of ventriculoscope would be significantly easier with the robot, particularly when several tracks are needed"* [5]. After, a growing experience on robotic endoscopy has been reported, concerning not only endoscopic third ventriculostomy (ETV) procedures, but also other treatments, such as trans-nasal endoscopic approaches, more difficult ventriculoscopies, and endoport tubular accesses for intracerebral hemorrhage or tumor resection [6, 7].

At the Bambino Gesù Children's Hospital, we adopt the ROSA (Robotized Surgical Assistant, Zimmer Biomet Inc.) system. According to the classification of Nathoo et al., that distinguished robotic systems on the basis of interaction modality between the surgeon and the robot, ROSA belongs to both categories of supervisory-controlled and shared-controlled systems [8]. By these modalities, the surgeon, after off-line planning of specific trajectories, can either supervise the robot performing autonomously the motion or directly control and move the surgical instrument during the procedure.

Since 2011, 229 patients underwent 244 operations under robotic assistance, with different indications, including epilepsy (implantation of intracerebral electrodes for stereoelectroencephalography, disconnection of hypothalamic hamartomas (HH)), brain tumors (stereotactic biopsies, intratumor catheter placement), disturbances of CSF circulation (ETV, cyst fenestration), movement disorders (deep brain stimulation, pallidotomy) [1].

Concerning endoscopy, our experience concerns 71 ROSA-assisted procedures, including treatment of obstructive hydrocephalus (14 procedures), disconnection of HHs (36 procedures), management of intraventricular tumors (21 procedures).

In the following sections of this chapter, general methodological aspects of the ROSA system and main possible applications in endoscopic procedures will be described.

Methods

Preoperative Planning

All patients undergo MRI with acquisition of a Gd-enhanced three-dimension (3D) magnetization-prepared rapid gradient-echo (MP-RAGE) sequence on 1.5 or 3 T scanner. To optimize skin rendering, a preoperative volumetric CT scan is also performed. CT and MR images are imported to the dedicated planning software and co-registered using a rigid and linear algorithm. The registration accuracy is validated by checking the correspondence of anatomical landmarks (ventricles, bone, venous sinus) between the selected sequences.

The entry and target points and the trajectory are selected on different possible views (axial, coronal, sagittal, perpendicular, and along the trajectory).

Once completed, the planning is copied into the same software on the robotic device (Fig. 10.1).

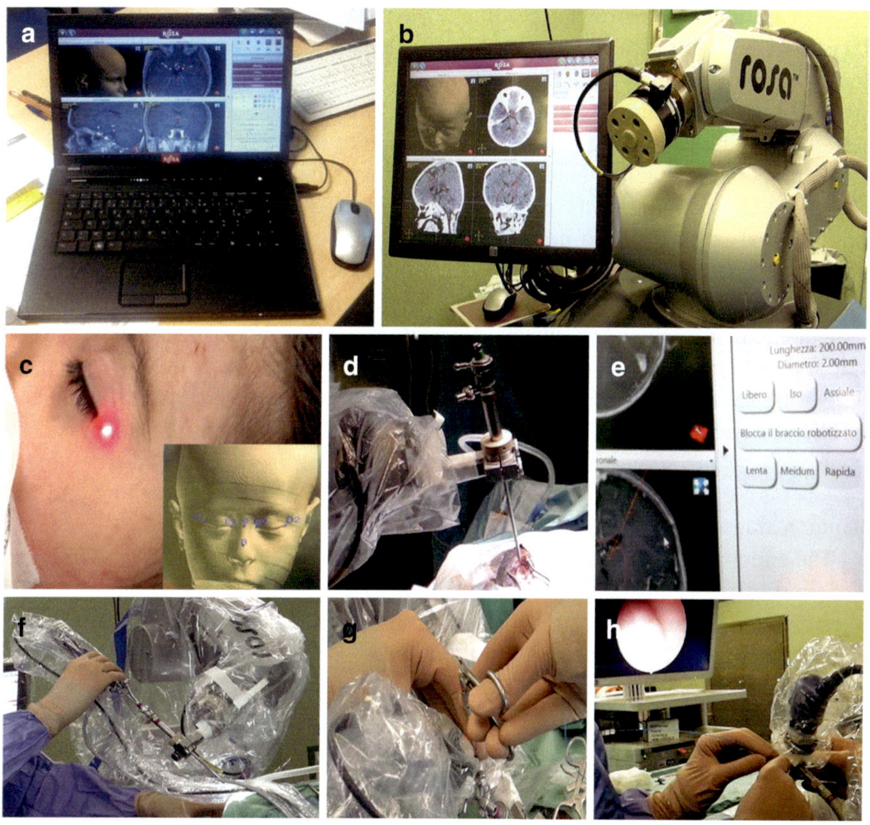

Fig. 10.1 Main characteristics and setting steps of the ROSA system. (**a**) The preoperative trajectory is planned on a dedicated software using volumetric MRI and CT sequences; (**b**) The planning information is transferred to the robot system, which is composed of a platform, including a compact robotic arm and a touch screen, mounted on a mobile trolley; (**c**) Registration is performed by laser scanning system, starting from standard reference points on the face (inset); (**d**) Positioning of the endoscope held at the extremity of the robotic arm to the entry point, according to the planned trajectory; (**e**) Possible movement control modalities, including 3 modes (axial, isocentric, and free) and 3 speeds (slow, medium, or fast); (**f**) Intraoperative control of the endoscope; (**g**, **h**) The robot provides stable support to the endoscope, enabling the surgeon to manage the different instruments, such as pincers (**g**) or laser probe (**h**)

Intraoperative Phase

The ROSA system is composed of a platform, including a compact robotic arm and a touch screen, mounted on a mobile trolley. A mechanical arm fixes the robot to the 3-pin support applied on the patient's head. Position of the head depends on the specific procedure. For endoscopic procedures, the head orientation can be neutral, slightly flexed or extended, according to target location.

Registration is performed according to frameless laser scanning of the patient's face. This includes different steps, namely: (1) arm calibration; (2) acquisition of facial landmarks by a contactless distance sensor held by the robot arm (midline frontal, bilateral lateral fronto-orbital region, internal and external eye canthus, nasion, and tip of the nasal bone); (3) correction of registration errors by matching the intraoperative scanned landmarks of step 2 with the preoperative 3D MRI data; (4) automatic scanning of the relevant areas of the patient's face; (5) manual scanning (lateral surface of the nose and lateral fronto-orbital region bilaterally); (6) trajectory feasibility verification according to the selected tool (sensor of distance, endoscope holder); and (7) final verification of the correspondence between the patient and neuroimaging, by manually positioning the robot arm at the level of the initial facial landmarks.

During the operative phase, the robot arm moves to the selected entry point and is oriented according to the corresponding trajectory. The arm movement can be controlled by the surgeon in 3 possible modes (axial, isocentric, and free) and 3 speeds (slow, medium, or fast). The robot arm has 6 degrees of freedom and has haptic features, based on force sensing and feedback.

The endoscope is inserted into a specific holder at the end of the arm. After performing skin incision and burr hole, according to the planned entry point, a rigid 30° endoscope (medium size, Karl Storz) integrated with the robot arm is moved from the cortex to the intraventricular or intracystic space under navigation iso-axial control.

After, the endoscope is moved to the target point by switching to the cooperative or free mode. The following procedure is performed by using the specific instruments needed through the endoscope, such as Fogarty balloon-tipped catheter, pincers, scissors, monopolar, laser fiber.

At the end of the procedure, the robotic arm is retracted, usually by axial mode, after aligning the endoscope to the trajectory.

Procedures

Management of CSF Circulation Disorders

Surgical management of CSF dynamics disorders is one of the most frequent situations in daily neurosurgical practice, especially in pediatric patients. Endoscopy is currently accepted as an effective treatment for obstructive hydrocephalus cases and the tendency to prefer this approach rather than shunt implantation increased over the last years.

The specific approach depends on the etiology and the level of obstruction, including foramen of Monro, aqueduct of Sylvius, fourth ventricle foramina, transition between spinal and cranial subarachnoid space, the age, the history, and the general medical condition of the patient [9].

ETV is a common procedure, boasting a solid tradition and a widespread practice. Standard indications for ETV include acquired aqueductal stenosis, adequate size of third ventricle, and potential patency of subarachnoid spaces. Other situations in which ETV might be indicated include myelomeningocele, Chiari malformation, congenital aqueductal stenosis, previous meningitis, age younger than 2 years, and prior ventriculo-peritoneal (V-P) shunt. On the other hand, the role of ETV in case of posterior fossa tumors, shunt malfunction, failure of previous ETV, neonatal patients is still debated [9].

In this context, neuroendoscopy for obstructive hydrocephalus constitutes one of the earliest applications of robotic technology. In 2002, Zimmermann reported preliminary data for 3 patients who underwent ETV procedures under robotic assistance. Surgeries were successfully completed, and a positive feedback concerning steering and precision of movement was acknowledged [7]. These positive results were confirmed in a subsequent series of 6 adults affected by triventricular obstructive hydrocephalus and in 9 children, who underwent robot-assisted ETV [10, 11].

We used the robot mainly for ETV, cyst fenestrations and coagulation, and septostomies. In all cases, the robotic system guided the endoscope to the planned target. After reaching the ventricular or intracystic space by axial mode, the control of the robotic arm was switched to the isocentric or manual mode according to freer trajectories, including rotations and axial translations. Moreover, endoscopic trajectories were marked out by a "safety zone," which allowed for more precise and stable control of the instrument, preventing the surgeon from risky movements.

We opted for robotic assistance to validate the technique in easier cases, especially at the beginning of our experience. Successively, more complex cases were considered. For example, in order to improve antibiotic efficacy in case of V-P shunt infection, removal of the device and robot-assisted ETV also without hydrocephalus can be proposed during the same procedure. In this circumstance, given the small ventricle size, the robotic arm provides a more stable support for the endoscope than freehand modality protecting the fornices and the thalamus from inadvertent excessive surgical maneuvering when reaching the floor of the third ventricle.

Furthermore, in patients with an excluded ventricle, due to previous shunt malfunction, or multiloculated hydrocephalus, a robot-guided endoscopic approach can be useful to perform a safe septostomy to restore the correct CSF circulation or to replace the catheter in a functioning position.

Finally, when multiple trajectories are necessary to perform different procedures during the same surgery, e.g., standard ETV and cyst shrinking, the robot system facilitates precise and stable navigation towards the area of surgical interest, preventing excessive brain manipulation and inappropriate adaptation of the endoscope angle to the specific trajectory needed (Fig. 10.2).

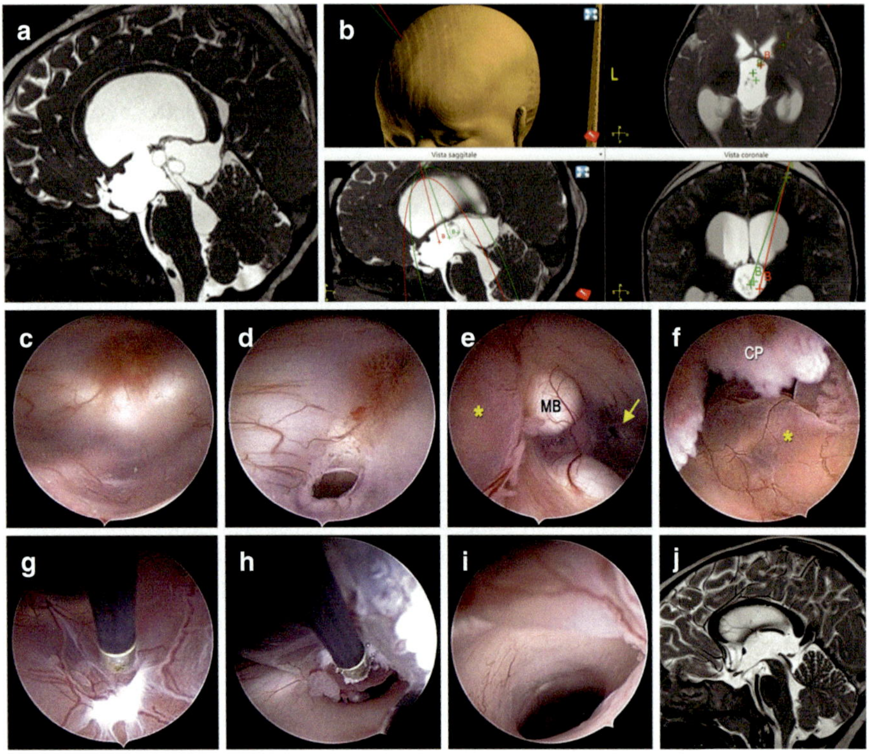

Fig. 10.2 Endoscopic ETV and intraventricular cyst coagulation. (**a**) Preoperative T2-weight MR sagittal sequence, showing a triventricular hydrocephalus, due to a cyst developing within the third ventricle and occluding the aqueduct of Silvius; (**b**) Endoscopic treatment was planned, including ETV (red trajectory) and cyst coagulation (green trajectory); (**c**, **d**) Endoscopic view of the third ventricle floor before (**c**) and after (**d**) ETV; (**e**, **f**) Using robotic neuronavigation, the endoscope is moved from anterior to posterior, according to the second trajectory. The ETV *(arrow)*, the mamillary bodies *(MB)*, the cyst *(*)*, and the choroid plexus *(CP)* are visualized; (**g**–**i**) Coagulation allows progressive shrinking of the cyst (**g**), until the aqueduct of Sylvius (**h**) is visualized and free; (**j**) Postoperative T2-weighted MRI, confirming the hydrocephalus' reduction

Disconnection of Hypothalamic Hamartomas

HHs are congenital benign lesions, centered in the hypothalamus and bulging into the third ventricle (intra-hypothalamic or sessile subtype), or attached to the *tuber cinereum* with an extraventricular extension (para-hypothalamic or pedunculated subtype) [12]. Intra-hypothalamic HHs may cause a typical drug-resistant epilepsy syndrome, characterized by gelastic seizures with an early infantile onset. Unfortunately, this disorder may evolve to a more severe condition, including epileptic encephalopathy, cognitive or behavioral impairments, and endocrinological disturbances [13].

The surgical management of HHs is of particular challenge, with no negligible risks of severe complications, mainly in relation to the deep location of the hypothalamic region, to its close relationships with eloquent neurovascular structures (thalamus, fornix, cerebral arteries), and to the physiological importance of the hypothalamus in several metabolic and functional aspects.

For these reasons, the best surgical treatment of HHs has been largely debated during the last decades, with the ultimate aim of optimizing the epilepsy outcome, while minimizing postoperative morbidity [14].

In this state of mind, transventricular endoscopic management has been proposed as effective and safer alternative, compared to the traditional microsurgical transcranial resection, especially when the lesion bulges into the third ventricle [15–18].

The first case of partial resection of a HH by an endoscopic approach was described by Akai in 2002 [19]. In 2003, based on the concept of an intrinsic epileptogenic activity within the HH, Delalande introduced the concept that simple HH disconnection from the surrounding hypothalamus, instead of total mass removal, is sufficient to prevent thalamic activation, which is mediated by propagation of seizure through the mammillothalamic tract. Moreover, he proposed a renewed classification of HHs (type 1–4), based on implant orientation and relationships with the third ventricle and recommended the use of endoscopic approach, a safer method for cases with endo- or peri-ventricular implantation (i.e., type 2 and type 3) [17].

Following case series reported positive results, by using an endoscopic approach for resection or disconnection of HHs, in terms of both seizure outcome and long-term morbidity [16, 20–22]. Further surgical improvement was also promoted by the introduction of laser and ultrasound aspirator techniques [23, 24].

During the presurgical planning of the trajectory, the entry point should be chosen on the opposite side to the main hypothalamic attachment of the HH (Fig. 10.3). As supported by other authors, the robot is useful to safely access the lateral ventricle and to easily guide the laser (2-μm thulium laser device, RevoLix®) or the monopolar system, not only to disconnect the HH along its implant on the hypothalamus, but also to perform multiple intralesional thermal ablations by radiofrequency or laser probe, under direct view and through a single intraparenchymal trajectory [15].

Moreover, considering that the size of the ventricular system of HH patients is usually normal, using an integrated system of neuronavigation combined with robotic arm for supporting the endoscope allows to optimize intraoperative orientation, limiting excessive intraventricular movement, and tissue manipulation [17, 22, 25].

Finally, as indicated by previous authors, thanks to minimally invasive robot-guided approach, repetition of procedure can be safely proposed, to improve the epilepsy outcome in case of persistent seizures [17, 20].

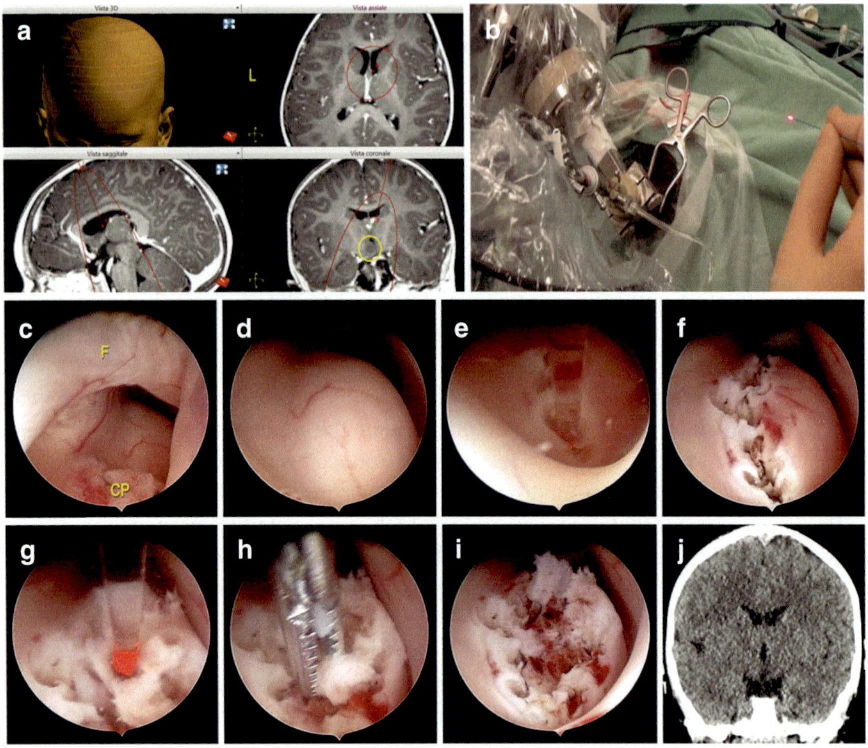

Fig. 10.3 Endoscopic disconnection of a HH. This case concerns a 4-year-old child with history of gelastic seizures starting from the first month of life. (**a**) MRI showed a T2-weigthed hyperintense lesion in the left hypothalamic region bulging in the third ventricle, compatible with HH type 2, according to Delalande classification *(yellow circle)* [17]. A robot-guided trajectory to the right lateral ventricle was planned; (**b**) The patient underwent endoscopic transventricular laser disconnection of the HH under robot assistance; (**c**) The ventricle is reached following the planned trajectory, by axial modality. The foramen of Monro, delimitated by the fornix *(f)* and the choroid plexus *(CP)* is identified; (**d**) The HH and its implant at the lateral wall the third ventricle are identified; (**e**, **f**) Using the laser system, the disconnection follows the whole implant line of the HH; (**g–i**) Laser coagulation is applied directly to the HH (**g**), to facilitate multiple samplings for histopathology (**h**), and to reduce the residual lesion (**i**); (**j**) Postoperative CT scan showed no complications

Management of Intraventricular Tumors

Endoscopy is becoming an increasingly common option for the management of intraventricular brain tumors, mainly due to instrumentation evolution, clarification of indications, and improvement of surgical expertise and results. Moreover, in comparison with traditional open neurosurgical approaches to the ventricular system, endoscopy allows to perform less invasive but effective surgeries, which is particularly important in childhood, in terms of surgery-related morbidity, blood loss, and hospitalization time.

Most frequently reported applications of endoscopic approach include tumor cyst fenestration, tumor biopsy, and tumor removal [26]. In all these procedures, the use of a robotic assistant may offer a valuable advantage in respect to traditional neuroendoscopic techniques (e.g., by freehand modality or using mechanical arms), by improving precision of endoscope movements, while reducing the surgeon fatigue, thanks to stable support for the instrument provided by the robotic arm.

Different tumors, frequently occurring during childhood, such as craniopharyngiomas, colloid cysts, suprasellar pilocytic astrocytomas, and gangliogliomas are frequently associated with a cystic component that may induce compression on the visual system and obstructive hydrocephalus, due to development within the third ventricle. Symptomatic cases can benefit from a transventricular endoscopic cyst fenestration, with consequent permanent or temporary decompression, before or instead carrying on with direct resection of the main tumor. As a consequence, since the long-term success of this procedure is related to the quality of cystic wall opening, which often requires a laborious work of coagulation, balloon expansion, and cutting, robotic assistance may facilitate managing the different surgical steps.

Endoscopic biopsy of tumors developing within the ventricle system is a common minimally invasive technique to obtain a reliable histological diagnosis. Moreover, in case of hydrocephalus due to tumor obstruction of CSF circulation, an ETV can be performed during the same surgery to normalize intracranial pressure.

The surgical trajectory is planned according to the lesion location, to provide the most direct access and easiest handling of surgical instruments. For this reason, while a standard precoronal access is appropriate for tumors harboring the region of the foramen of Monro (Fig. 10.4), a most anterior frontal route is preferred in case of more posterior location, such as the pineal region, so avoiding excessive traction of the foramen of Monro during the approach to the target. Robotic guidance may be useful, especially when multiple trajectories are planned, or in cases without significant ventricle dilatation, due to absence of CSF circulation obstruction or previously performed ETV (Fig. 10.5).

Removal of intraventricular solid tumors through an endoscopic approach may be indicated in selected cases, depending on tumor characteristics (size, density, vascularity, relationships with surrounding structures), adequate instrumentation, and familiarity of the surgical team to the procedure. According to these criteria, best candidates usually include tumors smaller than 2 cm, without calcification, avascular, and well-defined or pedunculated at the ependymal surface [26].

In childhood, one of the most frequently reported lesions requiring a neuroendoscopy treatment is the colloid cyst. This is a rare benign cystic tumor, normally located within the third ventricle, causing obstructive hydrocephalus by occlusion of the foramens of Monro [27]. Although the primary aim of treatment is removal of the lesion, an endoscopic approach can be effective in achieving decompression by evacuation of the cyst content, possibly followed by standard traditional open transcallosal route, in case of incomplete removal or relapse [27].

Also for the colloid cysts management, the robotic system offers the possibility of verifying the position of the endoscope through MRI, in addition to the direct endoscopic view and during the entire procedure and allows to constantly adjust the

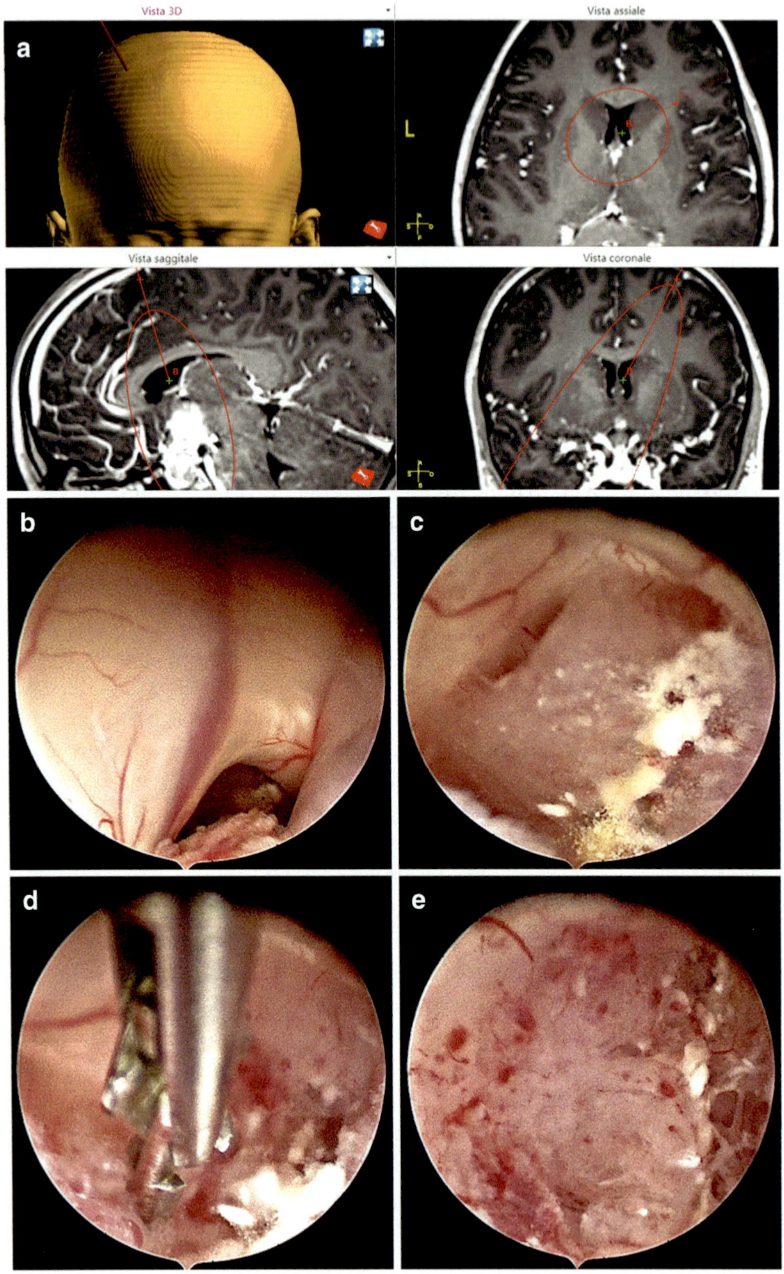

Fig. 10.4 Endoscopic biopsy of a sellar/suprasellar germinoma within a 10-year-old girl. (**a**) Preoperative planning of a trajectory to the right lateral ventricle; (**b**) As shown by neuroradiological images, the size of ventricles and the foramen of Monro were normal. The robot allowed to safely approach the lesion by controlled and stable movements; (**c**) Tumor bulging within the third ventricle; (**d**, **e**) Multiple samplings of the lesion, which was characterized by soft, bleeding tissue

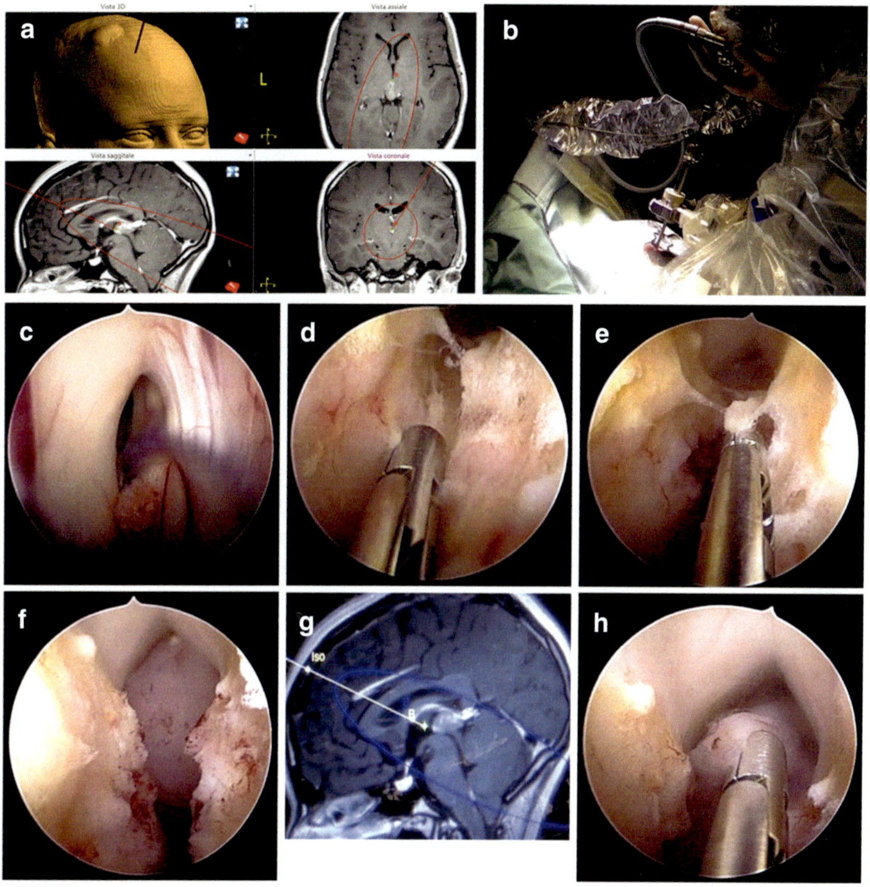

Fig. 10.5 Endoscopic biopsy of a pineal region tumor. A 14-year-old girl was referred to our hospital, coming from another center, where she had already undergone an ETV for an obstructive hydrocephalus, due to a lesion located within the pineal region. (**a**) Because of the small size of the ventricular systems, a robotic-assisted procedure was indicated. In order to correctly reach the lesion, a right frontal trajectory was planned; (**b, c**) the robotic arm improved accuracy of the approach (**b**), especially by avoiding to inappropriately stress the fornices (**c**); (**d–f**) The inter-thalamic adhesion was cut (**d**, **e**), allowing to sufficiently expose the tumor (**f**); (**g**) Intraoperative sagittal MRI sequence, showing the target achievement along the planned trajectory *(yellow line, B)*. In order to accurately manage the endoscope, the isocentric modality was set, allowing fine movements around a fixed fulcrum *(iso)*. (**h**) The tumor sampling allowed to conclusive histo-pathological diagnosis of pineal parenchymal tumor with intermediate differentiation

endoscope position in respect to the target by gentle controlled movements. In parallel with neuronavigation function, the robotic support to the endoscope enables the surgeon to use both hands and facilitates a more fluent sequential use of different instruments (electrocautery or laser, cupped biopsy forceps, and suction aspiration, ultrasound aspiration), without the need of continuously holding and stabilizing the endoscope.

Conclusions

In this chapter, we described the main possible applications of robotic technology in different neuroendoscopy procedures, including treatment of CSF disturbances and management of intraventricular malformations and tumors. Robotic assistants combine accuracy of image-guided neuronavigation with human decision-making, by enhancing haptic ability, ergonomics, and visualization capacity.

As a consequence, even at neurosurgery Centers with strong neuroendoscopy expertise, robotic guidance may improve precision and safety of minimally invasive surgeries, also extending the spectrum of indications to more complex approaches, such as in case of small sized or distorted ventricles, multiple trajectories, narrower corridors, and long-lasting procedures. These situations require the highest level of stability, which is not equally achievable by conventional free-hand technique, especially in pediatric patients.

Bioengineering research will contribute in optimizing the application of robotic technology to neuroendoscopy, with the aim of reducing the instrument size, while improving maneuverability of the robotic system, working angles, and possibility of using multiple instruments simultaneously, including flexible endoscopic systems.

Finally, since robot-assisted approaches are complex and require a well-trained team, systematic planning of sharing expertise and education programs by more experienced centers should be encouraged to promote robotic culture within the neurosurgical community.

References

1. De Benedictis A, Trezza A, Carai A, Genovese E, Procaccini E, Messina R, et al. Robot-assisted procedures in pediatric neurosurgery. Neurosurg Focus. 2017;42(5):E7.
2. Doulgeris JJ, Gonzalez-Blohm SA, Filis AK, Shea TM, Aghayev K, Vrionis FD. Robotics in neurosurgery: evolution, current challenges, and compromises. Cancer Control. 2015;22:352–9.
3. Miller BA, Salehi A, Limbrick DD Jr, Smyth MD. Applications of a robotic stereotactic arm for pediatric epilepsy and neurooncology surgery. J Neurosurg Pediatr. 2017;20:364–70.
4. Constantini S, Sgouros S, Kulkarni A. Neuroendoscopy in the youngest age group. World Neurosurg. 2013;79:S23.e1–11.
5. Benabid AL, Lavallee S, Hoffmann D, Cinquin P, Demongeot J, Danel F. Potential use of robots in endoscopic neurosurgery. Acta Neurochir Suppl. 1992;54:93–7.
6. Pillai A, Ratnathankom A, Ramachandran SN, Udayakumaran S, Subhash P, Krishnadas A. Expanding the spectrum of robotic assistance in cranial neurosurgery. Oper Neurosurg (Hagerstown). 2019;17:164–73.
7. Zimmermann M, Krishnan R, Raabe A, Seifert V. Robot-assisted navigated endoscopic ventriculostomy: implementation of a new technology and first clinical results. Acta Neurochir. 2004;146:697–704.
8. Nathoo N, Cavuşoğlu MC, Vogelbaum MA, Barnett GH. In touch with robotics: neurosurgery for the future. Neurosurgery. 2005;56:421–33.
9. Enchev YP, Shizuo O. The application of neuroendoscopic techniques in improving altered CSF physiology. In: Sgouros S, editor. Neuroendoscopy. London: Springer Heidelberg New York Dordrecht; 2014. p. 11–30.

10. Hoshide R, Calayag M, Meltzer H, Levy ML, Gonda D. Robot-assisted endoscopic third ventriculostomy: institutional experience in 9 patients. J Neurosurg Pediatr. 2017;20:125–33.
11. Zimmermann M, Krishnan R, Raabe A, Seifert V. Robot-assisted navigated neuroendoscopy. Neurosurgery. 2002;51:1446–52.
12. Freeman JL, Coleman LT, Wellard RM, Kean MJ, Rosenfeld JV, Jackson GD, et al. MR imaging and spectroscopic study of epileptogenic hypothalamic hamartomas: analysis of 72 cases. AJNR Am J Neuroradiol. 2004;25:450–62.
13. Debeneix C, Bourgeois M, Trivin C, Sainte-Rose C, Brauner R. Hypothalamic hamartoma: comparison of clinical presentation and magnetic resonance images. Horm Res. 2001;56:12–8.
14. Rosenfeld JV. The evolution of treatment for hypothalamic hamartoma: a personal odyssey. Neurosurg Focus. 2011;30:E1.
15. Bourdillon P, Ferrand-Sorbet S, Apra C, Chipaux M, Raffo E, Rosenberg S, et al. Surgical treatment of hypothalamic hamartomas. Neurosurg Rev. 2021;44(2):753–62.
16. Chibbaro S, Cebula H, Scholly J, Todeschi J, Ollivier I, Timofeev A, et al. Pure endoscopic management of epileptogenic hypothalamic hamartomas. Neurosurg Rev. 2017;40:647–53.
17. Delalande O, Fohlen M. Disconnecting surgical treatment of hypothalamic hamartoma in children and adults with refractory epilepsy and proposal of a new classification. Neurol Med Chir (Tokyo). 2003;43:61–8.
18. Mittal S, Mittal M, Montes JL, Farmer JP, Andermann F. Hypothalamic hamartomas. Part 2. Surgical considerations and outcome. Neurosurg Focus. 2013;34(6):E7.
19. Akai T, Okamoto K, Iizuka H, Kakinuma H, Nojima T. Treatments of hamartoma with neuroendoscopic surgery and stereotactic radiosurgery: a case report. Minim Invasive Neurosurg. 2002;45:235–9.
20. Ferrand-sorbets S, Fohlen M, Delalande O, Zuber K, Chamard P, Taussig D, et al. Seizure outcome and prognostic factors for surgical management of hypothalamic hamartomas in children. Seizure. 2020;75:28–33.
21. Ng YT, Rekate HL, Prenger EC, Wang NC, Chung SS, Feiz-Erfan I, et al. Endoscopic resection of hypothalamic hamartomas for refractory symptomatic epilepsy. Neurology. 2008;70:1543–8.
22. Rekate HL, Feiz-Erfan I, Ng YT, Gonzalez LF, Kerrigan JF. Endoscopic surgery for hypothalamic hamartomas causing medically refractory gelastic epilepsy. Childs Nerv Syst. 2006;22:874–80.
23. Calisto A, Dorfmüller G, Fohlen M, Bulteau C, Conti A, Delalande O. Endoscopic disconnection of hypothalamic hamartomas: safety and feasibility of robot-assisted, thulium laser-based procedures. J Neurosurg Pediatr. 2014;14:563–72.
24. Lekovic GP, Gonzalez LF, Feiz-Erfan I, Rekate HL. Endoscopic resection of hypothalamic hamartoma using a novel variable aspiration tissue resector. Neurosurgery. 2006;58:ONS166–9.
25. Shim KW, Chang JH, Park YG, Kim HD, Choi JU, Kim DS. Treatment modality for intractable epilepsy in hypothalamic hamartomatous lesions. Neurosurgery. 2008;62:847–56.
26. Souweidane MM. Endoscopic management of intraventricular brain tumors in children. In: Sgouros S, editor. Neuroendoscopy. London: Springer Heidelberg New York Dordrecht; 2014. p. 117–26.
27. Yadav YR, Yadav N, Parihar V, Kher Y, Ratre S. Management of colloid cyst of third ventricle. Turk Neurosurg. 2015;25:362–71.

Chapter 11
Robot-Assisted Stereotactic Biopsy

Marc Zanello, Giorgia Antonia Simboli, Marc Harislur, and Johan Pallud

Introduction

Since the appearance of modern neurosurgical stereotaxy in the early 1950s, numerous procedures have become stereotactic and brain biopsy followed this trend [1, 2]. Despite the development of alternatives such as frameless navigation-based biopsy, stereotactic biopsy remains the gold standard to obtain histomolecular data for a particular brain lesion and remains one of the most frequent neurosurgical stereotactic procedures [3, 4]. It is mandatory to clearly define what is a stereotactic neurosurgical procedure. The use of a stereotactic frame is no longer the only way to define a procedure as stereotactic or not, and a neurosurgical procedure is stereotactic when the mechanical precision is as high as possible [5, 6].

The evolution of stereotactic biopsy benefited from the refinement of neuroimaging and of the development of robot-based surgical assistance. Since the seminal works by Kwoh et al. and by Benabid et al., the robotic surgical assistance has been slightly improved but the core of the system remains unchanged: a robotic arm with various degrees of freedom and a computer workstation [7, 8]. Until now, more sophisticated robotic surgical assistances are not well-fitted for neurosurgical

M. Zanello (✉) · J. Pallud
Service de Neurochirurgie, GHU Paris—Psychiatrie et Neurosciences—Hôpital Sainte-Anne, Paris, France

Université de Paris, Sorbonne Paris Cité, Paris, France

Inserm, UMR1266, IMA-Brain, Institut de Psychiatrie et Neurosciences de Paris, Paris, France

G. A. Simboli · M. Harislur
Service de Neurochirurgie, GHU Paris—Psychiatrie et Neurosciences—Hôpital Sainte-Anne, Paris, France

Université de Paris, Sorbonne Paris Cité, Paris, France

J. A. González Martínez, F. Cardinale (eds.), *Robotics in Neurosurgery*, https://doi.org/10.1007/978-3-031-08380-8_11

stereotactic procedures [9]. Robot-assisted neurosurgical stereotactic procedures are as accurate as classical frame-based ones [10]. This comparable precision with greater versatility led to the diffusion of robotic surgical assistance for deep brain stimulation, stereoelectroencephalography (SEEG), and biopsy.

Past Neurosurgical Procedure Before 3D Intraoperative Imaging

Figure 11.1 represents the neurosurgical procedure performed in Sainte-Anne hospital before September 2019.

The neurosurgical procedure detailed here is the procedure performed at the Sainte-Anne Hospital between 2004 and 2019. It is based on the seminal Talairach's methodology and it remains of interest as it is a reliable and accurate technique [2, 11].

The stereotactic biopsy was performed under general anesthesia along one trajectory. Serial biopsies were made to sample all components of the imaging abnormalities of a particular neoplasm. Preoperative stereotactic MRI (tridimensional T1-weighted sequence with and without contrast agent including midface, acquired

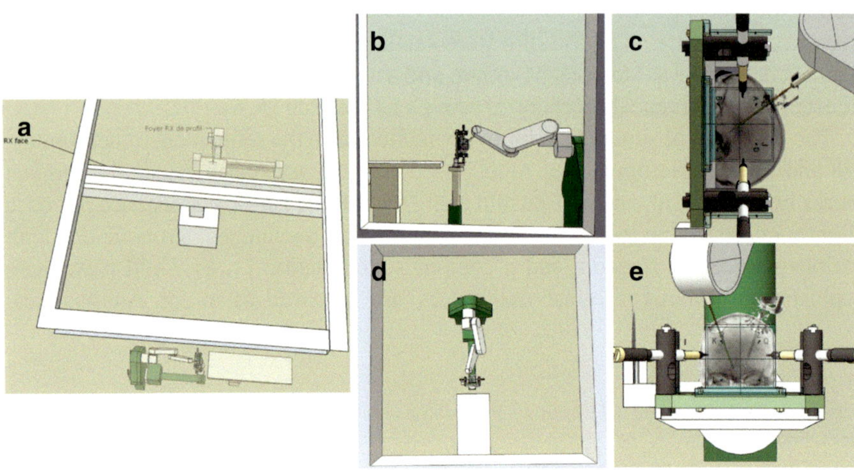

Fig. 11.1 Schematic presentation of the procedure performed before September 2019. From left to right: (**a**) general presentation of the stereotactic room with two flat-panel detectors localized at 5 m of the operating room table, (**b**) lateral view from the lateral flat-panel detector position showing the obtained plain X-ray in the operating room space, (**c**) close-up of lateral X-ray obtained with stereotactic positioning of the biopsy cannula, (**d**) front view from the front flat-panel detector position showing the obtained plain X-ray in the operating room space, (**e**) close-up of frontal X-ray obtained with stereotactic positioning of the biopsy cannula

the eve of surgery) was fused with preoperative oncological MRI including systematically a Fluid Attenuated Inversion Recovery (FLAIR) sequence and, whenever required and available, a perfusion sequence. The combined MRI was used for biopsy trajectory planning and sample selection. The biopsy trajectory was planned by the referring neurosurgeon using the iPlan Stereotaxy planning software (version 3.0, BrainLAB AG, Feldkirchen, Germany), in particular with the Probe's eye view, to reach the different tumor components as observed on MRI while avoiding critical structures, such as cerebral sulci, intracranial vessels, and eloquent brain areas. Trajectory coordinates were transmitted to the VoXim Neuromate software (version 6.0 to version 6.4, IVS Technology, Germany). The head of the patient was fixed in a Talairach base frame (Dixi, Besançon, France) fixed to the robot (Neuromate, Renishaw, New Mills, United Kingdom) holder. Bidirectional and orthogonal (anteroposterior and lateral) teleradiographic X-rays were acquired intraoperatively. The initial bidirectional 2D X-rays allowed preoperative 3D MRI images to be reformatted in the intraoperative stereotactic space using a co-registration between MRI images and these X-rays. This crucial step of 2D/3D co-registration was manually done by the radiology technician and carefully reviewed by the referring neurosurgeon using a module of fusion by points of the VoXim software. Therefore, the fiducials of the Talairach frame were not mounted on the frame: the Talairach base frame served only as a "stereotactic skull clamp." After the robot's arm deployment, a metallic punch was placed into the robot tool holder. The accuracy of the entry point and of the trajectory was confirmed, prior to the drilling of the skull, with bidirectional X-rays. The biopsy cannula was introduced under the guidance of the robotic arm following the defined trajectory through a drill hole made with a 2.5 mm diameter drill bit. Biopsy cannula movements were controlled by the robot ensuring the accurate positioning at each biopsy site. Biopsy samples were obtained using a 10 mm window side-cutting Sedan-Vallicioni biopsy cannula. Bidirectional X-ray images were taken at each biopsy site prior to collecting the samples in order to check the cannula's position. Typically, the first biopsy sampling site was located in seemingly normal brain parenchyma close to MRI-defined abnormalities, the second site was in areas of FLAIR-defined abnormalities, the third one in areas of contrast enhancement when present, and the fourth one in areas of necrosis when present. The act of biopsying starting from more superficial areas towards deeper areas (outwards-inwards) allows compression of an eventual small vessel, thanks to the presence of the cannula, in place that may have been trespassed in the trajectory and overlooked by preoperative MRI, which may reduce the risk of bleeding. Each biopsy sample was sent individually to neuropathology after detailing spatial orientation according to MRI-defined abnormalities. The extemporaneous histopathological analysis was frequently done. Postoperative CT scan was systematically performed on day one postoperatively.

Current Neurosurgical Procedure Using 3D Intraoperative Imaging

The neurosurgical procedure detailed here is the procedure currently performed at Sainte-Anne Hospital, GHU Paris Psychiatrie et Neurosciences, Paris, France. Figure 11.2 summarizes the principal steps of the neurosurgical procedure.

The main evolution compared to the previous method is the modification of the intraoperative imaging technique from bidirectional orthogonal teleradiographic X-rays to a mobile cone beam CT unit, the O-Arm (Medtronic, Inc., Littleton, MA). This evolution eases the co-registration process with automated 3D/3D fusion and shortens the imaging acquisition time. The O-Arm consists in a modification of the standard C-arm fluoroscope: a mobile segment allows closure of the ring (from C-Arm to O-Arm) enabling a 360° rotation of the flat-panel detector. Due to its architecture, O-Arm shows bone details with a great precision (it directly outputs a 3D dataset precisely depicting the skull) but is actually unable to reveal brain details. It is also possible to take plain X-rays.

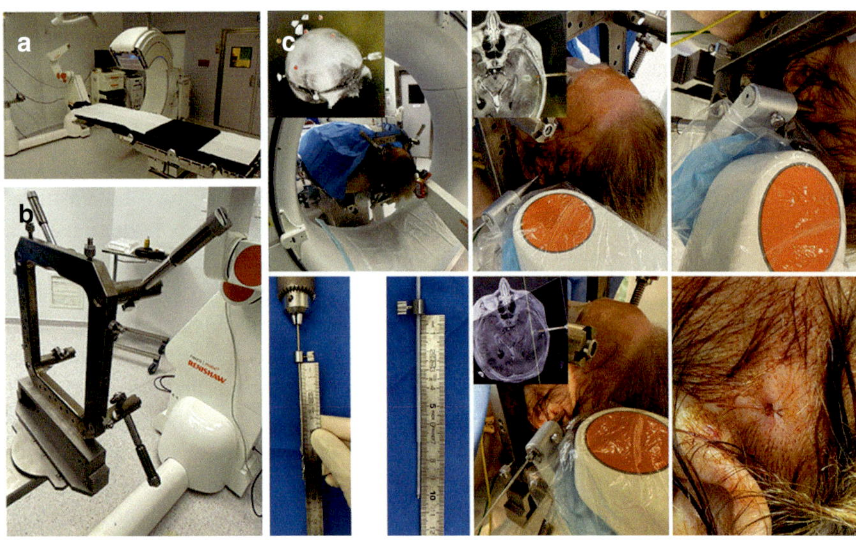

Fig. 11.2 Presentation of the current surgical procedure of robot-assisted stereotactic biopsy. From left to right and top to bottom: (**a**) general presentation of the operating room with the mobile CT unit O-Arm and the robot NeuroMate, (**b**) close-up on the Talairach stereotactic head clamp composed by the base of the Talairach frame, (**c**) first step of the procedure with a 3D series acquisition of the Neurolocate tool locked on the robot arm and moved close to the patient's head, control of the correct robot's positioning with a new 3D series and a metallic punch, robot arm positioned against the patient's skin to minimize the mechanical deviation, fine adjustment of the drill with a mechanical stop, adjustment of the monopolar coagulation 10 mm below the dura mater plane, intraoperative control of the needle position into the patient head with a third O-Arm acquisition, puncture wound closed with absorbable suture (minimal shaving)

All the preoperative steps remain unchanged (stereotactic MRI acquisition and trajectory using BrainLAB iPlan Stereotaxy planning software). The "Talairach stereotactic head clamp" and the updated Neuromate robot are still used. Tridimensional images are acquired intraoperatively with the O-Arm. The initial 3D acquisition is made with the Neurolocate tool of the robot. This tool has five carbon fiber branches: each branch supports a synthetic ruby sphere and the tool is fastened to the robot arm by a secured magnet. The neurosurgeon is required to bring together as close as possible the Neurolocate to the patient's head. A 3D series is acquired with the O-Arm: this imaging series allows to co-register preoperative MRI with intraoperative acquisition via a dedicated module of Neuroinspire software (Renishaw Mayfield SA). This planning software was specifically developed for the NeuroMate robot: the automated recognition of the five ruby spheres of the Neurolocate tool on the 3D series allows the registration of the O-Arm dataset space to the robotic working space. Preoperative MRI is registered to intraoperative 3D series, and then the cartesian coordinates of the entry and target points are copied from iPlan software coordinates and manually input in Neuroinspire. Following the safety check—the agreement between a test trajectory and the robot's arm actual movement—the robot's arm is moved until the tool holder touches the skin. This point is of practical importance as it reduces mechanical inaccuracy of the drill bit's trajectory as much as possible. The entry point and the biopsy trajectory are checked prior to the initialization of any invasive procedure thanks to a second O-Arm acquisition. If required, fine adjustments of the robot's arm position are easily made. The drill hole is performed with a 2.5 mm diameter drill bit: the drilling movement has to be as smooth as possible and the bit as sharp as possible (favor the single-use drill). Biopsy cannula movements are controlled by the robot, ensuring accurate positioning at each biopsy site. Biopsy samples are obtained using a 10 mm window side-cutting Sedan-Vallicioni biopsy cannula. Due to the ability of the O-Arm to perform 2D X-rays as 3D acquisitions, each biopsy site can still be checked prior to sampling. Biopsy sampling sites are chosen according to MRI-defined abnormalities. Postoperative CT scan is still performed at postoperative day one.

Literature Review of Robot-Assisted Stereotactic Biopsy

Robot-assisted biopsy remains scarcely reported in scientific literature. It probably relies on the slow diffusion of the robotic assistance prior to the broader use of SEEG [12]. In fact, the multiple stereotactic trajectories required for a SEEG are better performed using a robotic assistance. The increasing frequency of SEEG in North American neurosurgical departments should lead to a multiplication of robotic assistance use in functional neurosurgery in the near future. Prior to our series of 337 cases of robot-assisted stereotactic biopsy for supratentorial gliomas, the larger series consisted in 102 cases reported by Yasin et al. [13, 14]. A review of the literature made by Marcus et al. identified 15 studies published before December 31st 2017 [15]. All these studies were retrospective and did not compare frame-based and robot-assisted stereotactic biopsy procedures. Nevertheless, the diagnostic yield varied from 75% to 100% in individual series. By considering the two series of 100 patients or more, published before the one from Sainte-Anne Hospital, the rate of radiological defined postoperative hematoma was found to be equal or superior to 10%, which is in line with our findings. However, it is important to note that this frequent radiological finding of postoperative hematoma does not correlate to severe clinical outcomes (i.e., permanent severe morbidities, death) in the majority of cases: only one patient who suffered from a postoperative hematoma deceased. The accuracy was rarely studied due to scarcely performed intraoperative imaging. At the present era of facilitated 3D intraoperative imaging, the comparison between planned and actual trajectories is simplified. When reported, the average target accuracy stayed in the "stereotactic" range: 0.9–4.5 mm.

The Sainte-Anne Experience of Robot-Assisted Stereotactic Biopsy

Using a prospective database, we recently performed an in-depth analysis of our robot-assisted stereotactic biopsy practice with a particular focus on patients harboring a supratentorial diffuse glioma [14]. A total of 377 patients (60.5% men, mean age 59.9 ± 14.0-year-old) were included. No technical failure leading to the biopsy arrest occurred. We performed serial biopsies: a mean of 4.2 ± 1.9 (range, 1–14) biopsy samples were obtained at a mean of 2.6 ± 1.2 (range, 1–6) biopsy sites. Biopsy sampling was performed at various sites encompassing the different MRI-defined abnormalities with a decreasing frequency: area of contrast enhancement (mean 1.5 ± 1.2 (range, 0–7) samples), area of hypersignal on FLAIR sequence (mean 1.0 ± 1.1 (range, 0–6) samples), necrotic area, in a cystic component if any, and in the seemingly normal brain parenchyma. An extemporaneous histopathological analysis was performed intraoperatively in 324 (85.9%) cases with a decreasing frequency over time. The diagnostic yield of our stereotactic procedure was very high: the histopathological diagnosis of a diffuse glioma and the glioma grade were obtained in 98.7% and in 92.6% of cases, respectively. In multivariate analysis, a male sex (adjusted Odds ratio (aOR) 3.2, $p = 0.004$) and a ring-like pattern of contrast enhancement with central necrosis on MRI (aOR 4.9, $p = 0.002$) were independent predictors of a conclusive diffuse glioma grading. Postoperative clinical complications included new neurological deficit in 7.7%, epileptic seizures in 2.7%, systemic thromboembolic events in 1.3%, and intracerebral hematoma requiring surgical evacuation in 0.8%. No infection was observed. A KPS decrease ≥20 points postoperatively was observed in 4.0%. Eleven (2.9%) patients died during the first postoperative month, and four (1.1%) of them died during hospital stay. Of these four deceased during hospital stay, three of these passed for rapid evolution of the lesion's mass effect, while the fourth for preexisting bleeding of the glioblastoma prior to biopsy. None of these deaths was, hence, directly related to surgery.

Postoperative imaging revealed some complications including cerebral hemorrhage ≥10 mm in 14.6% (<20 mm in 10.6%, and ≥ 20 mm in 4.0%), increased mass effect in 4.4%, and cerebral ischemia in 0.5%. In multivariate analysis, a preoperative neurological deficit (aOR 4.0, $p = 0.030$), a cerebral hemorrhage ≥20 mm on postoperative imaging (aOR 7.1, $p = 0.004$), and an increased mass effect on postoperative imaging (aOR 5.4, $p = 0.014$) were independent predictors of a new postoperative neurological deficit. Only a preoperative anticoagulant therapy (although stopped preoperatively according to guidelines) (aOR 4.3, $p = 0.017$) was an independent predictor of a cerebral hemorrhage ≥20 mm on postoperative imaging. The number of biopsy sites and the number of biopsy samples were not independent risk factors of new postoperative neurological deficit, postoperative disability, cerebral hemorrhage, and increased mass effect on postoperative imaging. We identified five independent predictors of an inability to discharge at home postoperatively in multivariate analysis: 1/a preoperative neurological deficit, 2/a preoperative KPS <70, 3/a subventricular zone contact, 4/presence of contrast enhancement on preoperative MRI, and 5/a steroid use at the time of surgery. When stratifying the rate of inability to discharge at home postoperatively by the number of predictors present in a particular patient, the rate of discharge to home reduced from 100% to 20.0% with the increase from 0 to 5 of the presence of the predictors identified above.

The Complications of Robot-Assisted Stereotactic Biopsies

Following the analysis of our series of robot-assisted stereotactic biopsies, we decided to investigate further the cases with severe postoperative hemorrhage [16]. We selected the 12 patients presenting a postoperative intracerebral hematoma ≥20 mm of whom 3 required surgical evacuation. The preoperative MRI was performed at a mean 7.6 ± 11.4 (median 1; range, 1–31) days before the surgery. No technical problem led to the procedure abortion. A mean of 4.1 ± 2.1 (range, 2–9) biopsy samples were performed at a mean of 2 ± 1.4 (range, 1–6) biopsy sites. An intraoperative bleeding through the biopsy cannula was observed in six (54.5%) cases and precluded additional biopsy sampling to be performed. The mean neurosurgeon's experience was 16.4 ± 10.6 years (five involved neurosurgeons, range, 3–31). Two patients required the surgical evacuation of the intracerebral hematoma based on first imaging evaluation (21.0 and 20.4 cm^3), and a third patient required the surgical evacuation after clinical worsening related to an increase of the intracerebral hematoma (from 1.4 to 25.8cm^3). None of these three patients presented postoperative complications after the surgical evacuation of the hematoma, and no stereotactic biopsy related death occurred in this series of 12 patients.

We took advantage of Sainte-Anne Hospital's surgical procedure to reconstruct the actual trajectory. In fact, the actual position of the biopsy cannula was captured intraoperatively thanks to X-rays systematically obtained: (1) before skull drilling to control the entry point and the trajectory; (2) at each biopsy site before biopsy sampling to control the position of the biopsy cannula. We used a homemade Flash software (Rulsirah, version 2.0) plus BrainLab iPlan Stereotaxy software (version 3.0, BrainLAB AG, Feldkirchen, Germany) to co-register 2D plain X-rays obtained during surgery with 3D preoperative images. We then reviewed the biopsy trajectory to search for a possible conflict between the actual biopsy trajectory and an anatomical structure at risk (cerebral blood vessels and cerebral sulci) [17]. The matchings between the actual biopsy trajectory, the intracerebral hematoma, and anatomical structures at risk revealed that in eight (72.7%) cases, an anatomical structure at risk was identified along the actual biopsy trajectory: a vessel located within a sulcus outside biopsy sampling site in four cases, a sulcus without identification of any vessel outside biopsy sampling site in two cases, a cortical vessel outside biopsy sampling site in one case, and a vessel located in the tumor and corresponding to a biopsy sampling site in one case. In all cases, the actual trajectory matched with the planned trajectory. This work illustrates the scarcity of severe complications following robot-assisted biopsies and, at the same time, the need to be extremely vigilant during the planning procedure. The fact that even trained neurosurgeons experienced severe hemorrhagic complications, and that hemorrhage can occur in any part of the brain, highlights the requirement of assistance software to lower the complication rate.

Classical Pitfalls in Robot-Assisted Stereotactic Biopsies

Figure 11.3 details two cases enduring hemorrhagic complications after robot-assisted stereotactic biopsies.

Based on our experience, some neurosurgical complications are favored by poor preoperative conditions required to achieve a successful surgical procedure. The two following cases illustrate two classical pitfalls in robot-assisted stereotactic biopsies: intratumoral vessel and poor preoperative imaging. Interestingly, despite large postoperative hematoma, none of the patients died postoperatively.

The first case is a 30-year-old female with no particular medical history, suffering from headaches and cognitive-motor slowing for 15 days before consulting medical attention, discovered a lesion in the pineal gland with MRI imaging. Primary surgical indication for ventriculostomy in view of obstructive hydrocephalus was executed, without any postoperative complications and without conclusive histological diagnosis on the CSF analysis. Indication for stereotactic biopsy was proposed as a second intervention and accepted. During the procedure, intraoperative bleeding through the biopsy cannula occurred, without clinical repercussions. At day one postoperatively, the patient was found in the morning GCS 9 (E2 V1 M6), where immediate brain CT scan depicted a hematoma at the tumor site. Patient hospitalized in neurointensive care unit. An external ventricular drain was placed. During the subsequent weeks, the patient slowly continued to improve. Patient was eventually transferred for oncological care and treatment. The patient had only a Parinaud syndrome (i.e., pretectal syndrome) after complete resorption of the

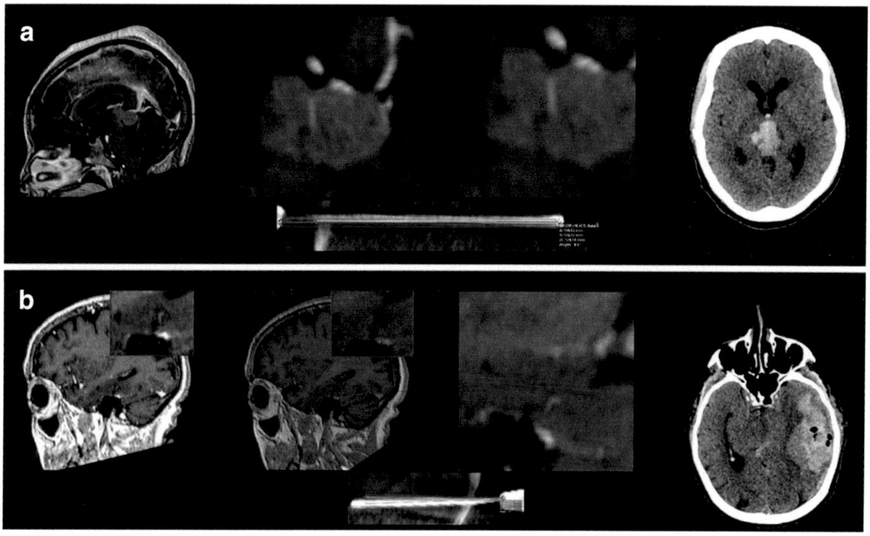

Fig. 11.3 Two cases of robot-assisted biopsies enduring complications. (**a**) From left to right, upper line: sagittal slice of preoperative 3DT1 with gadolinium enhancement MRI of a 30-year-old woman suffering from a pineal tumor, close-up on the tumoral vessel, co-registration of preoperative MRI and intraoperative O-Arm series showing a good overlap of planned trajectory (angular error: 0.5°, target error: 0.3 mm), close-up on the vascular conflict, postoperative CT scan acquisition showing the intratumoral bleeding. (**b**) From left to right, lower line: sagittal slice of first preoperative 3DT1 with gadolinium enhancement MRI of a 83-year-old woman suffering from a left temporo-mesial tumor, sagittal slice of second preoperative 3DT1 with gadolinium enhancement MRI, co-registration of preoperative MRI and intraoperative O-Arm series showing a good respect of planned trajectory (angular error: 2.6°, target error: 2.0 mm), close-up on the vascular conflict, postoperative CT scan acquisition showing the intraparenchymal and the subdural hematoma

hematoma. This case illustrates the need to check the planned trajectory until the end: intratumoral vessel largely visible on preoperative MRI is as prone to bleed as another physiological vessel.

The second case demonstrates a basic prerequisite of uneventful stereotactic procedure: an appropriate preoperative imaging. This 83-year-old female without cardiovascular comorbidities and hence no pro-bleeding therapy harbored a probable high-grade glioma located in the right temporo-mesial cortex. Indication for stereotactic biopsy was proposed and accepted. The procedure was planned based on a preoperative MRI performed at the eve of surgery in order to exclude any tumor progression before biopsy. This MRI was poorly enhanced, leading to a difficult visualization of the intraparenchymal vessels. This patient presented intraoperative bleeding through the biopsy cannula, motivating an immediate brain CT scan, depicting an important left temporo-insular hematoma with bradycardia and left anisocoria. Multidisciplinary discussion concluded no indication for evacuation of such hematoma in view of the patient's age, clinical state, and suspected aggressive and malignant histology. After 1 week in neuro intensive care unit, the patient recuperates with persistent right hemiparesis and mixed aphasia. A brain CT scan executed 2 weeks post-biopsy, demonstrated the chronicization of the hematoma. During the subsequent weeks, the patient continued to improve on a clinical level, which allowed for a transfer in a neuro-rehabilitation center. The patient harbored a severe hemiparesis, language disorder, and somnolence after complete resorption of the hematoma. This patient had a previous MRI leading to the neurosurgical appointment.

In both cases, intraoperative control ensured a correct positioning of the needle, respectively, with the preoperatively planned trajectory. This demonstrates how human-based preoperative preparation, i.e., good quality imagery, and anesthesia patient preparation preoperatively are essential for good surgery planning by the neurosurgeon to then execute the surgery assisted by the robot. This case analysis also proves the usefulness of intraoperative imaging: during the surgical procedure, the neurosurgeon can adapt his surgery if the trajectory seems deviated, and after the surgical procedure, the fusion between intraoperative image and preoperative MRI allows to understand the surgical complication, if any.

Perspectives

The trend in neurosurgical robotic assistance is towards smaller, faster, and cheaper tools. This trend is comprehensible in view of the cost and size of classical surgical robots, which look like poorly modified industrial robots. The democratization of robotic assistance will certainly fasten the adoption of robot-assisted stereotactic biopsy by numerous neurosurgical teams worldwide. From the authors' point of view, this evolution has to be carefully evaluated by the neurosurgical community. One of the main advantages of classical surgical robots over arms positioned via neuronavigation, such as Vertek and Varioguide arms (respectively, Medtronic and Brainlab systems), is their mechanical stability and reliability through thousands of arm deployment [18–20]. It remains unclear if the thinner robot's arms will be able to keep this mechanical accuracy, reducing the benefit of the robot-assistance compared to MRI-based neuronavigation [21, 22].

The same type of warning could be made regarding intraoperative imaging. Intraoperative imaging verification could be judged as a superfluous precaution in front of the numerous registration modes proposed in modern robot-assisted platforms (surface, marker-based, frame-based). However, it remains the only way to be certain of the trajectory. In agreement with seminal works of the Sainte-Anne school, we still think that performing intraoperative imaging acquisition is mandatory. This affirmation is reinforced by the new intraoperative imaging tools: 3D acquisition is now easily performed and fused with preoperative imaging. The time lost in intraoperative checking is no longer an argument to not perform such quality control. The classical 2D X-rays still maintain their purpose, as the acquisition is even faster than 3D series and has less of a radiant effect. In this way, the interest of a 2D/3D platform such as O-Arm for functional neurosurgery seems obvious: 3D datasets for automatic registrations and 2D projective X-rays for control. This will lower the patient irradiation and shorten the surgical procedure.

Robot-assisted biopsy is a safe and efficient neurosurgical procedure. Nevertheless, the current complication rate is similar to those of the first reported series [15]. The main axis of improvement is the development of new planning tools. The main source of potentially life-threatening complications, including cerebral hematoma, is the human error during trajectory planification. Errors can be made by the most experienced neurosurgeon despite adequate preoperative brain imaging. The assistance tool will probably be assistance software. It has to be kept in mind that the neurosurgeon is not a computer scientist and, in many cases, has limited time to perform trajectory planning. In this way, future software should be simplified and offer fast results. Sainte-Anne Hospital's group is currently working on finding simplified solutions to be easily incorporated into the surgical procedure, considering the limitations discussed thus far.

References

1. Spiegel EA, Wycis HT, Marks M, Lee AJ. Stereotaxic apparatus for operations on the human brain. Science. 1947;106(2754):349–50.
2. Daumas-Duport C, Szikla G, Vedrenne C. Stereotactic serial cerebral biopsies. Methodology (author's transl). Arch Anat Cytol Pathol. 1979;27(3):135–9.
3. Callovini GM, Telera S, Sherkat S, Sperduti I, Callovini T, Carapella CM. How is stereotactic brain biopsy evolving? A multicentric analysis of a series of 421 cases treated in Rome over the last sixteen years. Clin Neurol Neurosurg. 2018;174:101–7.
4. Kongkham PN, Knifed E, Tamber MS, Bernstein M. Complications in 622 cases of frame-based stereotactic biopsy, a decreasing procedure. Can J Neurol Sci J Can Sci Neurol. 2008;35(1):79–84.
5. Maciunas RJ, Galloway RL, Latimer JW. The application accuracy of stereotactic frames. Neurosurgery. 1994;35(4):682–94; discussion 694–695.
6. Galloway RL, Maciunas RJ. Stereotactic neurosurgery. Crit Rev Biomed Eng. 1990;18(3):181–205.
7. Kwoh YS, Hou J, Jonckheere EA, Hayati S. A robot with improved absolute positioning accuracy for CT guided stereotactic brain surgery. IEEE Trans Biomed Eng. 1988;35(2):153–60.
8. Benabid AL, Cinquin P, Lavalle S, Le Bas JF, Demongeot J, de Rougemont J. Computer-driven robot for stereotactic surgery connected to CT scan and magnetic resonance imaging. Technological design and preliminary results. Appl Neurophysiol. 1987;50(1–6):153–4.
9. Marcus HJ, Hughes-Hallett A, Cundy TP, Yang G-Z, Darzi A, Nandi D. da Vinci robot-assisted keyhole neurosurgery: a cadaver study on feasibility and safety. Neurosurg Rev. 2015;38(2):367–71; discussion 371.
10. Neudorfer C, Hunsche S, Hellmich M, El Majdoub F, Maarouf M. Comparative study of robot-assisted versus conventional frame-based deep brain stimulation stereotactic neurosurgery. Stereotact Funct Neurosurg. 2018;96(5):327–34.
11. Talairach J. Destruction of the anterior ventral thalamic nucleus in the treatment of mental diseases. Rev Neurol (Paris). 1952;87(4):352–7.
12. Bancaud J, Angelergues R, Bernouilli C, Bonis A, Bordas-Ferrer M, Bresson M, et al. Functional stereotaxic exploration (SEEG) of epilepsy. Electroencephalogr Clin Neurophysiol. 1970;28(1):85–6.

13. Yasin H, Hoff H-J, Blümcke I, Simon M. Experience with 102 frameless stereotactic biopsies using the neuromate robotic device. World Neurosurg mars. 2019;123:e450–6.
14. Zanello M, Roux A, Senova S, Peeters S, Edjlali M, Tauziede-Espariat A, et al. Robot-assisted stereotactic biopsies in 377 consecutive adult patients with supratentorial diffuse gliomas: diagnostic yield, safety, and postoperative outcomes. World Neurosurg. 2021;148:e301–13.
15. Marcus HJ, Vakharia VN, Ourselin S, Duncan J, Tisdall M, Aquilina K. Robot-assisted stereotactic brain biopsy: systematic review and bibliometric analysis. Childs Nerv Syst. 2018;34(7):1299–309.
16. Zanello M, Roux A, Debacker C, Peeters S, Edjlali-Goujon M, Dhermain F, et al. Postoperative intracerebral haematomas following stereotactic biopsies: Poor planning or poor execution? Int J Med Robot Comput Assist Surg MRCAS. 2021;17(2):e2211.
17. Zanello M, Carron R, Peeters S, Gori P, Roux A, Bloch I, et al. Automated neurosurgical stereotactic planning for intraoperative use: a comprehensive review of the literature and perspectives. Neurosurg Rev. 2021;44:867–88.
18. Bradac O, Steklacova A, Nebrenska K, Vrana J, de Lacy P, Benes V. Accuracy of VarioGuide frameless stereotactic system against frame-based stereotaxy: prospective, randomized, single-center study. World Neurosurg. 2017;104:831–40.
19. Verploegh ISC, Volovici V, Haitsma IK, Schouten JW, Dirven CM, Kros JM, et al. Contemporary frameless intracranial biopsy techniques: might variation in safety and efficacy be expected? Acta Neurochir. 2015;157(11):2011–6.
20. Li QH, Zamorano L, Pandya A, Perez R, Gong J, Diaz F. The application accuracy of the NeuroMate robot—a quantitative comparison with frameless and frame-based surgical localization systems. Comput Aided Surg Off J Int Soc Comput Aided Surg. 2002;7(2):90–8.
21. Vakharia VN, Rodionov R, Miserocchi A, McEvoy AW, O'Keeffe A, Granados A, et al. Comparison of robotic and manual implantation of intracerebral electrodes: a single-centre, single-blinded, randomised controlled trial. Sci Rep. 2021;11(1):17,127.
22. Krieg SM, Meyer B. First experience with the jump-starting robotic assistance device Cirq. Neurosurg Focus. 2018;45(VideoSuppl1):V3.

Chapter 12
Robot-Assisted Drug Delivery to the Brain

Neil Barua, Alison Bienemann, and Angelo Pichierri

A Brief History of Drug Delivery to the Brain

For many years, neurosurgeons have endeavoured to develop methods of direct drug delivery to the brain in order to bypass the blood–brain barrier (BBB). The BBB represents a physical and physiological barrier to the transfer of many therapeutic molecules from the bloodstream into the brain, thus limiting the efficacy of systemic treatments for a wide range of neurological conditions including neurodegenerative diseases and brain tumours.

Much of the historical research focus has been directed towards developing neuroprotective and neurorestorative strategies for Parkinson's Disease and chemotherapeutic innovations for high grade glioma. Direct drug delivery to the brain has particular relevance for the amelioration of Parkinson's Disease and intrinsic brain tumours, where there is an apparent surgical target. However, this novel method of drug delivery has potential applications to a wide range of neurological disorders including Huntington's disease, Alzheimer's disease and drug-resistant epilepsy.

N. Barua (✉) · A. Pichierri
Department of Neurosurgery, Southmead Hospital, Bristol, UK
e-mail: Neil.Barua@nbt.nhs.uk; Angelo.Pichierri@nbt.nhs.uk

A. Bienemann
Functional Neurosurgery Research Group, Learning and Research, University of Bristol, Bristol, UK
e-mail: Alison.Bienemann@bristol.ac.uk

J. A. González Martínez, F. Cardinale (eds.), *Robotics in Neurosurgery*,
https://doi.org/10.1007/978-3-031-08380-8_12

Intraventricular Infusion

Initial investigations focused on intraventricular infusion of neurotrophins including glial cell line-derived neurotrophic factor (GDNF) and neurturin (NTN) in rodent and non-human primate (NHP) models of Parkinson's disease (PD) [1–3]. Infusion of GDNF into the ventricles of rats results in widespread diffusion of GDNF into surrounding brain parenchyma including the cerebral cortex, striatum, substantia nigra, hypothalamus, and the ventral tegmental area. In rat models of PD, intraventricular infusion of GDNF successfully induced both locomotor improvements and increased striatal dopamine turnover. However, these early studies also identified one of the major potential pitfalls of intraventricular infusion—off-target side effects; increased hypothalamic dopamine led to cachexia and weight loss in experimental animals. In order to determine whether this was simply a consequence of the small volume of the rodent brain, intraventricular infusion therapies were tested in NHP models.

The neuroprotective and neurorestorative effects of intraventricular infusion of neurotrophins were once again confirmed in NHP models of PD. However, analysis of the intraparenchymal distribution of the infused therapy following intraventricular administration revealed the second potential pitfall and potential barrier to clinical translation—the large molecular size of the GDNF neurotrophin limited diffusion through the ependyma, thus preventing effective delivery to the caudate nucleus or putamen in NHP models. Again, these experimental studies identified weight loss and dyskinesias as off-target side effects of drug delivery into the ventricle.

Not surprisingly the first randomised double-blind placebo-controlled trial of intraventricular infusion of GDNF in 50 patients failed to achieve its primary end point with participants reporting significant side effects (hyponatraemia, anorexia, weight loss, nausea, vomiting, and Lhermitte's phenomenon), without improvements in the clinical manifestations of PD [4].

Intraparenchymal Drug Injection

Direct injection of therapies into the brain has also been extensively investigated in the pursuit of neuroprotective and neurorestorative treatments for PD. Intrastriatal injection of GDNF in rodents and intraputamenal injection of GDNF have both been shown to induce histological, biochemical and locomotor improvements in experimental models of PD.

Chronic intraputamenal infusions of GDNF and NTN in NHP models have been shown to result in substantial improvements in locomotor scores over a 3-month period when compared to control. However, analysis of drug distribution within the putamen again highlighted the challenges of achieving consistent, predictable and clinically relevant drug delivery with volumes of distribution ranging from less than 30% to over 90% of the entire putamen.

This variability and unpredictability has been implicated in the subsequent failure of clinical trials of intraputamenal infusion of GDNF. In a multicentre randomised controlled trial of intraparenchymal infusion of GDNF, 34 trial participants were randomised to either bilateral infusions of GDNF or placebo. The trial again failed to meet its primary endpoint as at 6 months, the GDNF cohort had failed to demonstrate the required improvement in clinical scores. Furthermore, neutralising antibodies were detected in 3 subjects, and the other 3 experienced serious device-related adverse events. The disappointing results of clinical trials of intraputamenal infusion of GDNF led to a re-appraisal of the state-of-the-art and a concerted effort to identify causative factors. Inadequate drug distribution within the target structure (the putamen) was again identified as a primary cause for the trial's disappointing results.

Contemporaneously, parallel studies of direct delivery of therapeutics into malignant gliomas were underway in a number of centres around the world. A wide range of therapeutics have been investigated including conventional chemotherapies, targeted toxins, viral vector-mediated gene therapies, radioisotopes and immunomodulators. To date, the tremendous potential of direct intratumoural drug delivery is yet to be realised in clinical studies. The results of the PRECISE phase 3 trial of intratumoural delivery of the targeted toxin IL13-PE38QQR (cintredekin besudotox) for Glioblastoma were reported in 2010 and again showed no benefit over standard treatment. The subsequent analysis of causative factors identified poor drug distribution, catheter design and infusion parameters as major contributors to the failure of the trial [5].

These factors led our group, and other groups around the world, to dedicate a programme of laboratory, preclinical and clinical research to the understanding and improvement of convection-enhanced drug delivery (CED), a novel method of direct drug delivery to the brain. By establishing a pressure gradient at the tip of an intraparenchymal microcatheter rather than relying on drug diffusion, CED offers a number of potential advantages over conventional drug infusion methods—homogeneous and highly targeted distribution of drug delivery to the brain through large and clinically relevant brain volumes, reduction in off-target side effects and minimisation of tissue trauma induced by catheter insertion and drug infusion. However, clinical translation of CED for the treatment of neurodegenerative and neuro-oncological disorders poses a number of significant challenges.

The Challenges of CED

Minimisation of Tissue Trauma

Analysis of the failed trials of intraputamenal neurotrophin infusion for PD and intratumoural drug delivery for GBM identified drug reflux as a major contributor to poor drug distribution and off-target side effects. Reflux describes the escape of infusate into the potential space at the catheter/brain interface, resulting in loss of therapeutic effect at the target site and uncontrolled dissemination of infusate into the various intracranial compartments. Reflux has been implicated in the development of adverse events in CED trials for glioblastoma such as skin irritation, and also in the development of neutralising antibodies against GDNF. Our own preclinical analysis of catheter design and implantation technique identified catheter materials, design and metrics (outer and inner diameter) as major drivers of optimal catheter performance. However, equally important was the method of catheter implantation—minimisation of tissue disruption at the brain/device interface proved of vital importance to the prevention of reflux.

Our early preclinical studies of catheter design and implantation in large animal (porcine) models utilised the Pathfinder image-guided neurosurgical robot (Armstrong Healthcare Ltd., UK) in order to provide a highly stable and accurate platform for delivery of catheters and instruments into the brain. Prior analysis of targeting accuracy in a brain phantom with the Pathfinder robot identified an application accuracy of 0.5 mm compared with 0.98 mm for conventional stereotactic frames.

Achieving Drug Distribution Through Clinically Relevant Brain Volumes

The success of clinical trials of direct drug delivery to the brain has been consistently undermined by inadequate drug delivery within the target structure. The distribution of a drug administered via CED is dependent upon a range of variables, in addition to the elimination of drug reflux:

- The physicochemical properties of the infusate
- The proximity of the catheter outflow to low resistance pathways (such as a necrotic tumour centre or perivascular space)
- Infusion parameters (rate and length of infusion)
- Clearance of the infusate through innate drainage pathways of the brain
- The ratio of the volume of infusion to the volume of drug distribution (Vi:Vd).

Whilst many of these variables are beyond the scope of this chapter, the final variable—Vi:Vd—can to a certain extent be optimised with the assistance of robotics. The volume of the human putamen is approximately $4cm^3$, whereas the target volume for a glioblastoma can range from anywhere from 10 to 300 cm^3. Infusion rates also have to be limited to the microlitres/minute range in order to prevent tissue trauma from excessively high flow rates. It quickly becomes apparent that in order to achieve homogeneous and predictable drug distribution through these large brain target volumes within clinically acceptable timeframes either very high flow rates (thus risking tissue trauma and reflux) or multiple catheters must be utilised. Although conventional stereotactic frames can be used to perform multiple catheter trajectories, this can be time-consuming, cumbersome and prone to human error. In our clinical trials of CED for Parkinson's disease, two catheters were implanted in each putamen with robotic assistance with the intention of addressing the pitfalls of prior studies of GDNF infusion. Robotic assistance facilitated rapid, highly accurate and reproducible implantation of multiple catheters in a software-driven surgical process [6, 7].

Robot-Assisted CED—Application in Parkinson's Disease and Neuro-Oncology

A Randomised Trial of Intermittent Intraputamenal Glial Cell Line-Derived Neurotrophic Factor in Parkinson's Disease

In 2019, we reported the results of a double-blind randomised trial of CED of GDNF in 42 subjects with moderately severe PD. In order to address the deficiencies of previous studies of intraputamenal drug delivery, we developed a novel implantable catheter system comprising four independent catheters and a transcutaneous bone-anchored port. The skull mounted port facilitated chronic intermittent drug delivery to the brain at 4 week intervals for 40 weeks.

Two catheters were implanted into each putamen using the Neuromate surgical robot (Fig. 12.1. Renishaw Plc., Gloucs., UK). Using this robotic system, we achieved highly accurate catheter targeting with a mean distance between the planned and actual target for the catheter tips of 0.6 ± 0.5 mm (range 0–2 mm). Test

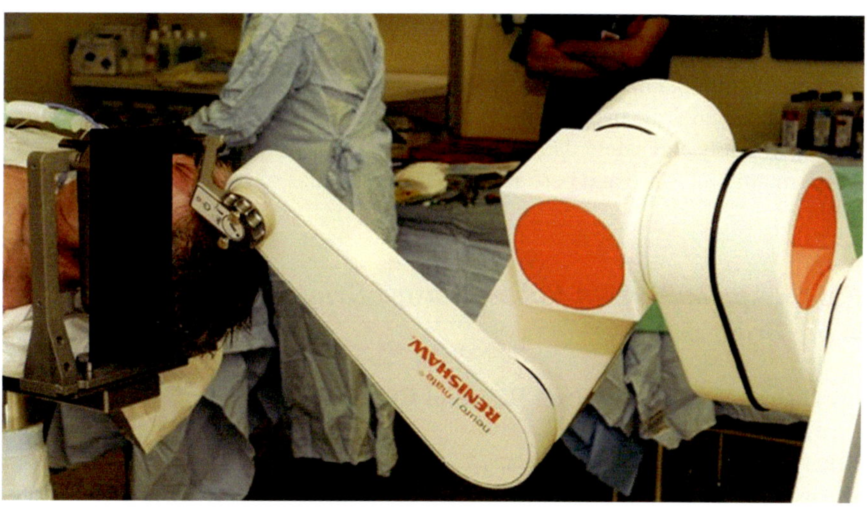

Fig. 12.1 Neuromate robot (Renishaw Plc., Gloucs., UK)

infusions of gadolinium were performed to ensure sufficient drug distribution before randomisation. Coverage of the total putamenal volume ranged from 47.8 to 55%. This distribution compares very favourably to estimates from prior trials of intraputamenal infusion in which the bioavailability of GDNF was estimated to be limited to less than 10% of the total putamen. No ischaemic or haemorrhagic events related to catheter implantation were identified, however, one participant suffered a mildly symptomatic ischaemic stroke, and one suffered an asymptomatic haemorrhage during their first infusions.

Despite these technological advances in catheter design and robot-assisted implantation, the trial failed to meet its primary endpoint of a predetermine reduction in mean OFF state UPDRS motor scores at week 40. However, 18F-DOPA imaging suggested a widespread biological effect from GDNF distribution throughout the putamen, indicating that the limitations of drug distribution seen in earlier trials had been overcome.

The same catheter system, skull-anchored port and robot-assisted implantation method were also used to deliver carboplatin to adults with recurrent and progressive glioblastoma and children with progressive diffuse intrinsic pontine glioma. One patient underwent re-resection of a recurrent left parietal GBM, followed by robot-assisted implantation of four catheters and a skull-anchored port. The trajectories for the catheters were planned to target areas of tumour enhancement and the infiltrated peri-tumoural penumbra. All catheters were implanted to within 1.5 mm of their planned target. The patient was recovered from anaesthetic, and a total volume of 27.9 mL of carboplatin was infused on two consecutive days. Further infusions were administered after an interval of 4 weeks on three consecutive days. Drug distribution was inferred from real-time T2-weighted MRI scans performed at multiple time points during and after infusions and indicated drug distribution throughout the targeted tumour volume and infiltrated peri-tumoural penumbra.

Follow-up imaging at 4 and 8 weeks post-infusion demonstrated a reduction in volume of enhancing tumour by almost 50%. Unfortunately, this response was short lived and further imaging confirmed significant tumour recurrence. We believe that the failure to achieve a sustained response was more likely attributable to the deficiencies of carboplatin as an anti-tumour agent than to the methodology of catheter implantation and drug distribution. The procedure did however confirm the feasibility of accurately and safely delivering microcatheters with robotic assistance to the peri-tumoural interface and performing repeat infusions of chemotherapy [8].

Future Applications of Robot-Assisted Drug Delivery to the Brain

Local Drug Delivery for Drug-Resistant Epilepsies

Drug-resistant epilepsies (DRE) may—in fact—not necessarily be drug resistant in all cases. The suggested mechanisms for medically refractory epilepsies include (amongst others) alterations of drug uptake into the brain, inadequate passage across a BBB in response to the chronic drug administration, pharmacokinetic alterations in the periphery [9]. Increasing AED dosage can only be done up to a point after which systemic or neurological adverse effects arise.

Systemic DRE (sysDRE) would be therefore more accurate in describing these cases [10]. For many patients with sysDRE, surgical resection is not an option at all due to a poorly localised or undefinable seizure focus, the occurrence of a mirror focus in the contralateral hemisphere, the existence of multiple seizure foci, too widespread an epilepsy network, generalised onset epilepsy, unacceptable surgical risks or expected unwanted postoperative adverse effects [10]. New ways of systemic delivery—such as nose-to-brain [11] and closed-loop "smart" intermittent drug release [12]—are under investigation. Delivering drugs directly to the brain (local drug delivery, LDD) seems to be a more promising and all-around way to bypass the issues causing sysDRE: a PubMed query about the topic "Brain drug delivery" returned 8000 papers in the last decade, of which about 300 are related to epilepsy. Most of them are at a preclinical stage. Generalised or focal onset epilepsies differ from each other for pathways and mechanisms: two distinct research lines would be required, but current experimental studies on LDD concentrate on focal onset epilepsies [10].

What emerges from these studies is that the beneficial effect of LDD comes from a combination of symptomatic seizure suppression (short-term) and neuromodulation of seizure networks (long-term) [10]. LDD is the chemical/biological response to electrical open-(DBS/SANTE, VNS) and closed-loop (RNS) solutions, with the promise of a higher versatility and control [13–15].

Silencing an epileptogenic zone (EZ)—instead of resecting it—is an attractive option due to the reversibility of the effect and the possibility to selectively suppress the regional hyperexcitability while maintaining the possible useful residual function of the involved neurons, particularly for EZ within the so-called eloquent brain areas [13].

While most of the literature investigates the feasibility of LDD to neocortical and limbic sites, another promising group of targets is represented by subcortical structures, particularly basal ganglia, for their crucial involvement in seizure propagation and remote modulation on seizure initiation [16]; it is remarkable that these structure are involved not only during secondary generalisation, but even during focal seizures [17]. The substantia nigra (pars reticularis) and the subthalamic nucleus seem to be particularly relevant targets for their non-selective role in the control and propagation of different types of epilepsies/seizures [18–20]; other possible targets include the ventral midbrain (via GABA modulation), the dorsal striatum (via dopamine modulation); and selected thalamic nuclei [10]. The concept of neuromodulation, as opposed to a simple seizure disruption, is even more relevant in this context. These targets may be effective for the treatment of cases where the EZ cannot be identified or extends to multiple nodes/extended networks [18]. They also represent an attractive field of research for generalised onset epilepsy [18].

Experimental challenges remain regarding the appropriate drug selection, type of administration (acute vs intermittent vs on demand), bi- vs unilateral targeting and, not least important, side effects (due to the complex and overlapping networks regulated by these structures).

Main Directions of Research

LDD research lines have forked in different strategies:

- Wafers/Bioceramics: bulky and only suitable for diffusible compounds; offer a highly non-uniform, limited extend of delivery; they are burdened from the issue of pharmacological tolerance due to the continuous drug release [13].
- Nanoparticles (polymers, nanotubes, liposomes, dendrimers): some of the solutions can be administered systemically (orally/intravenously/intranasally), with the associated drugs or prodrugs being released directly into the brain. Advantages include increase of systemic circulation half-life; reduction of side effects; suitability for poorly soluble drugs and lipid-soluble molecules larger >1 kDa that wouldn't otherwise cross the BBB. Drawbacks include rapid clearance from bloodstream and accumulation in liver/spleen, with toxicity issues for non-degradable particles [21].
- Passive diffusion using epidural, subdural, transmeningeal, intracerebroventricular (ICV) or intraparenchymal systems, via implants or acute injections. Main common disadvantages of these systems are related to the fluid dynamics that govern the passive diffusion process [13]: slow effect due to highly tortuous and inhomogeneous brain tissue (e.g. pial surfaces); small and inconsistent distribution volume (a few millimetres); non-uniform concentration distribution; rapid clearance due to CSF and capillary efflux; thus suitability is limited to diffusible and small substances. The ICV route has the hypothetical advantages of being easier to realise (non-robotic procedures) and of offering a widespread diffusion through CSF, which could be desirable if a whole-brain effect is wanted and an appropriate drug is found to be effective and non-toxic at the same time. In practice, though, its efficacy and applicability are limited by the exponential concentration decay of the infused compound, its rapid CSF clearance (4–5 h) and the challenge of finding such an ideal drug [13].
- Closed-loop devices: the most known closed-loop device is the responsive neurostimulator for seizures (RCS). This is a FDA-approved, commercially available device which employs electrical impulses to disrupt the seizure propagation after having detected its onset [14]; it is therefore crucial that the electrode(s) is/are inserted as near as possible to the seizure onset zone(s). At an experimental preclinical level, similar closed-loop technologies are being coupled with focal cooling [22] and some drug delivery solutions [10, 23] to provide an "on demand" delivery which seems to be effective in resolving the drug tolerance issue linked to the continuous infusion.
- Gene therapy: attractive perspective for biological molecules that would need frequent refilling or would be unstable if kept in subcutaneous reservoirs (at body temperature). It opens the way to modulations with a higher level of complexity and micro-environmental feedback (e.g. epigenetic pathways, multi-gene regulation, regional neural networks interactions) [24].
  - ex vivo: Embryonic or neuronal stem cells can be cultured, engineered to secrete neurotransmitters, neuromodulators and/or peptides. The enriched

phenotypes cells are then screened for transduction-induced defects prior to transplantation in the host, where they will modulate the hyperexcitability of the nearby cells (bystander effect) [25]. The transplant can be encapsulated (encapsulated cell biodelivery, ECB), to allow more control and possible removal of the grafted cells, or freely released into the targeted neural environment with the possibility of integration for a more complex interaction [25].

A relevant advantage is the lack of reservoirs, pumps, polymers, carriers, batteries, or electric devices, but several issues still remain open [25]: efficiency of integration with the surrounding environment; incorrect migration to target position, possible apoptosis/necrosis (enhancement with anti-apoptotic/neurotrophic factors is being studied), possible inflammatory reaction (ECB should reduce this risk); unstable action and lack of control, especially for unencapsulated cell grafts, for which rescue strategies must be found prior to any clinical application. Gene therapy would also be suitable for biological compounds only (e.g. GABA, adenosine, recombinant growth factors, peptides).

- in vivo: host cells can be engineered to release therapeutic substances via viral vectors. This method overcomes the problems related to integration/rejection of ex vivo manipulated cells. Concerns exist regarding the possibility of inflammatory response to the host cells; transduction efficiency and precision; insertional/transduction-induced mutagenesis; complex transgene regulation effects; undesired transduction of several neural phenotypes or off-target cells [25].

- Convection-enhanced delivery (CED): the potential advantages of this technique and the application to robotics described above also apply to LDD in epilepsy where target structure may have complex shapes and require multiple catheters. The ability of combining it with other methods (nanoparticles, gene therapy, stem cells closed-loop devices) further enhances its potentials [10, 13, 21].
- MicroFIP (microfluidic electrophoretic ion pump): a very promising line of research which also offers precise spatial-temporal drug delivery and overcomes the problems related to catheter clogging and fluid reflux, common to both passive diffusion and CED. The associated reservoir would have a long lifespan as it would only deliver the drug without its solvent, with negligible local pressure increase. The concentrated drug also provides a powerful action that allows a discontinuous infusion. Association to a closed-loop actuation would also allow on demand delivery [23].

Promising Studies

A number of papers have been published using various molecules such as growth factors, peptides, hormones (progesterone), phenytoin, valproate, inhibitory substances (GABA, muscimol, adenosine), systemically toxic substances (omega-conotoxin, botulinum), tiagabine, carisbamate [13, 21, 24, 26]. We will briefly summarise the ones we think more illustrative of the potentialities of LDD.

ω-conotoxins have been used in rat amygdala-kindling models (CED infusion), targeting their temporo-mesial structures. The depressant effect of these toxins on the calcium influx in presynaptic terminals suppresses presynaptic transmission, inhibiting spontaneous and evoked epileptiform discharges [13].

Botulinum neurotoxins A/B: rat amygdala-kindling models received a unilateral hippocampus infusion via CED, based on the rationale that these toxins cause a long-lasting inhibition of glutamate release. This resulted in an inhibition of focal seizures and their generalisation and in a neuroprotective action toward the hippocampal cells [10].

Dynorphins: These neuropeptides act as endogenous modulators of neuronal excitability. An adeno-associated virus has been used as a vector to deliver preprodynorphin into the mTLE of rodents models, resulting in a long-term suppression of seizures to up to 6 months (until the end of the observation period) after a single application [27].

Adenosine stem cells: Adenosine is an endogenous neuromodulator, whose intra- and extracellular concentrations are regulated by a passive nucleoside transporter. Extracellular adenosine concentration rapidly rises during seizures and binds to the inhibitory presynaptic A1 receptor that has a role in the termination of the seizure through a pathway which modulates the Ca^+ and K^+ channels. Adenosine is metabolised by the adenosine kinase (ADK) which increases with epilepsy progression, causing a relative depletion of the adenosine levels. Adenosine cannot be given systemically because its severe side effects (bradycardia, hypotension and hypothermia). Experiments targeting rat hippocampi using various delivery systems (osmotic mini-pumps, "ex-vivo" and "in-vivo" cell-base therapies) led to seizure reduction of 33% with no side effects [28].

Valproate: An ICV device (continuous CSF infusion) has been used to chronically administer valproate in patients already on oral valproate and poor seizure control. The study reported a recovered anticonvulsant effect with a reduced systemic toxicity, although burdened from adverse effects such as nausea and loss of appetite [29]. While this contribution confirms the concept of sysDRE, it also confirms the limitations of LDD using ICV systems.

Muscimol microparticles were administered intraparenchymally in various animal models with various strategies, including "on demand" systems using closed-loop devices. Diffusion to nearby regions was noted, with both toxicity and improved seizure control due to the seizure modulation of the tissue surrounding the EZ. A clinical study was carried out on three patients, using a temporary (12/24 h) infusion via CED, mostly for testing its safety rather than for establishing a therapeutic benefit, due to the short-living nature of the trial, the infusion didn't cause any adverse reaction and caused significant seizure reduction effect in one patient [30].

Benefits and Drawbacks of Robotics in Drug Delivery to the Brain

Our experience of convection-enhanced drug delivery to the brain in neurodegenerative and neuro-oncological conditions supports the use of robotic assistance in achieving rapid, highly accurate, reproducible and minimally traumatic implantations of multiple catheters. The high cost nature of these technologies remains a potential barrier to widespread use. However, the tremendous potential of CED is yet to be realised in clinical trials, highlighting the urgent need to identify and develop more effective therapeutics which will facilitate application to a wide range of neurological conditions.

References

1. Gimenez F, Krauze MT, Valles F, Hadaczek P, Bringas J, Sharma N, et al. Image-guided convection-enhanced delivery of GDNF protein into monkey putamen. NeuroImage. 2011;54(Suppl 1):S189–95.
2. Taylor H, Barua N, Bienemann A, Wyatt M, Castrique E, Foster R, et al. Clearance and toxicity of recombinant methionyl human glial cell line-derived neurotrophic factor (r-metHu GDNF) following acute convection-enhanced delivery into the striatum. PLoS One. 2013;8(3):e56186.
3. Gasmi M, Herzog CD, Brandon EP, Cunningham JJ, Ramirez GA, Ketchum ET, et al. Striatal delivery of neurturin by CERE-120, an AAV2 vector for the treatment of dopaminergic neuron degeneration in Parkinson's disease. Mol Ther. 2007;15(1):62–8.
4. Nutt JG, Burchiel KJ, Comella CL, Jankovic J, Lang AE, Laws ER, et al. Randomized, double-blind trial of glial cell line-derived neurotrophic factor (GDNF) in PD. Neurology. 2003;60(1):69–73.
5. Kunwar S, Chang S, Westphal M, Vogelbaum M, Sampson J, Barnett G, et al. Phase III randomized trial of CED of IL13-PE38QQR vs Gliadel wafers for recurrent glioblastoma. Neuro-Oncology. 2010;12(8):871–81.
6. Whone A, Luz M, Boca M, Woolley M, Mooney L, Dharia S, et al. Randomized trial of intermittent intraputamenal glial cell line-derived neurotrophic factor in Parkinson's disease. Brain. 2019;142(3):512–25.
7. Whone AL, Boca M, Luz M, Woolley M, Mooney L, Dharia S, et al. Extended treatment with glial cell line-derived neurotrophic factor in Parkinson's disease. J Parkinsons Dis. 2019;9(2):301–13.
8. Barua NU, Woolley M, Bienemann AS, Johnson DE, Lewis O, Wyatt MJ, et al. Intermittent convection-enhanced delivery to the brain through a novel transcutaneous bone-anchored port. J Neurosci Methods. 2013;214(2):223–32.
9. Löscher W, Potschka H, Sisodiya SM, Vezzani A. Drug resistance in epilepsy: clinical impact, potential mechanisms, and new innovative treatment options. Pharmacol Rev. 2020;72(3):606–38.
10. Gernert M, Feja M. Bypassing the blood-brain barrier: direct intracranial drug delivery in epilepsies. Pharmaceutics. 2020;12(12)
11. Musumeci T, Bonaccorso A, Puglisi G. Epilepsy disease and nose-to-brain delivery of polymeric nanoparticles: an overview. Pharmaceutics. 2019;11(3).

12. Yadav KS, Kapse-Mistry S, Peters GJ, Mayur YC. E-drug delivery: a futuristic approach. Drug Discov Today. 2019;24(4):1023–30.
13. Rogawski MA. Convection-enhanced delivery in the treatment of epilepsy. Neurotherapeutics. 2009;6(2):344–51.
14. Sisterson ND, Wozny TA, Kokkinos V, Constantino A, Richardson RM. Closed-loop brain stimulation for drug-resistant epilepsy: towards an evidence-based approach to personalized medicine. Neurotherapeutics. 2019;16(1):119–27.
15. Salanova V, Witt T, Worth R, Henry TR, Gross RE, Nazzaro JM, et al. Long-term efficacy and safety of thalamic stimulation for drug-resistant partial epilepsy. Neurology. 2015;84(10):1017–25.
16. Sisterson ND, Kokkinos V. Neuromodulation of epilepsy networks. Neurosurg Clin N Am. 2020;31(3):459–70.
17. Blumenfeld H, McNally KA, Vanderhill SD, Paige AL, Chung R, Davis K, et al. Positive and negative network correlations in temporal lobe epilepsy. Cereb Cortex. 2004;14(8):892–902.
18. Vuong J, Devergnas A. The role of the basal ganglia in the control of seizure. J Neural Transm. 2018;125(3):531–45.
19. Gale K. Subcortical structures and pathways involved in convulsive seizure generation. J Clin Neurophysiol. 1992;9(2):264–77.
20. Gernert M. Intrasubthalamic cell transplants for epilepsy therapy: hopes and concerns. Neuroreport. 2013;24(18):1062–6.
21. Bennewitz MF, Saltzman WM. Nanotechnology for delivery of drugs to the brain for epilepsy. Neurotherapeutics. 2009;6(2):323–36.
22. Hata K, Fujiwara K, Inoue T, Abe T, Kubo T, Yamakawa T, et al. Epileptic seizure suppression by focal brain cooling with recirculating coolant cooling system: modeling and simulation. IEEE Trans Neural Syst Rehabil Eng. 2019;27(2):162–71.
23. Proctor CM, Slézia A, Kaszas A, Ghestem A, Del Agua I, Pappa A-M, et al. Electrophoretic drug delivery for seizure control. Sci Adv. 2018;4(8):eaau1291.
24. Kobow K, Auvin S, Jensen F, Löscher W, Mody I, Potschka H, et al. Finding a better drug for epilepsy: antiepileptogenesis targets. Epilepsia. 2012;53(11):1868–76.
25. Falcicchia C, Simonato M, Verlengia G. New tools for epilepsy therapy. Front Cell Neurosci. 2018;12:147.
26. Van Dycke A, Raedt R, Vonck K, Boon P. Local delivery strategies in epilepsy: a focus on adenosine. Seizure. 2011;20(5):376–82.
27. Agostinho AS, Mietzsch M, Zangrandi L, Kmiec I, Mutti A, Kraus L, et al. Dynorphin-based "release on demand" gene therapy for drug-resistant temporal lobe epilepsy. EMBO Mol Med. 2019;11(10):e9963.
28. Güttinger M, Padrun V, Pralong WF, Boison D. Seizure suppression and lack of adenosine A1 receptor desensitization after focal long-term delivery of adenosine by encapsulated myoblasts. Exp Neurol. 2005;193(1):53–64.
29. Cook M, Murphy M, Bulluss K, D'Souza W, Plummer C, Priest E, et al. Anti-seizure therapy with a long-term, implanted intra-cerebroventricular delivery system for drug-resistant epilepsy: a first-in-man study. EClinicalMedicine. 2020;22:100326.
30. Heiss JD, Argersinger DP, Theodore WH, Butman JA, Sato S, Khan OI. Convection-enhanced delivery of muscimol in patients with drug-resistant epilepsy. Neurosurgery. 2019;85(1):E4–E15.

Chapter 13
Robotics in Radiosurgery

Ajay Niranjan, Zaid A. Siddique, Cihat Ozhasoglu, and L. Dade Lunsford

Brief History of Radiosurgery

Lars Leksell proposed the concept of radiosurgery and how it could be accomplished in a landmark article published in 1951 [1]. The first prototype Gamma Knife was constructed in 1967, and the first Gamma Knife surgery (GKS) was carried out for a craniopharyngioma patient on October 25th of that year Even though Leksell's original concept of the Gamma knife was a functional tool for pain, movement disorders, and refractory behavioral disorders. Between this date and the 1983 installation of a new gamma knife in Buenos Aires, Argentina, Stockholm was the only place in the world where GKS was offered. Shortly afterwards in 1984, the fourth constructed Gamma Knife was installed in Sheffield, England. The fifth GK was installed in Pittsburgh in 1987. Prior to the establishment of the GK in Pittsburgh, the predominant indications for GKS were management of vascular malformations, acoustic neuromas, and pituitary tumors. With the installation in Pittsburgh and the subsequent proliferation of GK centers in the US and elsewhere, the published evidence in favor of SRS for benign tumors rapidly increased [2, 3]. In the first years of the 90s, the treatment of brain metastases with GK began, but initially only for solitary tumors. These lesions often regressed after the procedure and it wasn't long before neurosurgeons started treating multiple metastases with radiosurgery.

A. Niranjan (✉) · L. D. Lunsford
Department of Neurological Surgery, University of Pittsburgh Medical Center, Pittsburgh, USA
e-mail: niraax@upmc.edu; niranjana@upmc.edu; lunsld@upmc.edu

Z. A. Siddique · C. Ozhasoglu
Department of Radiation Oncology, University of Pittsburgh Medical Center, Pittsburgh, PA, USA
e-mail: siddiquiza@upmc.edu; ozhacx@upmc.edu

J. A. González Martínez, F. Cardinale (eds.), *Robotics in Neurosurgery*,
https://doi.org/10.1007/978-3-031-08380-8_13

In the late 80s, an increasing number of institutions started doing SRS with other technologies such as linear accelerators adapted for use in stereotactic conditions and later with dedicated linear accelerator such as CyberKnife®. This growing adoption of the methodology of SRS has helped in the exponential growth and adaptation if radiosurgery.

Several factors have contributed to the exponential growth of SRS. First and foremost is the developments in neuroimaging since the introduction of the CT scanner. Equally important is the contribution of advances in computers that led to improvement in the dose planning capabilities. And finally advances in robotics and its incorporation in dose delivery system led to improvements in safety and precision of delivery of focused radiation to a target in the head.

Introduction of Robotics in Radiosurgery

The difficultly of loading and reloading the original Gamma Unit (U type unit) led to redesign of the source configuration in more of donut type array. This configuration (B Unit) allowed cobalt source loading using a robotic arm and therefore significantly reduced the down time. Patient care with the B unit began in 1996. The patient set up for each target was still manual in the unit. The users not only needed to change the collimator helmets manually using a forklift but also needed to set stereotactic coordinate for each target which were triple checked (by another physician and a physicist). This needed time and resources form a dedicated GK team comprising of neurosurgeons, radiation oncologists, medical physicists, fellows, residents, and nurses. Because of time taken in change of collimator helmet changes (about 10 min) and isocenter targets (6 min), most dose plans were designed using the minimum possible isocenters and beam diameters (helmets). The addition of automated positioning system (APS), a robotic positioning technology allowed modification of the existing B unit to C unit and 4-C with the robotic retrofit. With the introduction of APS (Fig. 13.1), GK team only needed to set the patient for the first target and the APS would automatically move patients head to all the planned target to complete the treatment. Use of the APS lead to significant improvements in safety and reduced overall time spent in dose delivery. The APS also led to significantly improved dose plans (i.e., better 3D conformality and improved radiation fall off outside the target, a feature called selectivity). Now multi-isocenter plans could be created without worrying about the dose delivery time. The robotic APS represented huge improvement in GK SRS as it not only reduced radiation delivery time but also improved the SRS patient experience.

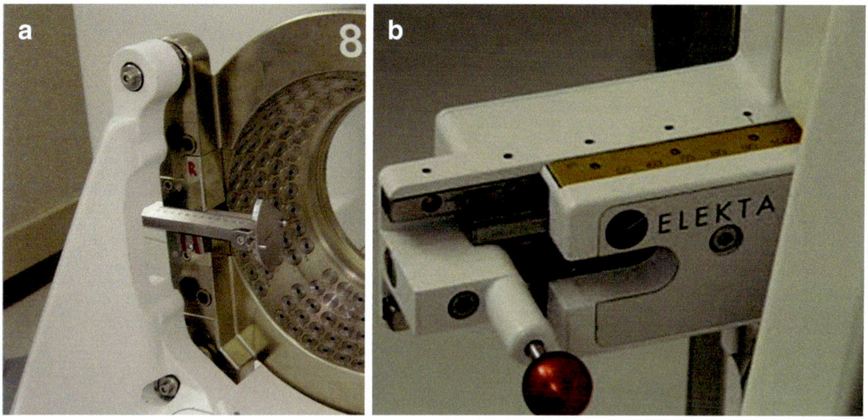

Fig. 13.1 In earlier versions of Gamma Knife manual set up of each isocenter using Trunnions (A) was required. In model C and 4 C, the first robotic isocenter set up (automated positioning system) was introduced (B)

Incorporation of Advanced Robotics

The care of patients with multiple brain metastases had become a fast-growing indication for radiosurgery by 2005. Two main problems associated with radiosurgery for these patients included the relatively long treatment times required to treat each patient and the difficulty of irradiating tumors located at the extreme limits of the brain. Although the APS technology obviated the need to manually adjust each set of coordinates for a multiple-isocenter plan, the APS had a reduced range in the X (59–141) and Y (40–160) dimensions. Because of these limitations, tumors located outside the central brain range needed treatment using a manual set up mode where trunnions were anchored to the stereotactic frame and adjusted to place the target isocenter at the focus of the 201 photon beams. Thus, in a patient with multiple metastases some tumors could be treated with the APS, but others required manual set up for x, y, and z coordinates using the standard trunnion mode. The changeover from APS to trunnion mode and manual coordinate set up on an average took 10 and 6 min, respectively, for each isocenter. This led to longer treatment times for patients who often had multiple medical comorbidities.

To solve these issues, a unique collaboration between industry and a brain trust of experienced and interested neurosurgeons, engineers, robotics experts, medical physicists, radiobiologists, and radiation oncologists was established under the direction of the Swedish manufacturer AB Elekta. A new model Leksell Gamma knife known as LGK- PERFEXION was designed to make all targets reachable in a fully robotic mode. The patient bed became the robot. This greatly facilitated the treatment of patients with multiple brain metastases.

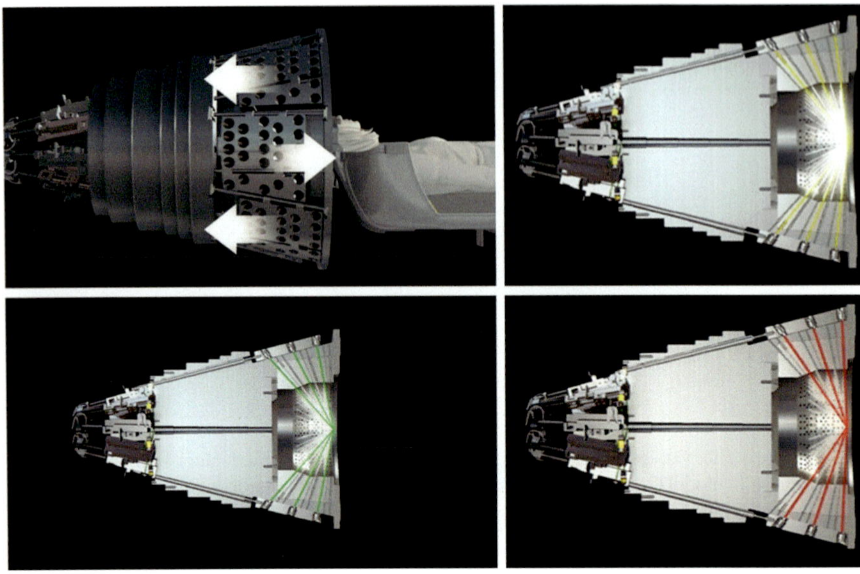

Fig. 13.2 The collimator body of LGK Icon has 8 sectors of 24 collimators. Robotic motors move the sectors to home, 4 mm, 8 mm, 16 mm and block positions. Photo courtesy of Elekta

The Leksell Gamma Knife PERFEXION or PFX (Elekta Instrument AB, Stockholm, Sweden) (LGK PFX) was introduced in 2006. This radiation unit was redesigned with entirely new beam geometry. A total of 192 60Co sources are arranged in a cylindrical configuration in five rings. In LGK PFX, primary and secondary collimators were replaced by a single large 120 mm thick tungsten collimator array ring (Fig. 13.2). Consequently, no external collimator helmets were needed for the LGK PFX system. The tungsten collimator array contained eight identical but independent sectors, each with 72 collimators (24 collimators for 4 mm, 24 collimators for 8 mm, and 24 collimators for 16 mm). Collimator size for each sector could be changed robotically by moving 24 sources over selected collimator set. A sector with 24 sources could be moved independently of other sectors to obtain five different positions: (1) home position when the system was in standby mode, (2) 4 mm collimator, (3) 8 mm collimator, (4) 16 mm collimator, and (5) sector off position—a position between 4- and 8-mm collimators providing blocking of all 24 beams for the sector (Fig. 13.3). Although the treatable volume was increased by more than 300% compared to previous models, the average distance from the cobalt source to focus was very close to previous models due to a better collimator system (120 mm tungsten ring). The enhanced treatment volume (more than three times) allowed for a greater mechanical treatment range in *X*/*Y*/*Z* dimension. The mechanical range in *X*/*Y*/*Z* dimension was 160/180/220 mm for LGK PFX system compared to 100/120/165 mm for other gamma knife models. This greater range allows treatment of tumors especially multiple metastatic tumors anywhere in the brain.

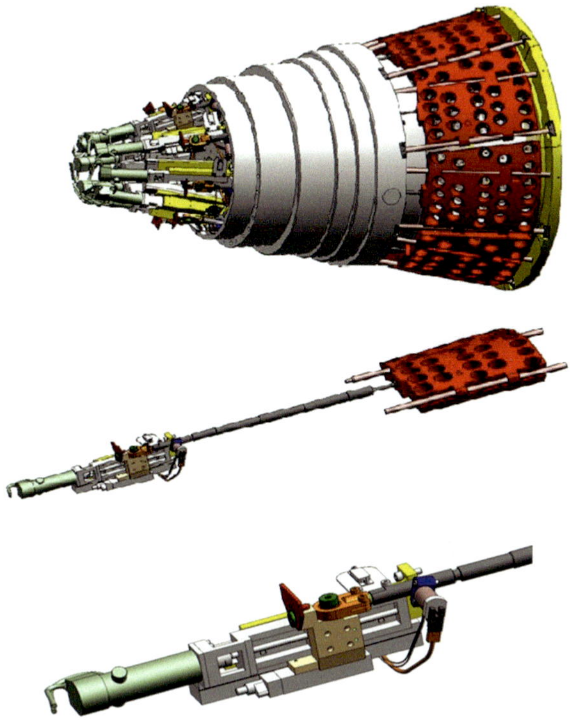

Fig. 13.3 Diagrammatic representation of collimator body showing individual sector and the motor that drives the sector to different positions. Photo courtesy of Elekta

The Automatic Positioning System (APS) of LGK earlier models C and 4C was replaced by a robotic Patient Positioning System (PPS) in the LGK PFX system. In PPS, instead of moving only the patient's head, the whole body of the patient lying on the PPS was moved into the pre-selected stereotactic coordinates. Manual stereotactic coordinate set up as used on LGK C and 4C was fully replaced by the robotic PPS in LGK PFX. The entirely redesigned hardware of LGK PFX also significantly impacted on the treatment planning performed by the Leksell GammaPlan. Robotics allowed creation of isocenters composed of different beam diameters. Such composite shots could optimize dose distribution shapes for each individual shot.

At the University of Pittsburgh Medical Center (UPMC), the efficient LGK PFX was installed in September 2007. Highly conformal plans comprising of many isocenters, each of differing collimator size and composition could be achieved with shortened treatment times. Over time, we noted a gradual increase in the number of isocenters used per plan. The treatment of multiple metastases with the LGK PFX particularly demonstrated its superior efficiency in treatment delivery [4, 5]. Patients with brain metastases also benefited from the increased treatment range.

The most recent GK device LGK Icon took the basics of LGK PFX and added a modification to include cone-beam CT technology (Fig. 13.4). This allowed in certain cases the standard G frame to be replaced with a mask-based fixation system (Fig. 13.5). A high-definition motion management system tracks the position of a

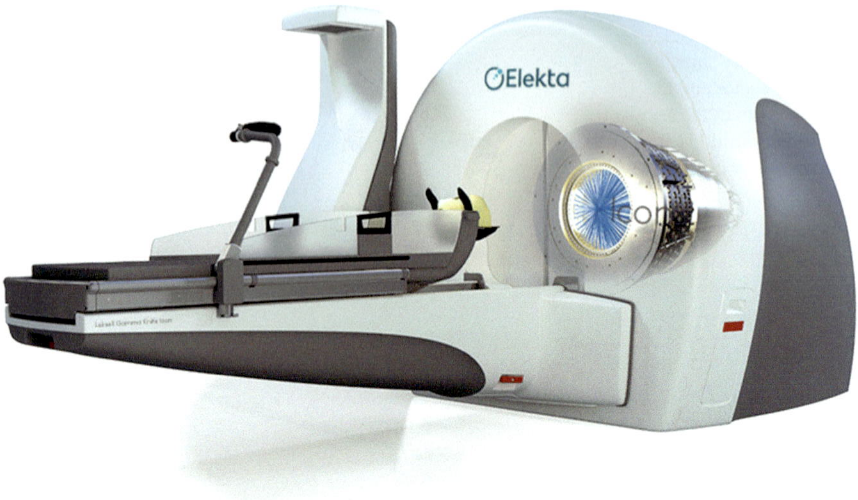

Fig. 13.4 Gamma Knife Icon model was introduced in 2017. Photo courtesy of Elekta

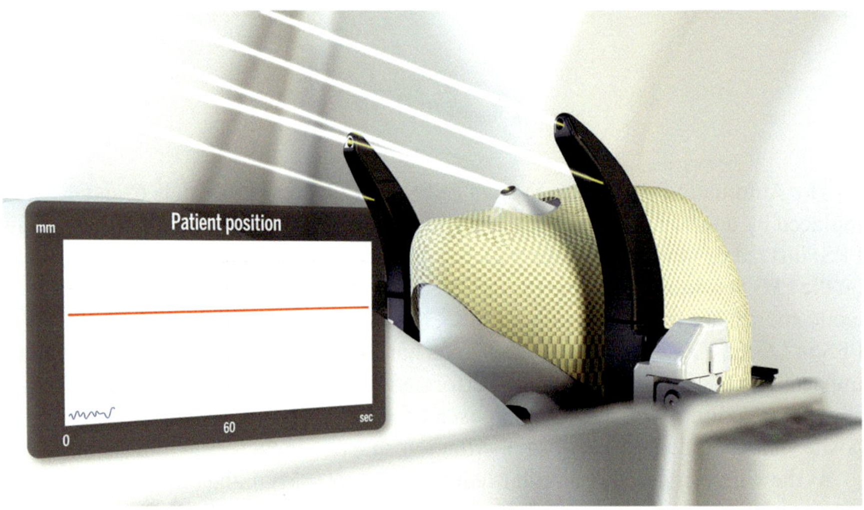

Fig. 13.5 Diagrammatic representation of mask-based radiosurgery with high-definition motion management system in LGK Icon. Photo courtesy of Elekta

reflective marker on the nose in real-time to make sure that there is no movement during mask-based SRS treatment. This technology has proven very valuable for a subset of patients with small tumors that can be treated quickly in a single treatment. It also allows selected patients to undergo 2–5 GK sessions for the same target (hypo-fractionated SRS) using the replaceable mask for head stabilization [6].

Role of Robotic in LINAC Radiosurgery

The proliferation of radiosurgery indications has led to multiple centers adapting conventional linear accelerators for stereotactic delivery. Robotics play a key role in modern linear accelerator gantries in the control of beam energy selection, dose-rate control, and precise delivery of total dose. Of special note with respect to radiosurgery is the role of robotics in automatic couch positioning, multi-leaf collimation aperture control, and gantry positioning.

Gantry LINAC tables are modified for stereotactic delivery to improve patient positioning, typically by adding three rotational degrees of freedom (pitch, yaw, and role) to the couch in addition to the three standard translational degrees of freedom in the *x*-, *y*-, and *z*-axes. In addition to allowing more precise manual control, most advanced tabletops allow for automated positioning based on online imaging done during the treatment session [7]. These registrations are not done in a live fashion, but rather at prespecified intervals—typically once with cone-beam CT alignment to planning CT alignment at the start of the SRS session. For typical SRS plans, there can be ~4 noncoplanar arcs delivered with the gantry, with each arc being (see Fig. 13.6- HyperArc) delivered at a different couch kick angle, with the position of the patient subsequently confirmed with flat-panel imagers. Typically, these couch kick angles are also controlled robotically from the plan delivery parameters.

The radiation dose delivery at the gantry head is modulated via a multi-leaf collimation system under robotic control. The treatment planning system (TPS) provides machine parameters controlling 2 paired sets of jaws as well as individual positions of the collimation leaf, which are tracked through servos with or without

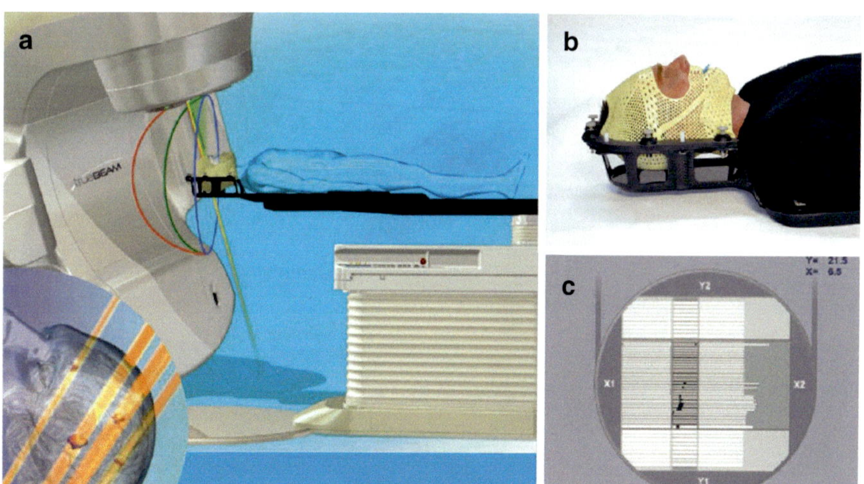

Fig. 13.6 HyperArc (**a**) is a frameless (**b**), multi-leaf collimator-based, (**c**) non-coplanar stereotactic radiosurgery system. Photo courtesy of Varian

optical tracking confirmation. The leaf positions and fluence pattern generated are second-checked prior to the patient's treatment session by measuring the output dose pattern and confirming that these highly modulated outputs match that estimated by the TPS (Figure—portal dosimetry). This second check represents a departure from prior step and shoot cone-based delivery, given the static geometries for the cones that are not controlled robotically. The combination of gantry movement and multi-leaf collimation is algorithmically controlled with a technique known as volumetric arc therapy, first introduced in 1995 by Cedric Yu [8]. A second noted development has been to allow the robotic MLC leaves to move beyond the midline of the aperture allowing for delivery away from the isocenter. This has allowed for multiple intracranial lesions to be treated in the same set of arcs, speeding delivery by at least four-fold [9]. A potential drawback of single isocenter, multiple target delivery is that the radial propagation of small positioning errors can cause large deviations in delivered dose at targets far from the isocenter.

CyberKnife Robotic Radiosurgery System

CyberKnife was introduced into clinical practice in 1997 [10]. It was the first radiosurgery device that utilized an industrial robot to direct a photon beam generated by a small on-board LINAC directly to the target. Some of its advantageous features included targeting of brain, spine, and body targets (Fig. 13.7). CyberKnife reported high mechanical precision and an innovative image-guided control loop with target-tracking capabilities, which allowed for the real-time tracking of target movement.

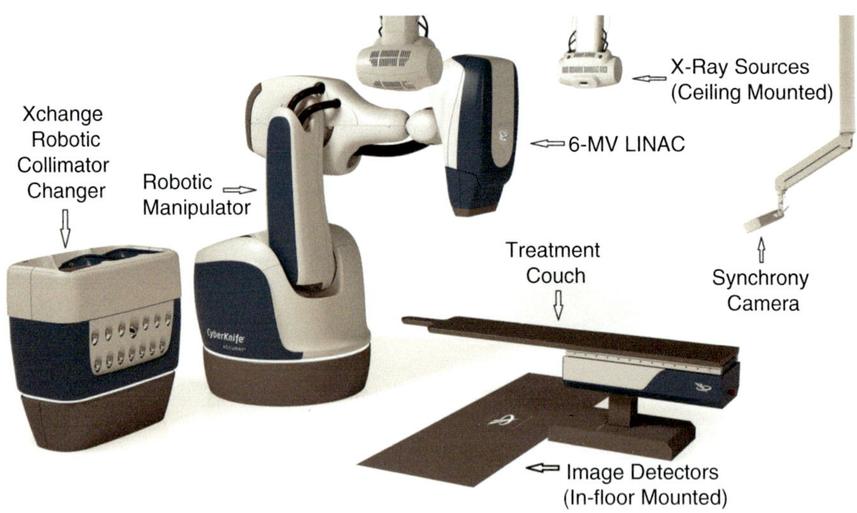

Fig. 13.7 The latest model of CyberKnife-S7. The new robot in S7 is faster compared to previous versions, and robot paths have been optimized for speed. Photo courtesy of Accuray

The CyberKnife system incorporates a miniature lightweight 6-MV LINAC, with circular secondary collimators of various diameters, mounted on an industrial robot with 6 degrees of freedom for movement. Treatment planning is based on an inverse planning system. A CT scan as well as MRI is used to generate pre- and intra-treatment digitally reconstructed neuroimages and is used for patient positioning and subsequent tracking.

For planning the dose delivery, the system chooses several nodes that lie on a sphere of 80 cm around the target volume. Guided by the dose and the constraints applied, the system chooses beam directions and weights for each node to reach optimal conformity with the planned dose distribution. A unique feature of the CyberKnife system is represented by the image-guided loop. Two flat-panel amorphous silicon X-ray cameras are used for intermittent patient positioning and treatment tracking. The system generates a sequence of digitally reconstructed radiographs from the pretreatment CT, which are matched with the orthogonal X-ray images acquired during treatment. The new target position is then compared with the target position at the planning phase, and the beam directions are corrected accordingly.

Various additions to the system have been introduced since its conception. The synchrony respiratory tracking system allows for continuous tracking and detection and correction for respiratory movements. This real-time detection is cross-checked by the system via digitally reconstructed radiographs to accommodate the robot's final position prior to treatment delivery. Another addition, the Xsight tracking system uses internal anatomy to directly track targets with accuracy and precision without the need for external frames or implanted fiducial markers. The CyberKnife is a device that represents the evolution of a concept radiosurgery with incorporation of robotic technology.

Summary

Stereotactic radiosurgery has transformed the practice of neurosurgery and is now considered mainstream neurosurgery. Current SRS techniques use real-time image guidance and robotic radiation delivery.

The application of robotic technologies has improved the accuracy, safety, and efficiency of radiosurgery. More complex and highly conformal dose plans can be created since the dose delivery is faster and does not require any manual set up. Robotics and image guidance have added more flexibility in treatment options as patients with multiple brain lesion can be treated with single or multiple sessions radiosurgery using frame based or frameless techniques.

Robotics systems have assumed greater control of all mechanical processes in the current radiosurgery technique, thereby automating the radiation delivery part of the radiosurgery procedure. In future, innovation in the radiosurgery treatment of epilepsy and certain psychiatric diseases could drive future technical innovation within robotic radiosurgery for brain applications.

References

1. Leksell L. The stereotaxic method and radiosurgery of the brain. Acta Chir Scand. 1951;102(4):316–9. https://www.ncbi.nlm.nih.gov/pubmed/14914373.
2. Lunsford LD, Maitz A, Lindner G. First United States 201 source cobalt-60 gamma unit for radiosurgery. Appl Neurophysiol. 1987;50(1–6):253–6. https://doi.org/10.1159/000100720.
3. Lunsford LD, Flickinger J, Lindner G, Maitz A. Stereotactic radiosurgery of the brain using the first United States 201 cobalt-60 source gamma knife. Neurosurgery. 1989;24(2):151–9. https://doi.org/10.1227/00006123-198902000-00001.
4. Novotny J, Bhatnagar JP, Niranjan A, et al. Dosimetric comparison of the Leksell Gamma Knife Perfexion and 4C. J Neurosurg. 2008;109(Suppl):8–14. https://doi.org/10.3171/JNS/2008/109/12/S3.
5. Niranjan A, Novotny J Jr, Bhatnagar J, Flickinger JC, Kondziolka D, Lunsford LD. Efficiency and dose planning comparisons between the Perfexion and 4C Leksell Gamma Knife units. Stereotact Funct Neurosurg. 2009;87(3):191–8. https://doi.org/10.1159/000222663.
6. Lunsford LD, Niranjan A, Fallon K, Kim JO. Frame versus frameless Leksell stereotactic radiosurgery. Prog Neurol Surg. 2019;34:19–27. https://doi.org/10.1159/000493046.
7. Meyer J, Wilbert J, Baier K, et al. Positioning accuracy of cone-beam computed tomography in combination with a HexaPOD robot treatment table. Int J Radiat Oncol Biol Phys. 2007;67(4):1220–8. https://doi.org/10.1016/j.ijrobp.2006.11.010.
8. Yu CX. Intensity-modulated arc therapy with dynamic multileaf collimation: an alternative to tomotherapy. Phys Med Biol. 1995;40(9):1435–49. https://doi.org/10.1088/0031-9155/40/9/004.
9. Ruggieri R, Naccarato S, Mazzola R, et al. Linac-based VMAT radiosurgery for multiple brain lesions: comparison between a conventional multi-isocenter approach and a new dedicated mono-isocenter technique. Radiat Oncol. 2018;13(1):38. https://doi.org/10.1186/s13014-018-0985-2.
10. Adler JR Jr, Chang SD, Murphy MJ, Doty J, Geis P, Hancock SL. The Cyberknife: a frameless robotic system for radiosurgery. Stereotact Funct Neurosurg. 1997;69(1–4 Pt 2):124–8. https://doi.org/10.1159/000099863.

Chapter 14
Robotic Navigated Laser Craniotomy: Current Applications and Future Developments

Fabian Winter, Julia Shawarba, and Karl Roessler

Abbreviations

AOT	Advanced Osteotomy Tools
CARLO	Cold ablation robot-guided laser osteotome
CT	Computed tomography
OCT	Optical coherence tomography

Introduction

Indications for laser in neurosurgery came a long way since its first introduction in 1960. A pulsed ruby laser lacked in desirable surgical procedures and at high powers damaged vital organs, including the brain [1]. A continuous wave CO_2 laser came along in 1967. Just to be replaced by more advanced Nd:YAG, Holmium:YAG, and Erbium:YAG lasers [1–3]. Nowadays, the most often used laser applications in neurosurgery include: (1) Laser ablation of brain tissue during open surgery [4, 5]; (2) Endoscopic laser applications [6]; (3) Laser assisted microanastomosis [3, 6, 7]; (4) Laser for intervertebral disc surgery [8, 9]; and (6) Novel laser-based applications for intraoperative tissue diagnosis (endomicroscopy, Raman spectroscopy) [1, 3, 10, 11]. However, laser application for craniotomies were not considered so far. Recently, we decided to investigate possible neurosurgical applications in bone cutting during craniotomy procedures after recognized studies for maxillotomies at the MedUniWien/AKH in Vienna. Thus, we first started to generate a model for

F. Winter · J. Shawarba · K. Roessler (✉)
Department of Neurosurgery, Medical University of Vienna, Vienna, Austria
e-mail: fabian.winter@meduniwien.ac.at; karl.roessler@meduniwien.ac.at

J. A. González Martínez, F. Cardinale (eds.), *Robotics in Neurosurgery*,
https://doi.org/10.1007/978-3-031-08380-8_14

precision bone channels for depth electrode placement in human cadavers at the Anatomical Institute of Basel, where the AOT (Advanced Osteotomy Tools, Basel, Switzerland) laser for maxillofacial developments was in use. Furthermore, we went into an animal model in a lab in Barcelona, to investigate the impact of the laser beam of the AOT System on the dura mater and the brain tissue while cutting the skull in an in vivo swine study. The goal was to perform hardware and software modifications which would allow more precise depth control and avoidance of dura and brain lesioning during laser craniotomies. Lastly, we have generated a sheep survival model to proof the concept of laser craniotomy as a standard procedure with no bleeding risk intracranially.

Methods and Materials

Ethical board approval was obtained from the Anatomical Institute of Basel for the cadaver study and by the local Department de Territori I Sostenibilitat for the in vivo non-recovery study in Barcelona. Also, ethical approval was obtained from the Medical University of Vienna and the Austrian Ministry of Education and Sciences for the sheep survival model. The surgeons performing the procedures are accredited with education and training courses in laboratory animal science with the EU Function A certificate.

Planning and Robotic Laser Device

Using surgical planning software (Suite Version 2.15.2, ImFusion GmBH, Munich, Germany), we planned multiple bone channels. Pre-planned trajectories allow a fully digital workflow and have the advantage to avoid cortical blodd vessels for safer craniotomies. In addition, the laser device integrates optical coherence tomography (OCT), allowing to detect the cut's shape and depth.

The robot is guided by a navigation system (Fig. 14.1) allowing exact procedures pre-planned on the software. It is integrated into one head which is mounted on a robotic arm (KUKA, Augsburg, Germany) which provides lateral repeatability with less than 0.15 mm variation. The non-contact, robotized cold laser device is a radically new cutting tool by employing robotics, laser, artificial intelligence, and a fully digital workflow (Fig. 14.2). Consequences of many disadvantages of mechanical instruments including but not limited to saws, files, and milling cutters used for osteotomies are long recovery time due to severe cases to non-unions, infections, and other complications. So far, hand-held mechanical instruments had the advantage of cutting any shape in any size spontaneously. Using a navigated laser mounted

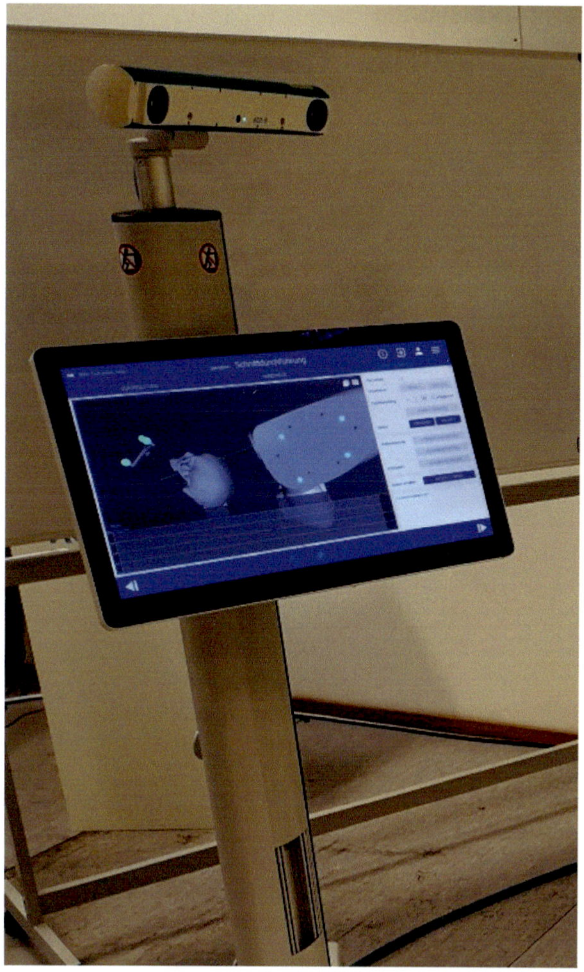

Fig. 14.1 Optical navigation system with two tracking cameras allowing exact procedures

on a robotic arm indication-specific planning tools allows shapes and sizes also to be configurated intraoperatively, and therefore spontaneously, with high precision and freedom of geometry. This is not to replace but to support the surgeon in his goal of ensuring the best possible treatment for each individual patient. Available laser systems are often not flexible and spacious enough to allow interactions between external devices and surgeons [12]. To facilitate symbiotic workflows, this device uses an in-room memory function of the robotic arm allowing a retraction of the arm at any time, re-entering the surgical field from the side (Fig. 14.3) so the surgeon could operate freely from the front.

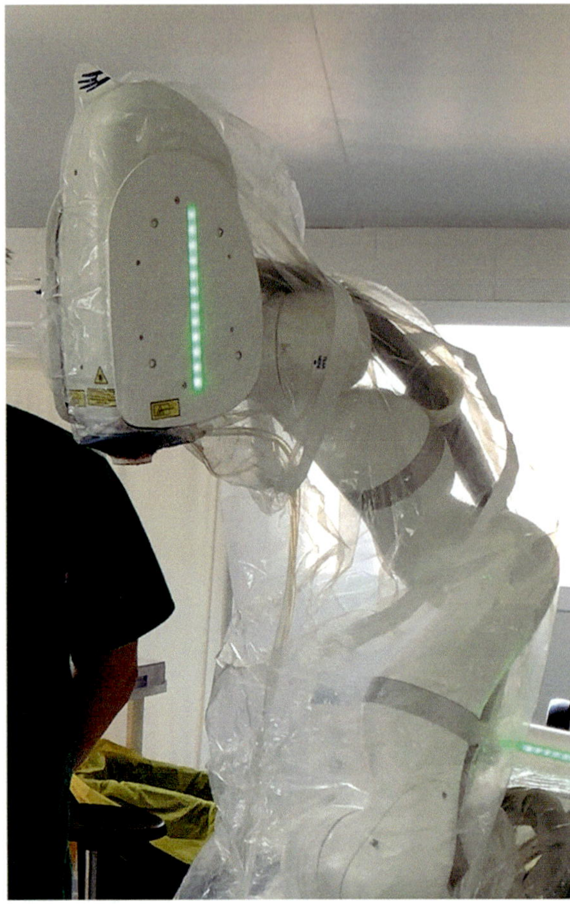

Fig. 14.2 The robotized cold laser, a tool by employing robotics, laser, artificial intelligence, and a fully digital workflow

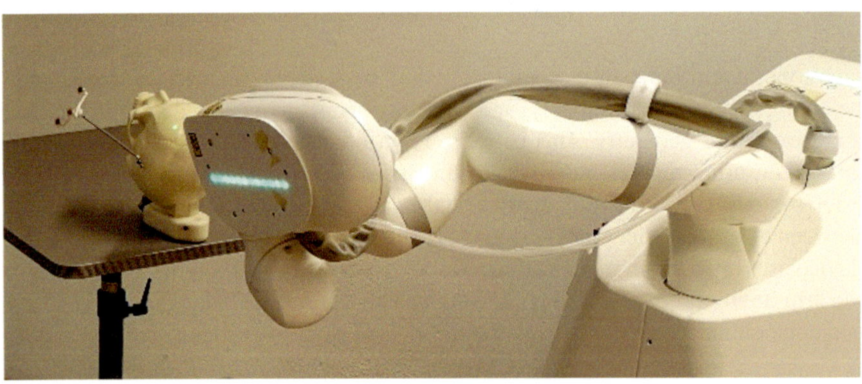

Fig. 14.3 The device uses an in-room memory function of the robotic arm allowing a retraction of the arm at any time, re-entering the surgical field from the side

Procedure

The cold ablation robot-guided laser osteotome (CARLO, AOT, Advanced Osteotomy Tools, Basel, Switzerland) uses a 2.94 μm Erbium:YAG laser with 0.8 mm focal diameter. The robotic arm provides safe speed and force while being tactile, designed to maximize human–machine collaboration. In the cadaver as well as in the in vivo study, the specimen was placed in a prone position. A registration marker fixated on the skull is necessary for optimal navigation as the robot is guided by a navigation system based on two tracking cameras (Fig. 14.4). The bone channels for depth electrodes were ablated fully autonomously by the robotic laser beam. Optical Coherence Tomography (OCT) is integrated within the laser device system, allowing the device to detect the shape and depth of the cut being performed.

Data Analysis

For the cadaver study, postoperative CT scans allowed comparison of pre-planned trajectories and performed bone channels. Distances were determined at the outer and inner surface of the cranial bone as well as at the target point.

Results

Building the drill hole for the implantation of depth electrodes is one of the crucial surgical steps for invasive monitoring in epilepsy surgery. Small drilling deviations due to hand-held instruments can cause large deviations in accuracy for the target point. With robot-guided non-contact laser craniotomy, small entry point deviations of 0.69 mm (+/– 0.63 mm SD) and target point deviation of 2.0 mm (+/– 0.64 mm

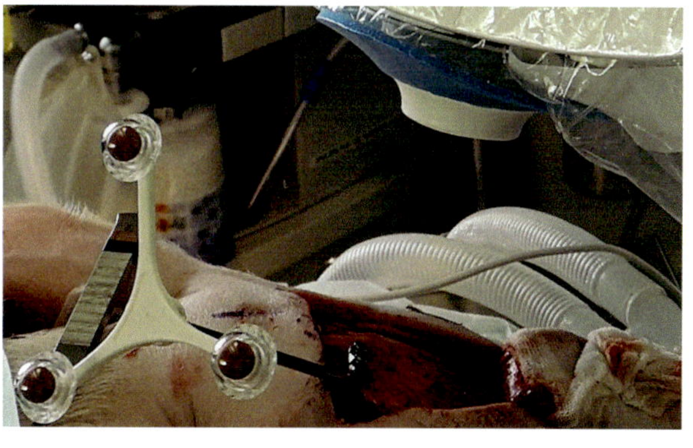

Fig. 14.4 A registration marker fixed on the skull was necessary for optimal navigation

SD) were achieved in a cadaveric model [13]. Implantation time per electrode is comparable to other published data using other techniques such as frame-based, frameless, and hand-held techniques [13–16].

The complete digital workflow allowed exact transfer of the digital plan in situ to avoid cortical blood vessels. The specimens were not fixed. However, spontaneous specimen movements had no consequences as this is a non-contact technique, and the device could detect and calculate variances with the aid of the fixed registration fiducial. Furthermore, the cutting process could be stopped at any time by the surgeon as there were no mechanical parts in contact. In an in vivo study cut through was obtained with a power of 1.1 W. However, due to inflowing cerebrospinal fluid, the power setting was raised up to 2.1 W. The dura was punctured but it did not result in bleeding. The cortex was not damaged after one beam, but further experimental pre-planned multiple beams resulted in cortical damage. Cutting debris could be ejected during the procedure without impairing the bone structure and allowed optimized visualization through the co-axial camera system within the device.

Discussion

Current craniotomy instruments require direct physical contact with the patient during the procedure. This results in heat up during friction and often does not allow clean precise cuts due to their mass. Mechanical in-contact instruments may bend under force, while robotic devices follow strict coordinates without being influenced from mechanical deformation as there is no contact and no friction. Robotic osteotomies corresponding exactly to pre-planned maneuvers. Pre-planned trajectories also have the advantage to avoid cortical blood vessels for safer craniotomies.

Laser osteotomies show high precision and freedom in geometry [17]. However, in the operating room, the freedom in geometry cannot be achieved as available laser devices lack in flexibility. In recent years, devices combining the laser and the navigation system to safe space and make it desirable for the operating room have emerged. A navigation system is crucial for exact placement of bone channels for pre-planned trajectories. The tested device using Er:YAG laser in these studies has already been successfully investigated in the oral and maxillofacial surgery [18, 19].

In a previous clinical setting, the studied autonomous laser device revealed cutting efficiency without any damage of adjacent soft tissue structures [20]. Er:YAG laser ablates bone while heating to the surrounding tissues is very limited [21]. Furthermore, blood circulation can be hindered from cutting debris which is often observed when cutting with mechanical instruments. With the integrated cooling spray, cutting debris can be held to a minimum. The cooling spray also brings the advantage of avoiding necrosis due to heat dissipation often observed in first generation medical lasers and mechanical instruments. Therefore, the aim is to ablate the hard tissue cold to not impair the bone's ability to grow back. The robotic arm also provides flexibility in the operating room, facilitating interactions between the surgeon and the laser device.

High entry and target point accuracy could be achieved with this device. The screws fitted so well, that there was no additional guidance system necessary to place the depth screws. Measured target point accuracies of 2.0 ± 0.64 mm is within the accepted accuracy range for frameless systems [13, 14, 22].

Recent studies using Er:YAG lasers observed limited visual inspection [20, 23]. The co-axial camera system within the CARLO allows visual inspection through the device itself. However, results in the in-vivo study were not satisfying due to inflow of liquids after dura perforation. Nevertheless, contrast differences could be observed. With optimization of these tools, damages to dura and more importantly cortex can be avoided.

Conclusion

Navigated robotic assisted laser precision osteotomies in neurosurgical procedures are a promising new method and may have many advantages over standard burr holes and saw craniotomies.

References

1. Stellar S, Polanyi TG. Lasers in neurosurgery: a historical overview. J Clin Laser Med Surg. 1992;10(6):399–411. https://doi.org/10.1089/clm.1992.10.399.
2. Ryan RW, Wolf T, Spetzler RF, Coons SW, Fink Y, Preul MC. Application of a flexible CO2 laser fiber for neurosurgery: laser-tissue interactions—laboratory investigation. J Neurosurg. 2010;112(2):434–43. https://doi.org/10.3171/2009.7.JNS09356.
3. Krishnamurthy S, Powers SK. Lasers in neurosurgery. Lasers Surg Med. 1994;15(2):126–67. https://doi.org/10.1002/lsm.1900150203.
4. Greenway MRF, Lucas JA, Feyissa AM, Grewal S, Wharen RE, Tatum WO. Neuropsychological outcomes following stereotactic laser amygdalohippocampectomy. Epilepsy Behav. 2017;75:50–5. https://doi.org/10.1016/j.yebeh.2017.07.033.
5. Youngerman BE, Save AV, McKhann GM. Magnetic resonance imaging-guided laser interstitial thermal therapy for epilepsy: systematic review of technique, indications, and outcomes. Neurosurgery. 2020;86(4):E366–82. https://doi.org/10.1093/neuros/nyz556.
6. Belykh E, Yagmurlu K, Martirosyan NL, et al. Laser application in neurosurgery. Surg Neurol Int. 2017;8:274. https://doi.org/10.4103/sni.sni_489_16.
7. Hendrikse J, van der Zwan A, Ramos LMP, Tulleken CAF, van der Grond J. Hemodynamic compensation via an excimer laser-assisted, high-flow bypass before and after therapeutic occlusion of the internal carotid artery. Neurosurgery. 2003;53(4):855–8. https://doi.org/10.1227/01.neu.0000083552.45265.46.
8. Ahn Y, Moon KS, Kang BU, Hur SM, Kim JD. Laser-assisted posterior cervical foraminotomy and discectomy for lateral and foraminal cervical disc herniation. Photomed Laser Surg. 2012;30(9):510–5. https://doi.org/10.1089/pho.2012.3246.
9. Brouwer PA, Brand R, Van Den Akker-Van Marle ME, et al. Percutaneous laser disc decompression versus conventional microdiscectomy for patients with sciatica: two-year results of a randomised controlled trial. Interv Neuroradiol. 2017;23(3):313–24. https://doi.org/10.1177/1591019917699981.

10. Ashraf O, Patel NV, Hanft S, Danish SF. Laser-induced thermal therapy in neuro-oncology: a review. World Neurosurg. 2018;112:166–77. https://doi.org/10.1016/j.wneu.2018.01.123.
11. Kim AH, Tatter S, Rao G, et al. Laser ablation of abnormal neurological tissue using robotic neuroblate system (laantern): 12-month outcomes and quality of life after brain tumor ablation. Neurosurgery. 2020;87(3):E338–46. https://doi.org/10.1093/neuros/nyaa071.
12. Augello M, Baetscher C, Segesser M, Zeilhofer H-F, Cattin P, Juergens P. Performing partial mandibular resection, fibula free flap reconstruction and midfacial osteotomies with a cold ablation and robot-guided Er:YAG laser osteotome (CARLO(®))—a study on applicability and effectiveness in human cadavers. J cranio-maxillo-facial Surg Off Publ Eur Assoc Cranio-Maxillo-Facial Surg. 2018;46(10):1850–5. https://doi.org/10.1016/j.jcms.2018.08.001.
13. Roessler K, Winter F, Wilken T, Pataraia E, Mueller-Gerbl M, Dorfer C. Robotic navigated laser craniotomy for depth electrode implantation in epilepsy surgery: a cadaver lab study. J Neurol Surg A Cent Eur Neurosurg. 2021;82:125–9. https://doi.org/10.1055/s-0040-1720998.
14. Dorfer C, Stefanits H, Pataraia E, Wolfsberger S, Feucht M, Baumgartner C. Frameless stereotactic drilling for placement of depth electrodes in refractory epilepsy: operative technique and initial experience. Neurosurgery. 2014;10(Suppl 4):582–91. https://doi.org/10.1227/NEU.0000000000000509.
15. Cardinale F, Casaceli G, Raneri F, Miller J, Lo RG. Implantation of Stereoelectroencephalography electrodes: a systematic review. J Clin Neurophysiol. 2016;33(6):490–502. https://doi.org/10.1097/WNP.0000000000000249.
16. Cardinale F. Stereoelectroencephalography: application accuracy, efficacy, and safety. World Neurosurg. 2016;94:570–1. https://doi.org/10.1016/j.wneu.2016.07.070.
17. Augello M, Baetscher C, Segesser M, Zeilhofer H-F, Cattin P, Juergens P. Performing partial mandibular resection, fibula free flap reconstruction and midfacial osteotomies with a cold ablation and robot-guided Er:YAG laser osteotome (CARLO((R)))—a study on applicability and effectiveness in human cadavers. J Craniomaxillofac Surg. 2018;46(10):1850–5. https://doi.org/10.1016/j.jcms.2018.08.001.
18. Baek K-W, Deibel W, Marinov D, et al. Clinical applicability of robot-guided contact-free laser osteotomy in cranio-maxillo-facial surgery: in-vitro simulation and in-vivo surgery in minipig mandibles. Br J Oral Maxillofac Surg. 2015;53(10):976–81. https://doi.org/10.1016/j.bjoms.2015.07.019.
19. Augello M, Deibel W, Nuss K, Cattin P, Jurgens P. Comparative microstructural analysis of bone osteotomies after cutting by computer-assisted robot-guided laser osteotome and piezoelectric osteotome: an in vivo animal study. Lasers Med Sci. 2018;33(7):1471–8. https://doi.org/10.1007/s10103-018-2502-0.
20. Stübinger S, Nuss K, Pongratz M, et al. Comparison of Er:YAG laser and piezoelectric osteotomy: an animal study in sheep. Lasers Surg Med. 2010;42(8):743–51. https://doi.org/10.1002/lsm.20946.
21. Berg B-I, Peyer M, Kuske L, et al. Comparison of an Er: YAG laser osteotome versus a conventional drill for the use in osteo-odonto-keratoprosthesis (OOKP). Lasers Surg Med. 2019;51(6):531–7. https://doi.org/10.1002/lsm.23053.
22. Dorfer C, Minchev G, Czech T, et al. A novel miniature robotic device for frameless implantation of depth electrodes in refractory epilepsy. J Neurosurg. 2017;126(5):1622–8. https://doi.org/10.3171/2016.5.JNS16388.
23. Stübinger S, Ghanaati S, Saldamli B, Kirkpatrick CJ, Sader R. Er:YAG laser osteotomy: preliminary clinical and histological results of a new technique for contact-free bone surgery. Eur Surg Res Eur Chir Forschung Rech Chir Eur. 2009;42(3):150–6. https://doi.org/10.1159/000197216.

Chapter 15
Small Footprint Stereotactic Robotic Devices

Sogha Khawari and Vejay Vakharia

Introduction The first reported robotic system to aid with neurosurgical procedures was the Programmable Universal Machine for Assembly (PUMA) 200 device to facilitate brain biopsy, in 1988. This and subsequent devices were modifications of industrial robotic arms. Consequently, the devices are heavy (circa 180 kg), free-standing and necessitate fixation of the robotic platform to the head holding frame or bed. For cranial procedures, they necessitate placement of a stereotactic frame and fiducial box before surgery so that a CT or MRI acquisition can be performed. The fiducial box markings that appear on the imaging are then subsequently identified by the device software for registration purposes. The frame is then attached to the robotic device, and positional information of the robotic arm relative to the patient is provided through absolute encoders within the articulations. Alternatively, an intraoperative CT can be acquired with the patient fixed to the device allowing for frameless registration. For spinal procedures, intraoperative imaging is required. Here, a portable CT scan is undertaken with the patient on the operative table, and a bone-anchored reference marker is usually included in the field of view for registration purposes. Due to the mobility of the spine, segmental registration with repeated acquisitions is usually required for extensive multi-level fixations.

Small footprint robotic devices are a more recent concept. The smaller and lighter nature of the devices allows for them to be affixed directly to the head holder or bed via an articulating multifunctional mechanical arm. Consequently, they require the surgeon to fix the device within a rough approximation (4 × 4 cm area)

S. Khawari · V. Vakharia (✉)
Victor Horsley Department of Neurosurgery, National Hospital for Neurology and Neurosurgery, London, UK

Department of Clinical and Experimental Epilepsy, Queen Square Institute of Neurology, University College London, London, UK
e-mail: sogha.khawari@nhs.net; v.vakharia@nhs.net

J. A. González Martínez, F. Cardinale (eds.), *Robotics in Neurosurgery*,
https://doi.org/10.1007/978-3-031-08380-8_15

of the predefined entry point. The articulations within the multifunctional mechanical arms are not robotic and do not move without manual manipulation. Once the mechanical arm is locked in place, the software utilises the guidance from the neuronavigation system to provide fine adjustments to align the working channel to the intended trajectory. Unlike their large footprint counterparts, the smaller devices require an external neuronavigation system that provides continuous guidance utilising an infrared system that tracks the location of fiducial markers attached to the device or tool. Consequently, any error acquired during or after registration is directly translated to the alignment of the device.

To date, there are two commercially available small footprint robotic systems: the Stealth Autoguide (Medtronic, USA, previously known as iSYS1, Interventional Systems Medizintechnik GmbH, Austria) and the Cirq (Brainlab AG, Munich, Germany). These devices have been used for CT guided percutaneous needle placement, brain and spine biopsies, stereoelectroencephalography (SEEG), laser interstitial thermal therapy (LITT) and spine pedicle screw fixation procedures. In this chapter, we will first provide an overview of both systems along with their comparative differences to larger footprint devices. We will then provide an evidence-based summary of the contemporary literature for both devices covering both cranial and spinal applications.

Small Footprint Devices

Both the Stealth Autoguide and Brainlab Cirq utilise a similar design concept, with a robotic positioning unit attached to a mechanical arm. The multifunctional mechanical arm for the Stealth Autoguide is derived from the Stealth Vertek system and requires the surgeon to manually tighten the articulations once in place. The Brainlab Cirq system, however, utilises the Medineering surgical base, a system that is attached to the bed frame and incorporates grip-lock sensors that secure the arm position once pressure on the arm is removed. Both the Stealth Autoguide and Cirq robotic arm systems were awarded FDA approved in 2019 through the 510K route due to substantial equivalence to previously approved (predicate) devices. Whilst both are approved for brain and spinal procedures, the Stealth Autoguide system has principally been used for cranial applications whilst the Brainlab Cirq for spinal procedures. Table 15.1 compares the similarities and differences between the two devices in relation to larger footprint devices.

Stealth Autoguide

The Stealth Autoguide (Medtronic, USA) robotic trajectory guidance system provides a working channel for use with invasive tools, such as biopsy needles, laser catheters and intracerebral electrodes. The device uses a predefined trajectory

Table 15.1 Comparison of small and large footprint robotic device attributes

Attribute	Stealth Autoguide (Medtronic)	Cirq (BrainLab)	Neuromate (Renishaw)	ROSA (Zimmer Biomet)
Footprint	Small	Small	Large	Large
Weight (kg)	1.2	11	180	150
Fixation method	Head clamp	Head clamp	Stereotactic frame	Stereotactic frame
Registration method	Optical	Optical	Fiducial markers Neurolocate Ultrasound	Fiducial markers Optical
Mechanical arm	Vertek multifunctional arm (manual tightening)	Medineering surgical base (grip lock sensors)	Integrated	Integrated
Motorised mechanical arm	No	No	Yes	Yes
Navigation software	StealthStation (S7 onwards)	Brainlab IGS Cranial and Spinal software	NeuroInspire	ROSA software
Localization method	Infrared camera	Infrared camera	Robotic arm absolute encoders	Robotic arm absolute encoders
Calibration	Intraoperative	Intraoperative	Factory calibration	Factory calibration
Instrument navigation	Real-time	Real-time	No	No
Immobilisation between patient and device	Not required as localiser attached to head holder as reference	Not required as localiser attached to head holder as reference	Yes	Yes
Verification of accuracy method	Pointer probe	Pointer probe	Laser pointer	Navigation probe and laser beam

derived from the Stealth neuronavigation system (StealthStation S7 and beyond) and incorporates this with live geospatial data from the optical tracking system to allow for precise alignment of the device's tool holder. Once the desired trajectory is obtained, the surgeon manually advances the instrument along the trajectory to the final target.

The Stealth Autoguide system consists of 3 main components: A robot-needle positioning unit (RPU) consisting of 2 flat modules allowing rotational and sliding movements with 4 degrees of freedom (DOF) to allow for precise alignment to the predefined trajectory, disposable tool guide extension and the control panel. In the early versions of the device, branded as the iSYS1, the control panel constituted a standalone computer panel that provided guidance information to the surgery along with a separate switch that was used to initiate movement of the RPU. Subsequent versions of the device, marketed as Stealth Autoguide, integrate the computer panel and screen on the back of the RPU.

The surgical workflow requires the patient to be placed in a Mayfield head clamp. The area for surgery is then prepared with a sterilising solution and draped in an aseptic fashion. A non-sterile multifunctional arm then provides a rigid connection to the bed or head clamp. The device is covered by a sterile plastic cover. The tool guide extension is the only part of the device that requires sterilisation and attaches through small holes in the plastic drape. The tool guide extension has reflective balls attached to it to allow for optical tracking of the working channel. Tools such as drill bits, biopsy needles, bone anchors, screwdrivers and electrodes along with their corresponding reduction tubes can then be passed through the working channels. The Stealth neuronavigation station is then used for registration, in the usual fashion. Once the trajectory has been chosen on the StealthStation, this information is relayed to the surgeon via the computer panel on the back of the device. The computer panel then guides the surgeon to roughly align the device to the predefined trajectory. Once the working channel is aligned to within a 4 × 4 cm area of the entry point, the device computer panel signals to the surgeon to manually lock the multifunctional arm (Fig. 15.1). A separate remote control is then used to control the movement of the RPU to mitigate against any unintended movement of the device. The remote control also can be used to manually control movements of the device

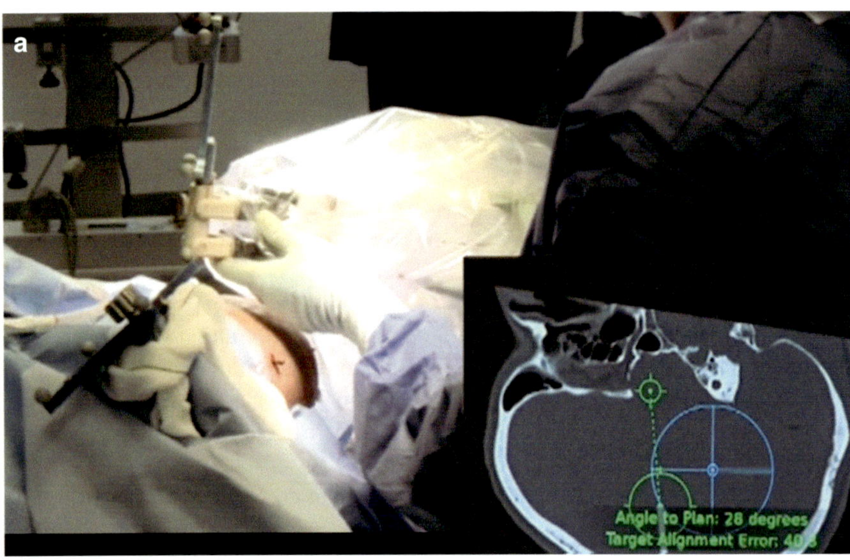

Fig. 15.1 Robotic alignment of device
The iSYS1 device is mounted to the Mayfield clamp. The Vertek probe can be seen positioned within the sterile tool guide extension providing navigation guidance via the StealthStation (inset). In image (**a**), the device is placed in rough proximity to the entry point and fixed in position. In image (**b**), the device has then automatically aligned to the trajectory with a target alignment error of 0.1 mm

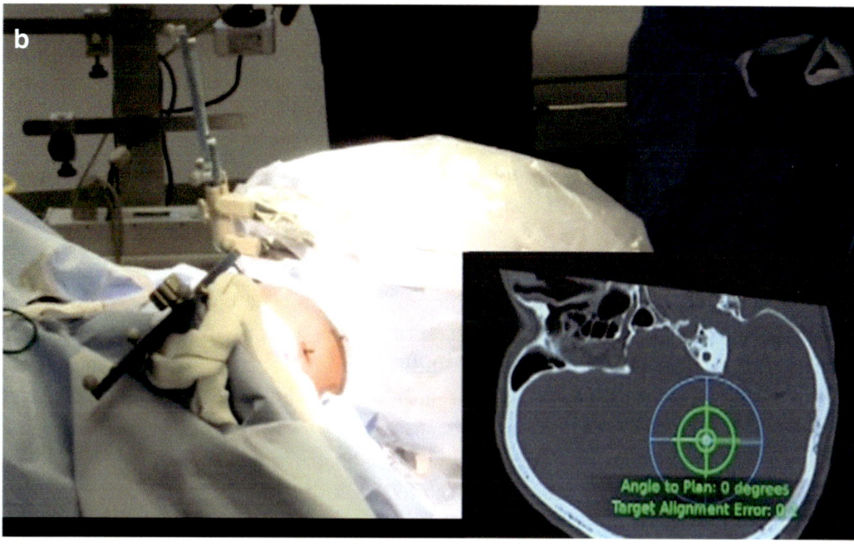

Fig. 15.1 (continued)

using the joystick. This is particularly important for performing procedures requiring manual adjustment or where planned trajectories cannot be defined such as CT guided spinal injections or biopsy procedures.

Percutaneous Interventional Radiological Procedures

The Stealth Autoguide system was initially called the iSYS1 system and was developed by Interventional Systems Medizintechnik, GmbH before acquisition by Medtronic Inc. The first clinical studies focused on the use during interventional radiological procedures as a means of allowing the physician to control the device remotely whilst performing CT scans. For this application registration or guidance from a neuronavigation system was not required as the CT scan images would provide up to date spatial information and the physician would manually control the RPU using the joystick.

In an ex vivo study, 5 copper wires were randomly inserted into a custom-made phantom torso [1]. A CT scan of the torso was then undertaken, and trajectories were planned to the outer tips of the wires. The system was mounted onto the side of the CT scanner bed. Registration was carried out using fiducial registration markers, and the RPU was positioned within proximity of the entry point. The iSYS1 device was then used to align to the planned trajectory. A needle was mounted within the working channel of the iSYS1 device, and the operator advanced the needle to the target depth. Target point accuracy between the needle tip and the wire (intended target point) was 2.3 ± 0.8 (range 0.9–3.7) mm. The median intervention time was 9.6 min. This marked the first study to demonstrate the utility of a small robotic system for CT guided injections.

In the following year, the successful use of the iSYS1 combined with a cone-beam CT for K-wires insertion during spinal procedures was also reported [2]. The robotic working channel was used to guide 20 K-wires into the thoracolumbar pedicles of a cadaver specimen. The mean distance from actual to planned target placement was as little as 0.35 mm, with a mean intervention time of 10 min 13 s per pedicle.

In a further study, the iSYS1 was utilised for stereotactic vertebral body biopsy [3]. Accuracy was first confirmed within an animal model before human use in 3 patients requiring biopsy of suspicious spinal bony lesions. In all 3 patients, the biopsies were taken from the desired pathological target and a histological diagnosis was obtained with no complications, although formal target point accuracy was not reported.

Larger case series and prospective comparison trials are still awaited to determine whether small footprint table-mounted robotic trajectory guidance devices offer advantages over freehand, navigated or larger footprint robotic devices for percutaneous interventional radiological procedures. Key metrics for comparison would include overall radiation dosage, total procedure time, target point accuracy and diagnostic yield of biopsy procedures.

Preclinical Cranial Studies

In all reported studies, large footprint devices were introduced into clinical practice without prospective comparison to the current gold standard technique used in that institution at the time. This raises a significant patient safety concern about the introduction of novel devices, especially when the surgeons have comparatively less experience with the device and it may take time to accrue sufficient clinical data to undertake a historical comparison study [4]. To mitigate the risk posed to patients, the iSYS1 trajectory guidance system underwent preclinical studies to assess the accuracy, learning curve and safety profile of the device before clinical use [5]. Three patients that had previously undergone a total of 21 SEEG electrode implantations using the conventional frameless Vertek biopsy method (Medtronic Inc.) were identified [6]. A 3D printed skull model was recreated for each patient and covered with synthetic skin substitutes. The same surgeons who implanted the electrodes into the patients replicated the SEEG implantation using the iSYS1 system to simulate the introduction of the device to clinical practice. Following placement, the accuracy of the robot-guided implantation was compared to actual implantation using the conventional frameless methods based on the post-implantation CT scans. The results revealed a statistically significant improvement in the mean entry point from 1.90 mm to 0.76 mm. The improvement in mean target point accuracy from 1.72 mm to 1.34 mm, however, did not reach statistical significance. Cumulative summation analysis was also utilised in this study to directly compare the real-time differences in accuracy, thereby acting as a quality assurance mechanism.

A similar preclinical study compared the use of the Stealth Autoguide to two commonly used conventional stereotactic systems for SEEG, the frameless Navigus biopsy system (Medtronic Inc.) and the Leksell (Eleksa Ltd) stereotactic frame [7]. The study initially used phantom cranial models filled with gelatin mixture to represent the brain and later used cadaveric specimens. The main finding from this study was that the Stealth Autoguide maintained accuracy when compared to both conventional models, despite being faster.

Brain Biopsy

One of the main applications of robotic technology in neurosurgery is for stereotactic brain biopsy procedures of deep-seated lesions. Brain biopsies require tissue sampling from a precise target to reduce possible complications and increase diagnostic yield. These procedures were historically performed using frame-based stereotaxy. Due to the cost and time-consuming nature, this was overtaken by the use of navigation-guided mechanical arm-based biopsies. Mechanical arm-based techniques are manually aligned to the predefined trajectory based on the information relayed by the neuronavigation system. Robot-guided biopsies help to combine the benefits of both high precision and speed.

Trajectory planning is carried out as standard utilising a neuronavigation system with the patient's head is fixed in a surgical clamp. The robotic guidance device is fixed onto the head clamp adapter and positioned manually over the entry point. The operator continually presses a button to allow the device to align to the planned trajectory. As a safety feature, robotic movement is stopped if the surgeon stops pushing the button. Once the trajectory is set, this is used as a fixed working channel. A small skin incision is made, and a K-wire is used to create a notch in the outer table of the skull. Drilling of the skull is performed through the working channel with the appropriately sized reduction tube based on the diameter of the drill bit. The surgeon then advances the biopsy needle along the trajectory to the depth defined by the real-time optical tracking system.

A prospective case series of the iSYS1 in 39 patients undergoing brain biopsy revealed a mean target error of 1.06 mm (range 0.1–4 mm), with no associated mortality or morbidity, and a diagnostic yield of 97.4% overall [8]. A comparison of the iSYS1 device in 32 patients to standard frameless burr-hole biopsy in 34 patients returned significantly better accuracy at entry, (median 1.5 mm [range 0.2–3.2 mm] vs 1.7 mm [range 0.8–5.1 mm], $p = 0.008$) and at target (median 1.5 mm [range 0.4–3.4 mm] vs 2.0 mm [range 0.8–3.9 mm], $p = 0.019$), respectively [9]. Of note, the iSYS1 biopsies were faster and required a significantly shorter incision length. The same findings were also confirmed in a further cohort of 40 patients reported by the same group. Additionally, it showed that the histological diagnostic yield and complication rates remained the same in both groups [10]. To date, there are no direct comparison studies between frame-based, frameless or robotic biopsy methods but a systematic review of both large and small footprint devices revealed a similar diagnostic yield (~95%) and complication profile [11].

Stereoelectroencephalography

The global shift in epilepsy practice from grid and strip implantations towards SEEG for invasive investigation of drug-resistant epilepsy has been a major force driving robotic installations in many institutions. SEEG consists of the implantation of up to about 20 electrodes into predefined areas of the brain to localise the seizure onset zone as well as the wider epileptogenic network. Conventionally, a stereotactic frame was used for this procedure. As described previously, the cost and time-consuming nature of frame-based systems led to the more widespread use of frameless systems, with acceptance of potentially worse accuracy [12]. Due to these limitations, there has been a boom in robot installations to guide insertion.

The choice of target points and the total number of SEEG electrodes implanted is case dependent and decided upon by an epilepsy multidisciplinary team based on the clinical, anatomical and electrophysiological hypothesis. Bone fiducials have been found to improve the accuracy of registration when used in combination with a neuronavigation system [13]. The Stealth Autoguide system is used to align the guide sheath to the predefined trajectory, with an accuracy of <0.1 mm. A skin incision is made, and a K-wire is inserted to create a divot in the bone. The skull is drilled, and an anchor bolt implanted through the working channel and respective reduction tube (Fig. 15.2). A styled is advanced by the surgeon to the target depth before insertion of the electrodes.

In an early series, 93 electrodes were placed in 16 patients. Compared with the manual frameless stereotactic approach, the iSYS1 resulted in an improved target point accuracy from 3.0 ± 1.9 mm to 1.7 ± 1.1 mm (mean ± SD) [14]. Additionally, the mean duration of depth electrode placement was significantly faster in the robot-guided group. The case series was the first to show that small footprint devices could provide comparable accuracy to large footprint devices. A comparative clinical study between different robotic devices has yet to be undertaken. The principal difficulty is that this would require a single institution to have more than one robot device, something which is cost-prohibitive and the need to have a surgeon that has similar experience with both devices. An alternative would be to compare implantations undertaken at different institutions that have different robotic devices but introduces both a surgeon and institutional bias.

To date, the highest level of evidence favouring robotic SEEG implantation is derived from a single-blinded randomised control parallel-group study of 32 patients (328 electrodes) comparing the iSYS1 system to manual frameless implantation utilising the Vertek biopsy arm [15]. Whilst the study sample size appears small, this sample size calculation revealed that as few as 11 subjects were required in each intervention arm to identify a reduction in bolt insertion time of 20%. The additionally recruited patients were to account for the possibility of patient dropout and cluster size variability. This study was undertaken over 2 years and baseline variables such as laterality of implantations as well as age were well balanced. Strict study criteria were implemented to ensure that the surgical workflow between the two implantation methods was identical except for the trajectory alignment method (see Fig. 15.3). To further prevent bias, the trajectory planning for both implantation

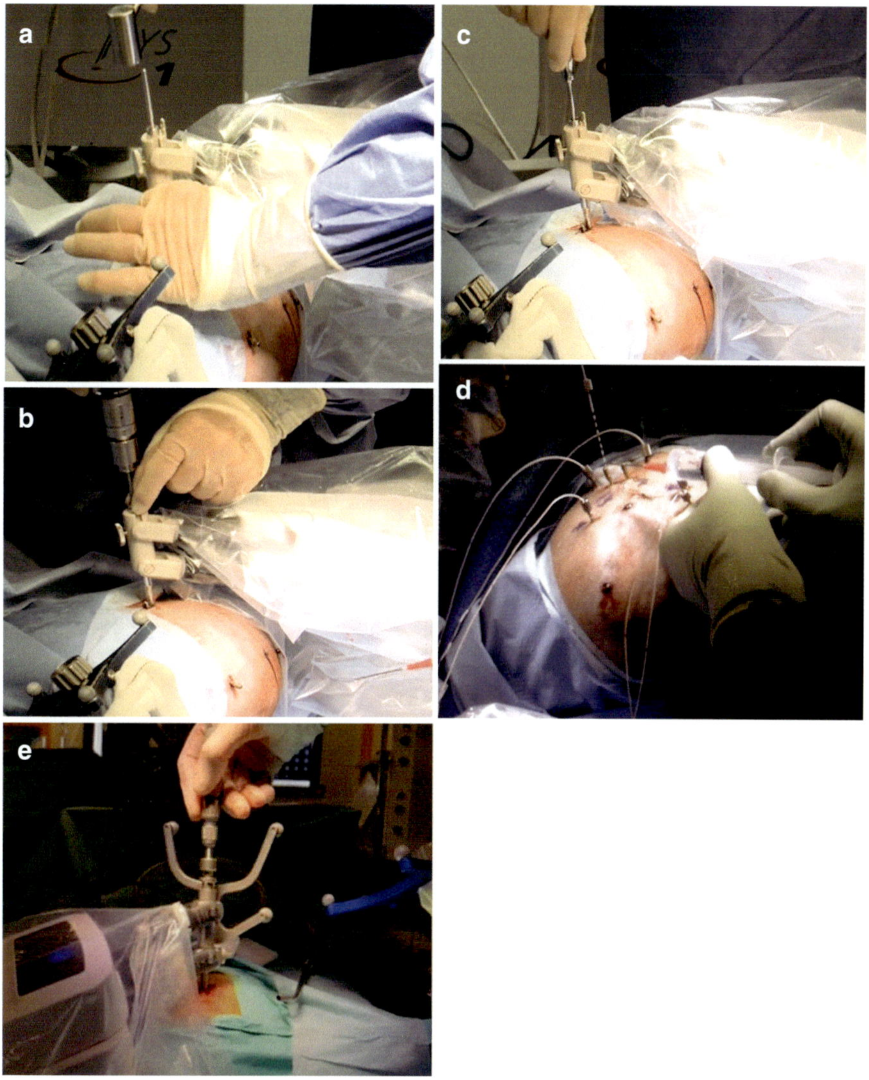

Fig. 15.2 SEEG implantation steps
Intraoperative images depicting the salient steps of an SEEG implantation utilising the iSYS1 device. (**a**) After alignment to the predefined trajectory the Vertek probe is removed, and a K-wire with the appropriate reduction tube is used to create a divot in the underlying bone after the skin has been incised. (**b**) The drill is then used through the working channel, (**c**) followed by the bolt. A stylet is passed through the bolt to the target pointed (**d**) followed by the electrodes. (**e**) Image of Autoguide device. In comparison to the iSYS1, there is no longer a need for the Vertek probe as the optical tracking spheres are mounted to the sterile tool guide. This allows for continuous tracking during drilling and bolt insertion which would alert the surgeon to any potential error introduced during these steps. The Autoguide also incorporates the guidance screen on the back of the device whilst previously with the iSYS1 this required a separate screen cart

<table>
<tr><th>Frameless technique</th><th>Robotic technique (Stealth Autoguide)</th></tr>
<tr><td colspan="2">Place bone fiducial
↓
Head CT scan
↓
Optic surface-based registration
(S7 neuronavigation system)
↓
General anaesthesia
↓
Place Mayfield Clamp
↓
Routine preparation and draping
↓
Mark entry point
↓</td></tr>
<tr><td>Align frameless guidance device to first electrode trajectory
↓</td><td>Roughly align robotic guidance device to first electrode trajectory
↓</td></tr>
<tr><td>Obtain target point accuracy of < 0.7 mm (current clinically accepted threshold)
↓</td><td>Precise alignment of robotic trajectory guidance device to final target point accuracy of < 0.1 mm (device threshold)
↓</td></tr>
<tr><td colspan="2">Incise skin
↓
Check trajectory with Vertek probe
↓
Insert intracranial bolt
↓
Remove mechanical arm
↓
Measure electrode trajectory length
↓
Insert stylet and electrode to predefined length
↓
Repeat previous 9 steps for each electrode
↓
Remove bone fiducials
↓
Close skin</td></tr>
</table>

Fig. 15.3 Workflow for SEEG placement of conventional frameless technique compared to robotic technique, using Stealth Autoguide
Comparative operative steps from randomised control trial comparing robotic (iSYS1) with manual frameless (Precision aiming device) SEEG electrode assisted insertion. Demonstrates that the operative techniques employed in the two arms of the only differed for trajectory alignment to mitigate against confounding factors

methods was undertaken before randomisation utilising a semi-automated planning software called EpiNav. The trajectories were then transferred to the StealthStation to control the iSYS1 implantation. The primary outcome of the study was to compare implantation time as previous studies and pilot data had revealed that entry and target point accuracy was similar. Overall, this showed that individual electrode insertion time fell by 30% from 9.06 min [95% CI 8.16–10.06] min with the frameless implantation arm to 6.36 min [95% CI 5.72–7.07]. On average 10 electrodes were inserted per patient translating into a reduction in overall operative time of 30 min. It should be noted, however, that target point accuracy was slightly worse with the robotic device with a median target point accuracy of 1.58 mm ([95% CI 1.38–1.82] versus 1.16 mm [95% CI 1.01–1.33], $p = 0.004$). For SEEG, the difference of 0.4 mm is not of clinical significance, but this may have a bearing on other stereotactic procedures such as deep brain stimulation. There was no difference in the incidence of radiological haemorrhages, post-operative infections or neurological deficits, although these parameters were underpowered to identify all but gross differences.

Differences in entry and target point accuracies between robotic devices and both frame-based and frameless systems can be found in Table 15.2. It should be noted, however, that accuracy measurements derived from these studies are measured in different ways with some authors calculating the Euclidean distance between the planning and achieved entry and target points and others choosing to measure lateral deviation. The difference between lateral deviation and Euclidean distance measurements is based on inclusion of the depth component. To date, all robotic devices align to the pre-planned trajectories, but the surgeon performs the insertion of the electrode. The depth component is, therefore, related to the accuracy of the surgeon and not the device so some authors argue that reporting the lateral deviation is more comparable.

Table 15.2 Entry point and target point accuracy (mean and 95% confidence interval) between robotic, frameless and frame-based systems for insertion of SEEG electrodes in clinical studies. Data derived from Vakharia et al. (2021) [15]

	Device	Entry point	Target point
Robotic systems			
Dorfer et al. (2017) [14]	iSYS1	1.54 (1.38, 1.79)	1.82 (1.60, 2.04)
Vakharia et al. (2021) [15]	iSYS1	1.20 (1.11, 1.29)	1.90 (1.72, 2.07)
Gonzalez-Martinez et al. (2016) [16]	ROSA	1.20 (−0.36, 2.76)	1.70 (−0.08, 3.62)
Cardinale et al. (2013) [4]	Neuromate + Talairach	0.78 (−0.09, 1.65)	1.77 (−0.08, 3.62)
Cardinale et al. (2017) [17]	Neuromate + Neurolocate	0.59 (−0.34, 1.52)	1.49 (−0.50, 3.48)
Mean group effect estimate		**1.06 (0.34, 1.80)**	**1.74 (0.87, 2.59)**
***I*-squared = 99.2% *P* < 0.001**			
Frameless systems			
Dorfer et al. (2017) [14]	Vertek	3.50 (3.21, 3.79)	3.00 (2.63, 3.37)

(continued)

Table 15.2 (continued)

	Device	Entry point	Target point
Roessler et al. (2016) [18]	Leyla retractor	1.40 (1.09, 1.71)	3.20 (2.63, 3.77)
Hou et al. (2014) [19]	Navigus	–	2.03 (1.88, 2.18)
Nowell et al. (2014) [6]	Vertek	–	3.66 (3.34, 3.98)
Mascott et al. (2006) [20]	Leyla retractor	–	2.40 (2.10, 2.70)
Mehta et al. (2005) [21]	Vertek	–	3.10 (2.95, 3.25)
Vakharia et al. (2021) [15]	Vertek	1.40 (1.29, 1.51)	1.40 (1.25, 1.55)
Mean group effect estimate		**2.23 (1.30, 3.17)**	**2.75 (2.18, 3.32)**
***I*-squared = 98.9% *P* < 0.001**			
Frame-based systems			
Hou et al. (2014) [19]	Leksell	–	1.79 (1.59, 1.99)
Cardinale et al. (2013) [4]	Talairach	1.43 (1.35, 1.51)	2.69 (2.58, 2.80)
Munyon et al. (2013) [22]	Leksell	–	1.00 (0.95, 1.05)
Ortler et al. (2011) [23]	Vogele-Bale-Hohner	2.17 (0.42, 3.92)	2.43 (1.65, 3.21)
Ortler et al. (2011) [23]	Fischer-Leibinger	1.37 (1.04, 1.70)	1.80 (1.57, 2.03)
Mean group effect estimate		**1.61 (1.36, 1.87)**	**1.93 (1.05, 2.81)**
***I*-squared = 99.2% *P* < 0.001**			

Laser Interstitial Thermal Therapy

The Stealth Autoguide system has been described in conjunction with laser interstitial thermal therapy (LITT) for the stereotactic placement of the laser catheter. LITT consists of implantation of a laser catheter to perform a thermal ablation of pathological tissue under MR thermography guidance. The MR thermography allows for real-time assessment of heat dissipation and is vital in preventing ablation of nearby critical structures. After an ablation is undertaken, the catheter can then be retracted and further ablations repeated. The success of the treatment is dependent on trajectory planning and accurate catheter placement to ensure that all of the pathological tissue is effectively ablated whilst sparing the surrounding normal tissue [24, 25]. Epilepsy interventions utilising LITT technology include ablation of hypothalamic hamartoma [26], mesial temporal sclerosis [27, 28], ablation of SEEG defined targets [29], ablation of deep epileptogenic lesions and corpus callosotomy [30, 31]. An overview of how LITT can be performed utilising the iSYS1 and step by step demonstration of the surgical workflow has been described by Casali et al. [32]. They advocate the use of robotic assistance in cases with multiple catheters, proximity to eloquent areas, complex lesion morphology and high-risk trajectories.

Experimental Indications

Finally, cadaveric studies have been undertaken to determine the utility of the iSYS1 for use in lateral skull base surgery [33]. The system was used as a hybrid guidance system to allow for navigated drilling and intraoperative structure localisation, that is compatible with microscope use and without obstructing the surgeon. The iSYS1 was modified to position a laser beam emitter onto the surgical field along a predefined trajectory to identify critical anatomy and guide drilling. The study revealed an accuracy of 1.2 mm ± 0.5 mm, which was deemed suitable for most lateral skull base procedures by the authors.

CIRQ

Spinal instrumentation surgery has seen advancement in recent years, due to the use of trajectory planning software and navigation, intraoperative CT scanning and robotic systems. The main use of robotics in spinal surgery has been around minimally invasive pedicle screw insertion. Cirq, Brainlab was first introduced into the US market in 2019. A lightweight (11 kg) and small robotic device attached to a table-mounted arm. The general method consists of registering the patient's intraoperative CT imaging with the Brainlab navigation system. The robotic arm is used to align to the predefined trajectory and provide a working channel for screw insertion. The platform acts as an assistive device to provide more accurate and consistent instrumentation in minimally invasive procedures of the spine.

Early experience with the device for lumbar instrumentation was described in 2018 in video format by Krieg and Meyer [34]. They used the robotic device for spinal L3-4 stabilisation using navigated pedicle screws and reported satisfactory outcomes. Additional experience of the Cirq for percutaneous cervical and thoracic pedicle screw fixation was described in 2020 [35]. The case series reported 7 patients undergoing insertion of 28 pedicle screws. Intraoperatively, a CT scan using the AIRO was acquired for registration and assessment of the intraoperative fracture morphology. The imaging was transferred to the Brainlab Curve navigation system, and a probe was used to identify the skin entry point. After the skin incision, the Cirq was aligned to the screw trajectory. A navigated drill was used through the Cirq arm to penetrate the layer of the bone, thereafter the surgeon placed a K-wire. The process was performed for all subsequent screw trajectories before the intraoperative CT scan was repeated to ensure satisfactory positioning of the K-wires. Finally, cannulated screws were inserted along the K-wires under image guidance and connected using rods. The case report highlighted minimal blood loss (20 ml), minimal pain reported by the patient and adequate screw positioning. Based on the Neo and Heary classification, 85.7% of the pedicles were rated as acceptable and the remaining 14.3% as poor.

A larger case series has now been reported including 714 thoracolumbar screws in 84 patients, with the Cirq [36]. The mean operative time per screw was 28 min, with a learning curve of median operative time improving from 32 min to 25 min when comparing the first and latter half of cases. They reported no intraoperative screw revisions, but a 2.4% (2/84 patients) instrumentation revision rate necessitating a return to theatre. Their experience highlighted the efficacy and safety of the Cirq system.

Although the use of Cirq has been reported in several case series, further evidence is awaited to assess the accuracy, patient outcomes and cost-effectiveness of pedicle screw placement compared to freehand, navigation and other robotic devices.

Conclusion

Robotics in neurosurgery has been reported for over 3 decades [37]. Although growth has previously been limited by cost and clinical utility, recent technological advancement has meant the use of robotics has exponentially grown. Many case series have been reported to compare the use of robotic systems to conventional methods, showing superiority in several areas. However, further level 1 evidence is required to assess accuracy, patient outcomes, clinical utility and cost-effectiveness. Two small footprint devices, the Autoguide (previously known as iSYS1) and the Brainlab Cirq, are currently commercially available. Small footprint devices have several advantages over larger robotic devices and are more likely to be used for wider indications due to their convenience, lower cost and speed. Nevertheless, comparative accuracy studies are now needed to ensure that results are comparable to large footprint devices, especially for procedures where high levels of accuracy and precision are needed, such as in deep brain stimulation.

References

1. Kettenbach J, Kronreif G, Figl M, Furst M, Birkfellner W, Hanel R, Ptacek W, Bergmann H. Robot-assisted biopsy using computed tomography-guidance: initial results from in vitro tests. Investig Radiol. 2005;40:219–28.
2. Czerny C, Eichler K, Croissant Y, et al. Combining C-arm CT with a new remote operated positioning and guidance system for guidance of minimally invasive spine interventions. J Neurointerv Surg. 2015;7:303–8.

3. Groetz S, Wilhelm K, Willinek W, Pieper C, Schild H, Thomas D. A new robotic assistance system for percutaneous CT-guided punctures: initial experience. Minim invasive Ther Allied Technol MITAT Off J Soc Minim Invasive Ther. 2016;25:79–85.
4. Cardinale F, Cossu M, Castana L, et al. Stereoelectroencephalography: surgical methodology, safety, and stereotactic application accuracy in 500 procedures. Neurosurgery. 2013;72:353–66.
5. Vakharia VN, Rodionov R, McEvoy AW, Miserocchi A, Sparks R, O'Keeffe AG, Ourselin S, Duncan JS. Improving patient safety during introduction of novel medical devices through cumulative summation analysis. J Neurosurg. 2018;130:213–9.
6. Nowell M, Rodionov R, Diehl B, Wehner T, Zombori G, Kinghorn J, Ourselin S, Duncan J, Miserocchi A, McEvoy A. A novel method for implementation of frameless stereoEEG in epilepsy surgery. Neurosurgery. 2014;10:525–34.
7. Brandman D, Hong M, Clarke DB. Preclinical evaluation of the stealth autoguide robotic guidance device for stereotactic cranial surgery: a human cadaveric study. Stereotact Funct Neurosurg. 2021;99:343–50.
8. Legnani FG, Franzini A, Mattei L, et al. Image-guided biopsy of intracranial lesions with a small robotic device (iSYS1): a prospective, exploratory pilot study. Oper Neurosurg. 2019;17:403–12.
9. Minchev G, Kronreif G, Martínez-Moreno M, Dorfer C, Micko A, Mert A, Kiesel B, Widhalm G, Knosp E, Wolfsberger S. A novel miniature robotic guidance device for stereotactic neurosurgical interventions: preliminary experience with the iSYS1 robot. J Neurosurg. 2017;126:985–96.
10. Minchev G, Kronreif G, Ptacek W, Kettenbach J, Micko A, Wurzer A, Maschke S, Wolfsberger S. Frameless stereotactic brain biopsies: comparison of minimally invasive robot-guided and manual arm-based technique. Oper Neurosurg. 2020;19:292–301.
11. Marcus HJ, Vakharia VN, Ourselin S, Duncan J, Tisdall M, Aquilina K. Robot-assisted stereotactic brain biopsy: systematic review and bibliometric analysis. Childs Nerv Syst. 2018;34:1299–309.
12. Vakharia VN, Sparks RS, O'Keeffe AG, Rodionov R, Miserocchi A, McEvoy A, Ourselin S, Duncan JS. Accuracy of intracranial electrode placement for stereoencephalography: a systematic review and meta-analysis. Epilepsia. 2017;58:921–32.
13. Rodionov R, O'Keeffe A, Nowell M, et al. Increasing the accuracy of 3D EEG implantations. J Neurosurg. 2020;133:35–42.
14. Dorfer C, Minchev G, Czech T, Stefanits H, Feucht M, Pataraia E, Baumgartner C, Kronreif G, Wolfsberger S. A novel miniature robotic device for frameless implantation of depth electrodes in refractory epilepsy. J Neurosurg. 2017;126:1622–8.
15. Vakharia VN, Rodionov R, Miserocchi A, McEvoy AW, O'Keeffe A, Granados A, Shapoori S, Sparks R, Ourselin S, Duncan JS. Comparison of robotic and manual implantation of intracerebral electrodes: a single-Centre, single-blinded, randomised controlled trial. Sci Rep. 2021;11:17127.
16. González-Martínez J, Bulacio J, Thompson S, Gale J, Smithason S, Najm I, Bingaman W. Technique, results, and complications related to robot-assisted stereoelectroencephalography. Neurosurgery. 2016;78:169–80.
17. Cardinale F, Rizzi M, d'Orio P, Casaceli G, Arnulfo G, Narizzano M, Scorza D, De Momi E, Nichelatti M, Redaelli D, Sberna M, Moscato A, Castana L. A new tool for touch-free patient registration for robot-assisted intracranial surgery: application accuracy from a phantom study and a retrospective surgical series. Neurosurg Focus. 2017;42:E8.
18. Roessler K, Sommer B, Merkel A, Rampp S, Gollwitzer S, Hamer HM, Buchfelder M. A frameless stereotactic implantation technique for depth electrodes in refractory epilepsy using intraoperative magnetic resonance imaging. World Neurosurg. 2016;94:206–10.
19. Hou Z, Chen X, Shi X, An N, Yang M, Yang H, Zhang D, Liu S. Comparison of neuronavigation and frame-based stereotactic system in implanting epileptic depth electrodes. Turk Neurosurg. 2016;26:574–81.

20. Mascott CR, Sol JC, Bousquet P, Lagarrigue J, Lazorthes Y, Lauwers-Cances V. Quantification of true in vivo (application) accuracy in cranial image-guided surgery: influence of mode of patient registration. Neurosurgery. 2006;59:146–56.
21. Mehta AD, Labar D, Dean A, Harden C, Hosain S, Pak J, Marks D, Schwartz TH. Frameless stereotactic placement of depth electrodes in epilepsy surgery. J Neurosurg. 2005;102:1040–5.
22. Munyon CN, Koubeissi MZ, Syed TU, Lüders HO, Miller JP. Accuracy of frame-based stereotactic depth electrode implantation during craniotomy for subdural grid placement. Stereotact Funct Neurosurg. 2013;91:399–403.
23. Ortler M, Sohm F, Eisner W, Bauer R, Dobesberger J, Trinka E, Widmann G, Bale R. Frame-based vs frameless placement of intrahippocampal depth electrodes in patients with refractory epilepsy: a comparative in vivo (application) study. Neurosurgery. 2011;68:881–7.
24. Vakharia VN, Sparks R, Kuo L, O'Keffee A, Miserocchi A. Automated trajectory planning for laser interstitial thermajl therapy (LiTT) in mesial temporal lobe epilepsy. Epilepsia. 2018;59:814–24.
25. Vakharia VN, Sparks RE, Li K, et al. Multicenter validation of automated trajectories for selective laser amygdalohippocampectomy. Epilepsia. 2019;60:1949–59.
26. Wilfong AA, Curry DJ. Hypothalamic hamartomas: optimal approach to clinical evaluation and diagnosis. Epilepsia. 2013;54:109–14.
27. Gross RE, Willie JT, Drane DL. The role of stereotactic laser amygdalohippocampotomy in mesial temporal lobe epilepsy. Neurosurg Clin N Am. 2016;27:37–50.
28. Li K, Vakharia VN, Sparks R, França LGS, Granados A, McEvoy AW, Miserocchi A, Wang M, Ourselin S, Duncan JS. Optimizing trajectories for cranial laser interstitial thermal therapy using computer-assisted planning: a machine learning approach. Neurotherapeutics. 2019;16:182–91.
29. Youngerman B, Oh J, Deepti A, et al. Laser ablation is effective for temporal lobe epilepsy with and without mesial temporal sclerosis if hippocampal seizure onsets are localized by stereoelectroencephalography. Epilepsia. 2018;59:595–606.
30. Vakharia VN, Sparks RE, Vos SB, Bezchlibnyk Y, Mehta AD, Willie JT, Wu C, Sharan A, Ourselin S, Duncan JS. Computer-assisted planning for minimally invasive anterior two-thirds laser corpus callosotomy: a feasibility study with probabilistic tractography validation: automated laser callosotomy trajectory planning. NeuroImage Clin. 2020;25:102174.
31. Palma AE, Wicks RT, Popli G, Couture DE. Corpus callosotomy via laser interstitial thermal therapy: a case series. J Neurosurg Pediatr. 2018;23:303–7.
32. Casali C, Del Bene M, Messina G, Legnani F, DiMeco F. Robot assisted laser-interstitial thermal therapy with iSYS1 and Visualase: how I do it. Acta Neurochir. 2021;163:3465–71.
33. Bárdosi Z, Plattner C, Özbek Y, Hofmann T, Milosavljevic S, Schartinger V, Freysinger W. CIGuide: in situ augmented reality laser guidance. Int J Comput Assist Radiol Surg. 2020;15:49–57.
34. Krieg SM, Meyer B. First experience with the jump-starting robotic assistance device Cirq. Neurosurg Focus. 2018;45:V3.
35. Farah K, Meyer M, Prost S, Albader F, Dufour H, Blondel B, Fuentes S. Robotic assistance for minimally invasive cervical pedicle instrumentation: report on feasibility and safety. World Neurosurg. 2021;150:e777–82.
36. Chesney K, Triano M, Dowlati E, Zhang I, Felbaum DR, Aulisi EF. Cirq robotic arm-assisted transpedicular instrumentation with intraoperative navigation: technical note and case series with 714 thoracolumbar screws. J Robot Surg. 2022;16:893–8.
37. Elsabeh R, Singh S, Shasho J, Saltzman Y, Abrahams JM. Cranial neurosurgical robotics. Br J Neurosurg. 2021;35:532–40.

Chapter 16
Robotics in Spine Procedures

Gordon Mao and Nicholas Theodore

Introduction

The field of spinal surgery has evolved over the past few decades and has become reliant on instrumentation to correct, stabilize, and fuse regional bony anatomy. Although there have been numerous updates in techniques and technology both to increase fixation durability and decrease hardware failure, adjunctive advanced technologies, such as image guidance and robotics to enhance the safety of instrumentation placement, have similarly evolved.

The term *robot* was originally introduced by Czech writer Karel Capek in his 1920 science fiction play R.U.R. (*Rossum's Universal Robots*). That play tells the story of a factory of living mechanical creatures that resemble human beings and have the capacity for consciousness and individual thought. These creatures ultimately rebel against their human masters in a dystopian ending. Outside the fictional setting, thankfully, robots have been much more predictable. Robotic systems were initially introduced to increase automation and efficiency in labor-intensive manufacturing industries and to improve safety in hazardous environments, such as working with radioactive material [1].

Today, the medical device industry has found more and more applications for robotics systems, including minimally invasive prostate tumor resections, placement of endovascular stents, intracranial brain biopsies, epilepsy surgery, and, more recently, spinal surgery. The adoption of robotic systems for surgical utilization has progressed quickly across different subspecialties, including urological,

G. Mao
Department of Neurosurgery, Indiana University, Indianapolis, IN, USA

Department of Neurosurgery, The Johns Hopkins School of Medicine, Baltimore, MD, USA
e-mail: gomao@iu.edu

N. Theodore (✉)
Department of Neurosurgery, The Johns Hopkins School of Medicine, Baltimore, MD, USA
e-mail: theodore@jhmi.edu

J. A. González Martínez, F. Cardinale (eds.), *Robotics in Neurosurgery*,
https://doi.org/10.1007/978-3-031-08380-8_16

gynecological, and orthopedic procedures, doubling between 2010 and 2017, and with an annual volume increase from 136,000 to 877,000 during the same period [2]. Spinal surgery procedures often require fine manipulation of vital structures that must be accessed via limited surgical corridors and can require repetitive tasks over lengthy periods of time—tasks for which robotic assistance is ideally suited to complement human ability [3].

In the United States, with the passage of the Affordable Care Act in 2012 and the subsequent Medicare Access and CHIP Reauthorization Act in 2015, payers have been increasingly emphasizing value-based compensation schema. During this same period, there has been increased demand from patients for minimally invasive surgery (MIS) procedures, which are perceived by patients as being safer and less expensive than their open procedure counterparts [4]. This perception is to some degree supported by economic analyses, which show increased cost-effectiveness of MIS procedures [5], and by clinical trial data, which show equivalent patient-reported outcomes regardless of procedure type (i.e., open or MIS) [6]. MIS is associated with smaller incisions, decreased rates of postoperative infections, shorter lengths of stay, and decreased duration of patient convalescence following surgery [7].

In the US, there are currently 7 FDA-cleared robotic spine surgery systems on the market, from 4 vendors: (1) Mazor SpineAssist® (Mazor Robotics), (2) Mazor Renaissance® (Mazor Robotics), (3) Mazor XTM (Mazor Robotics), (4) Mazor XTM Stealth Edition (Medtronic [acquired Mazor Robotics in 2018]), (5) ROSA® Spine (Zimmer Biomet), (6) ROSA® ONE Spine (Zimmer Biomet), and (7) ExcelsiusGPS® (Globus Medical).

Historical Foundation

The evolution of robotics in spinal surgery parallels the evolution of image guidance [1]. In 1908, Victor Horsley and Robert Clarke first coined the term "stereotaxis" to define a neurosurgery method utilizing the Cartesian coordinate system to locate points within the brain using external cranial landmarks [8]. The advent of robotics into neurosurgery began with the PUMA 560 system (Programmable Universal Machine for Assembly 560; Unimation) in 1985; this system was used for stereotactic intracranial procedures. Robotic arms evolved in terms of dexterity, precision, and decreased bulk all of which carry advantages for minimally invasive approaches. The concept of MIS was born in 1987, the year of the first-ever laparoscopic cholecystectomy. After the widespread success of this operation, a large effort in the medical community was initiated in order to promote and expand upon this novel concept toward all surgical disciplines.

The introduction of robotic systems into spinal surgery began in 1998, with Okada et al. describing the first use of a thoracoscope in transthoracic surgery [9]. Shortly thereafter, the first da Vinci system—funded by the military, with the goal of establishing telepresence surgery—premiered, allowing for intricate intracavitary surgeries for both general surgery and spinal approaches to the anterior spine. The da Vinci system, though not cleared by the FDA for spinal applications, has been used to perform anterior lumbar interbody fusions (ALIF) [10] and to remove benign nerve sheath tumors [11]. The first modern spinal robotic surgery system to gain FDA approval was the Mazor SpineAssist in 2004.

General Overview

The adoption of robotic assistance (RA) in spinal surgery provides many benefits for the patient, surgical staff, and surgeon, with studies demonstrating that robotic procedures have lower intraoperative complications than freehand (FH) surgeries [12, 13]. The technical considerations for a safe and well-placed pedicle screw are based on local spinal anatomy, understanding that the delicate neurovascular structures within the bony spinal canal are sensitive to injury from traction, compression, mechanical violation, or heat that can cause hemorrhage, as well as sensory and motor loss during either surgical dissection or screw placement.

Intraoperative navigation, which registers a patient's anatomy to a medical image, allows for a real-time understanding of anatomy that can be crucial when operating on patients with complex spinal and other skeletal deformities, osteoporosis, and tumors. Intraoperative navigation also requires a shift of the surgeon's attention from the patient to the screen with the registered image. Image-guided robotic systems allow the surgeon to access three-dimensional visualizations of the patient's imaging with a rigid arm, which can be locked on trajectory to decrease attention shift and could also enable the surgical team to view the operation remotely via telesurgery in some instances [14, 15].

Robots can offer a number of other benefits, including eliminating hand tremors, reducing surgeon fatigue, decreasing incision size, and providing up to 7 degrees of freedom while operating [16–18]. Studies have reported that, because of reduced muscle retraction, patients who undergo minimally invasive procedures may experience decreased postoperative pain [19]. Because spinal robots follow a precise plan, they have also been found to help avoid damaging the proximal facet joint, which may lead to a decreased rate of adjacent segment disease [20].

The bony landmarks used in the process of navigating to the surgical site often need to be visualized with fluoroscopy. This means that the patient, surgeon, and operating room staff are all exposed to large amounts of harmful radiation. This is especially important because spinal procedures can involve 10- to 12-fold higher amounts of radiation compared with non-spinal procedures [21]. Because surgeons and surgical staff exposed to these high doses of radiation have increased levels of malignancy later in life, many surgeons elect to avoid minimally invasive approaches because they use more fluoroscopy. A retrospective review of spine cases between 2004 and 2007 demonstrated that only 13.2% of spine cases were performed in a minimally invasive manner [22]. One significant aim of robotic technology is to reduce radiation exposure to both patients and providers, improve the safety profile of spinal surgery, and potentially promote the increased adoption of minimally invasive approaches.

Despite its intraoperative advantages, robotic surgery is still mostly confined to minor surgical procedures and has, to date, not seen wide adoption in neurosurgery or orthopedics compared with other surgical specialties [14, 23]. This may not be due to a lack of surgeon optimism regarding robotics, but instead may be due to the complexity of the surgical operations performed in these fields [23]. However, as robots are able to complete increasingly complex surgical tasks, the indications for RA surgery will continue to expand. For example, spinal tumor resections and ablations, revision procedures, vertebroplasties, and deformity corrections are just a few of its emerging indications [24].

Computer-Assisted Navigation

Both manual and robotic spine surgery have benefited from image guidance or computer-assisted navigation (CAN). Widely used by many surgeons, image guidance is included in most currently available robotic platforms [25]. Real-time image guidance, along with continuous computation and scan integration by the navigation system, allows the surgeon to visualize a comprehensive three-dimensional picture of the patient. Because of this, intraoperative computed tomography (CT) scans paired with infrared and other optical guidance systems have significantly increased surgeons' ability to accurately place screws [7]. Navigation is now widely used in spinal procedures ranging from fusions to resections of intradural tumors to spinal deformity correction [18].

There are many CAN options currently available for surgeons. These systems include the Brainlab Spine Navigation system, the Stryker Spinal Navigation system with the SpineMask Tracker and the SpineMap software (Stryker), the Stealth Station Spine Surgery Imaging and Surgical Navigation system (Medtronic), and the Ziehm Vision FD Vario 3-D system with NaviPort integration (Ziehm Imaging). For surgeons operating with robot assistance, several CAN systems can be integrated with currently available robots. The Mazor® and ROSA® robots can also have their native navigation software optimized for spinal operations [7].

Screw Placement Procedure

Current commercial systems are all semi-autonomous robots designed to assist the surgeon in the placement of various pedicle and iliac fixation screws (Fig. 16.1a). Most systems are now integrated with real-time image guidance to track the movement of the robotic arm, end effectors, spinal instruments, and implants or screws. The overall workflow depends on the capability of the system to utilize the preoperative CT for planning before the surgery (i.e., CT-fluoroscopy merge) versus the need to obtain intraoperative images first, with the patient positioned and secured on the OR table, before making surgical plans (the so-called scan and plan). The ability to make surgical plans before the case begins (Fig. 16.1b) reduces the patient's time under general anesthesia and can be a smoother workflow, especially for shorter segment cases. Intraoperative CT or fluoroscopic imaging may be beneficial for

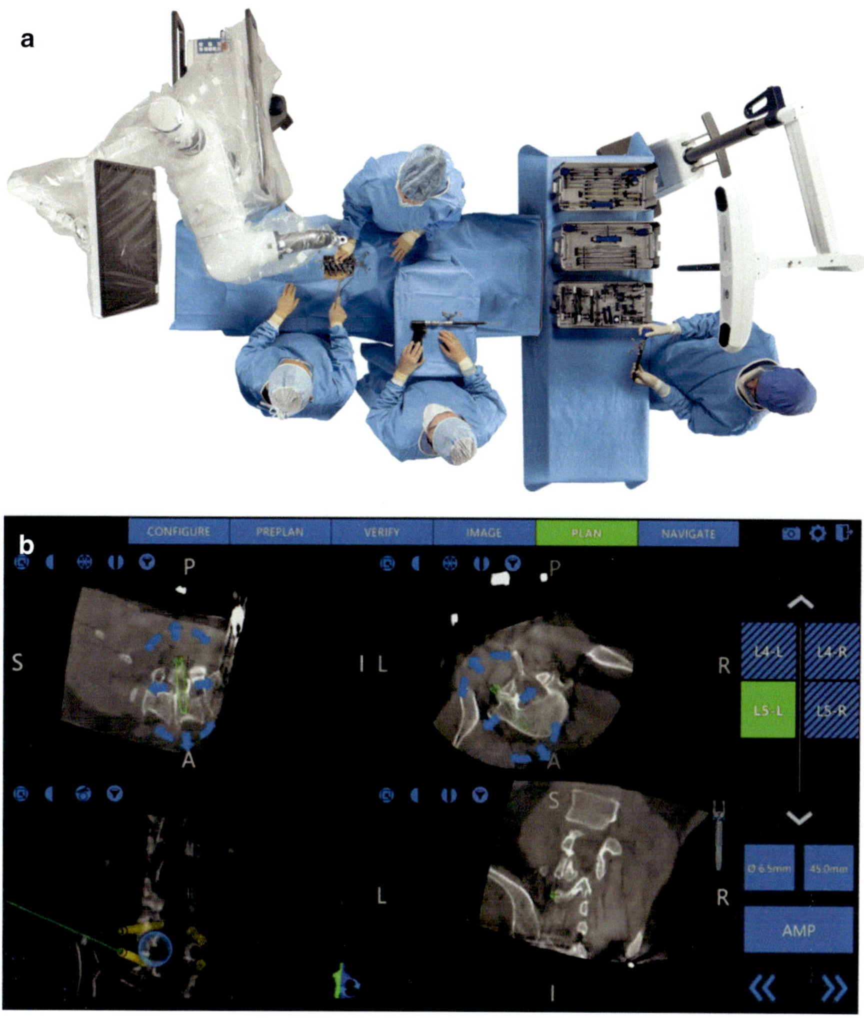

Fig. 16.1 (**a**) Overview of the general intraoperative arrangement of the patient, surgical staff, and surgical robot. (**b**) Preoperative planning of pedicle screw construct utilizing proprietary software technology with three-dimensional rendering demonstrated on the ExcelsiusGPS system. (**c**) Demonstration of patient positioning and placement of anatomic reference arrays to bilateral posterior superior iliac spine with the Globus ExcelsiusGPS system. (**d**) Intraoperative placement of pedicle screws with robotic assistance and real-time image guidance through the end effector arm

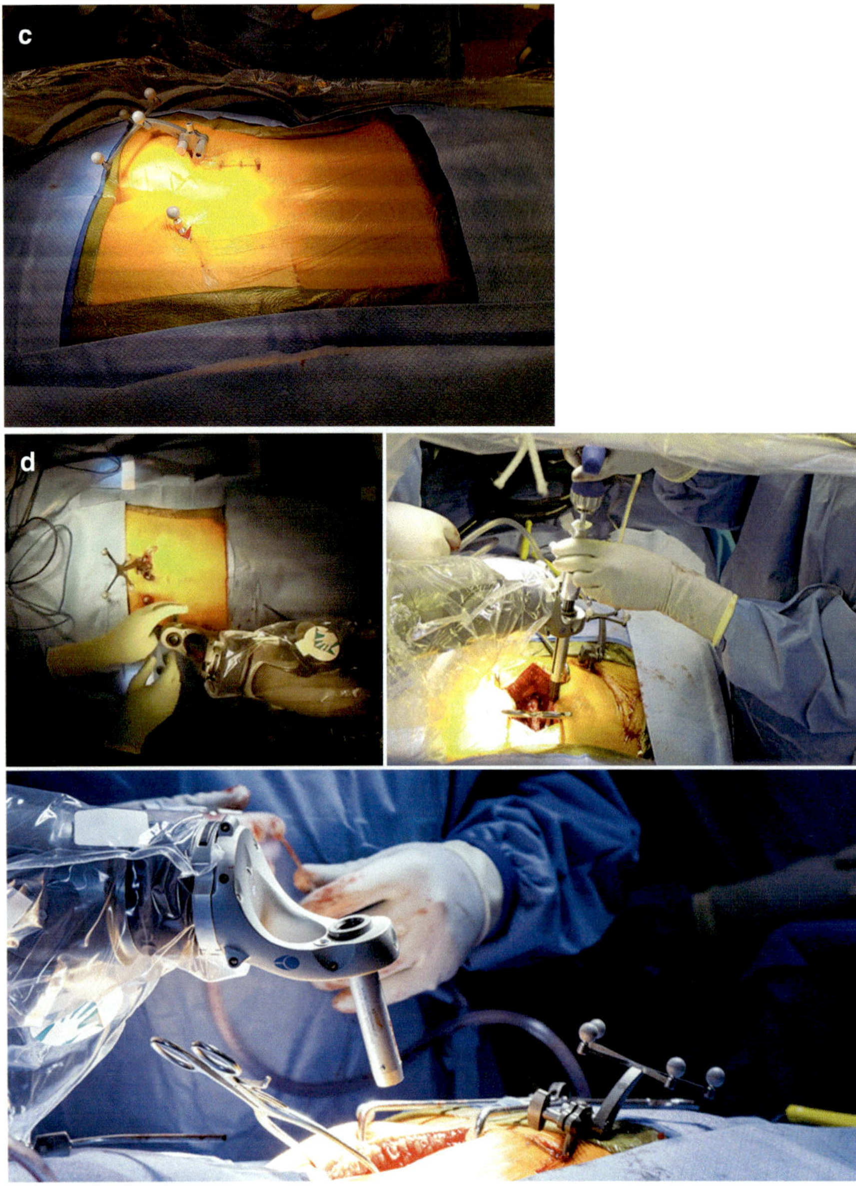

Fig. 16.1 (continued)

those concerned about major alignment shifts in the spine based on patient positioning or underlying instability or in morbidly obese patients. This can also be true in procedures in the upper thoracic spine, where imaging can be difficult secondary to the patient's arms and shoulders.

The more commonly used preoperative CT planning workflow obviates the extra time needed to plan out multiple pedicle screws in longer fusion constructs in the operating room. Once the patient is positioned on the table, one or more reference arrays or fiducials are placed on a stable, bony prominence that can be the spinous process, posterior superior iliac spine (PSIS), or any solid fixation point (Fig. 16.1c). The robot is then brought close to the surgical field to allow adequate reach of the arm to all planned levels and secured via a combination of fixation to the floor, OR table, and/or the patient, depending on which system is used. The robotic arm is typically connected to a base that may be directly fixated to the patient via a pin or clamp system, as is the Mazor X.

At this point, the workflow diverges based on the use of preoperative CT. If a preoperative CT has been obtained and uploaded to the robotic system, co-registration is then completed via two fluoroscopic images per vertebral segment that merge each vertebral segment independently and provide an updated three-dimensional reconstruction of the spine. A proprietary algorithm typically assigns internal validity scores to the merge, which is ultimately confirmed visually by the surgeon for each level. A second registration method includes mounting a rigid reference array either directly to the patient's bony anatomy or to the robotic arm so that intraoperative CT and subsequent planning can be performed. Finally, a third registration option is available on some systems, which allows registration with only 2 planar orthogonal (anteroposterior/lateral) radiographs to allow screw trajectory planning and robotic guidance. Some systems also use another parallel electromagnetic (EM)-based imaging system to map out the patient's torso and skin surface to avoid accidental collision of the arm against the patient during RA instrumentation.

After planning, the appropriate skin incisions can be easily planned using robotic guidance and soft tissue dissections can be made for MIS case. The end effector control arm can then be brought into the designated spinal level and pedicle entry site (Fig. 16.1d). At this point, manually operated instruments are typically brought in and introduced through the robotic arm end effector to drill a pilot hole, cannulate the pedicle, and place a screw of predetermined width and length. Newer robotic systems typically have reference arrays on each instrument that allow for real-time tracking of the precise movement of the instruments and implants as they are being placed, utilizing an optical tracking system as well.

Current Commercial Systems

Mazor SpineAssist

The oldest spine system on the market today, the SpineAssist (Fig. 16.2a), was first approved by the FDA in 2004. This is a shared-control robot that simultaneously allows both the surgeon and the robot control of instruments and motions. The system is mounted directly to the patient rather than to the OR bed or floor and uses a

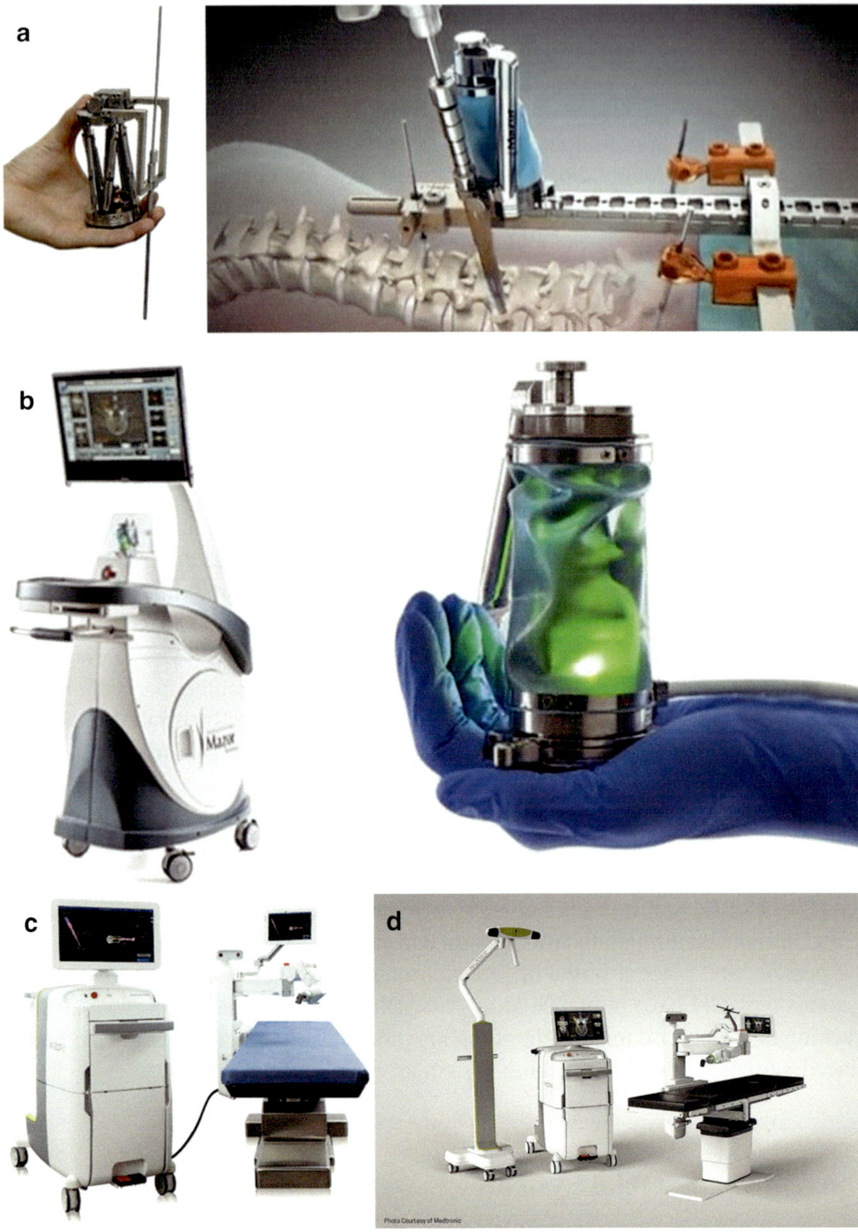

Fig. 16.2 (**a**) Medtronic SpineAssist robotic system. Image provided courtesy of Medtronic. (**b**) Medtronic Renaissance spine robotic system. Image provided courtesy of Medtronic. (**c**) Medtronic Mazor X spine robotic system. Image provided courtesy of Medtronic. (**d**) Medtronic Mazor X Stealth Edition robotic system. Image provided courtesy of Medtronic

Kirschner-wire cannulated screw technique. A small frame is initially mounted to the patient's spine via multiple Kirschner wires. After fiducial markers are attached to the frame, 6 intraoperative fluoroscopy images are taken. The small cylindrical robot is attached to the mounting frame, and the preoperative CT is then co-registered one vertebrae at a time. The robot automatically aligns its arm based on planned trajectory to allow for placement of the cannulated soft tissue dilator, drill guide, drill, K-wire, and final the cannulated pedicle screw.

Mazor Renaissance

Introduced in 2011 as the second-generation update to Mazor's SpineAssist, the Renaissance system (Fig. 16.2b) included both hardware and software updates, such as the ability for the surgeon to flatten the bony prominence around screw entry points before drilling [7]. This process assists in preventing the deflection of the guiding cannula on a sloped anatomy [26]. Both the SpineAssist and Renaissance have accuracy rates ranging from 85% to 100% [27]. The Renaissance has faced similar problems to its first-generation counterpart, the most significant of which is screw misplacement secondary to deflection [28].

Mazor X

The Mazor X (Fig. 16.2c) premiered in 2016 and represented improvements over the Renaissance system by introducing a completely new platform, which still requires attachment of the robot to the OR table. The workflow also changed compared with the prior systems, and this iteration involved (1) preoperative analytics, in which a preoperative or intraoperative CT is uploaded to the system and screw planning is performed; (2) intraoperative guidance, in which the robot is attached to the operating table and then mounted rigidly to the patient's spine, a 3D image of the surgical field is obtained, and the intraoperative anatomy is matched with the CT scan via two fluoroscopic images (anteroposterior and oblique); and (3) intraoperative verification, in which the robotic guidance arm is sent to the preplanned trajectory and real-time instrument tracking is afforded by the integrated 3D camera (Mazor X–Eye). The addition of preoperative CT planning streamlines the workflow by reducing the time spent in the OR planning screw trajectories and spinal alignment, which can be extensive for larger deformity constructs. Similar to its predecessor, screw placement still required guide wires following each cannulation. Unique to this system are its preoperative analytical features, including the Mazor XTM Align application, which can simulate the impact of a correction on the alignment of a patient's entire spine.

Mazor X Stealth Edition

The latest update to the Mazor robotics system family, the Mazor X Stealth Edition (Fig. 16.2d), received FDA approval in 2018. This version integrates the robotic base and arm with the Medtronic Stealth Station technology, allowing for real-time image-guided tracking of the various instrument tips and implants as they are used or inserted through the robotic arm. Although the SpineAssist could not properly account for movements by the patient intraoperatively, the Mazor X utilizes its camera to track patient movements and accordingly readjusts the robot position in real time. The Stealth Edition also eliminates the finicky K-wire system that had to be used on previous iterations, which often significantly crowded the surgical field.

ROSA Spine

The initial ROSA® BRAIN robot (Zimmer Biomet Robotics) was designed for cranial operations and was cleared by the FDA in 2012. The Rosa SPINE system (Fig. 16.3) was created based on the brain version and first approved in 2016 in the US. It comprises 2 mobile components—a floor-fixable cart with a mounted 6-axes robotic arm, and a second mobile base with optical tracking system attached. Preoperative CT cannot be used, so trajectory planning is achieved either with intraoperative fluoroscopy or with CT. Using a percutaneous reference pin placed in the iliac wing, a “fiducial box” held by the robotic arm, and images from an intraoperative cone beam CT, the ROSA performs automatic image registration and

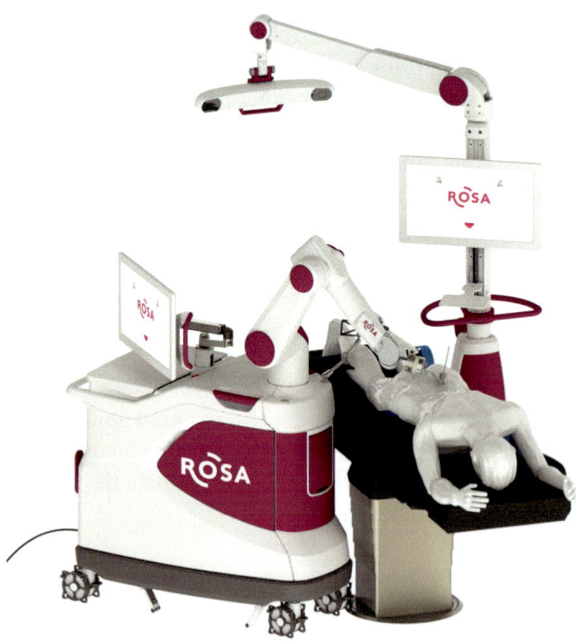

Fig. 16.3 ROSA ONE Spine System. Image provided courtesy of Zimmer Biomet

produces a 3D reconstruction. The surgeon then merges the preoperative and intraoperative scans in order to plan the 3D trajectory. Although instruments can be tracked in real time, guide wires have to be used following pedicle cannulations.

ROSA ONE Spine

The ROSA ONE Spine system is an update to the original robot in 2019 that is built upon the system platform as the ROSA ONE Brain and One Knee systems. Thus, this platform is the only commercial system on the market cleared for spine, intracranial, and orthopedic joint applications.

Globus Medical Excelsius

The ExcelsiusGPS™ (Globus Medical) is a floor-mounted, highly rigid robotic arm system fully integrated with real-time image guidance (Fig. 16.4). The robot is not attached to the patient for functionality. Screw trajectory planning can be performed

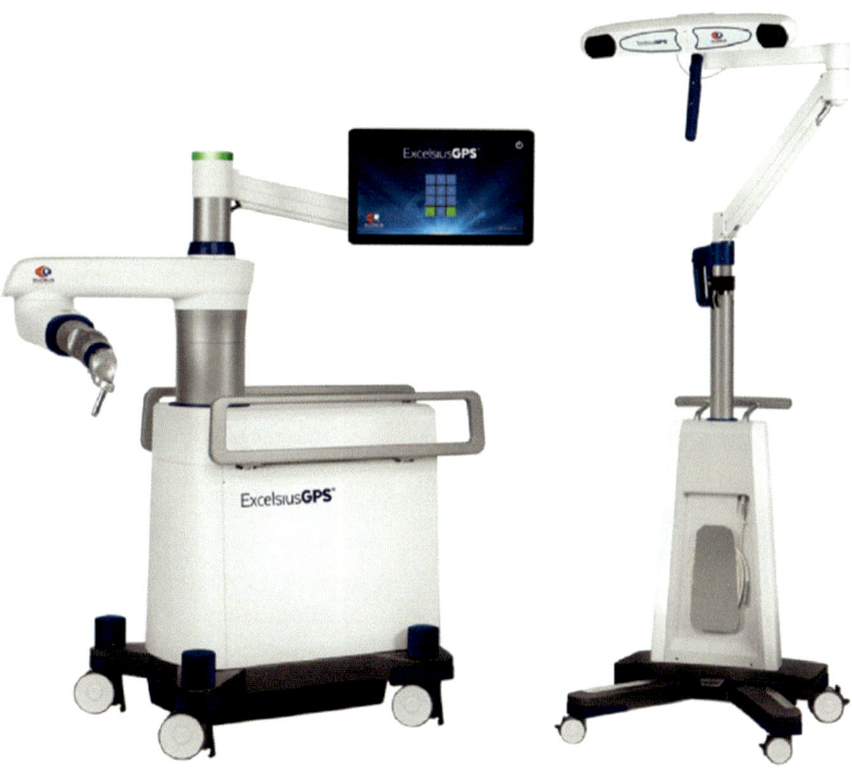

Fig. 16.4 Globus ExcelsiusGPS spine robotic system. Image provided courtesy of Globus Medical

using intraoperative cone beam CT, preoperative CT, or simple anteroposterior and lateral radiographs. Screws are deployed via the rigid tubular robotic arm, eliminating reliance upon patient-mounted frames and surgical guidewires (e.g., Kirschner) [29].

In addition, this system incorporates several features to ensure navigation integrity. These features include a shock-absorbing dynamic reference base, which can deflect forces and spring back to its original position; a separate minimally invasive surveillance marker with Quattro™ spike, which anchors securely into the iliac crest via four small spikes; and associated surveillance software, which can alert the surgeon to a loss of navigation integrity [30]. The ExcelsiusGPS™ system also integrates hardware and software to alert the surgeon of possible instrument deflection (i.e., skiving) during instrumentation placement [30].

Intuitive Surgical: da Vinci Surgical System®

The da Vinci Surgical System® (Fig. 16.5) was developed by Intuitive Surgical and was approved by the FDA in 2000 for general laparoscopic procedures [7]. The da Vinci utilizes a master–slave telesurgical model by which the surgeon operates the device from a remote telesurgical booth equipped with 3D vision screens, thereby allowing the robot to serve as an extension of the surgeon's arm. The da Vinci has been widely studied, yielding results that show superior visualization and magnification compared to traditional laparoscopy. Other benefits include control grips for the surgeon, 7 degrees of freedom, tremor filtering, high-definition video, and improved ergonomics.

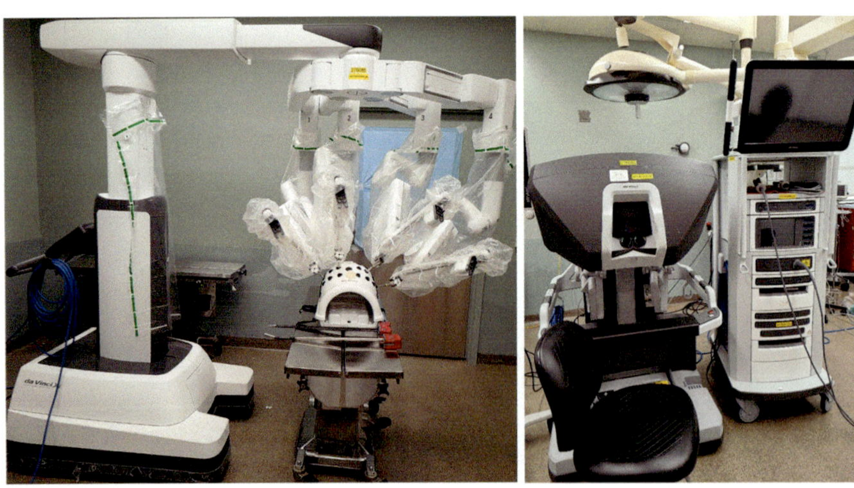

Fig. 16.5 Intuitive Surgical da Vinci Surgical System

In spinal surgery, the da Vinci robot has been utilized for numerous procedures, including ALIF, resection of thoracolumbar neurofibromas, resection of paraspinal schwannomas, and transoral odontoidectomies [24, 31–34]. Originally, laparoscopic ALIF showed no benefit compared to the traditional FH technique in terms of reducing patient blood loss, length of stay, complications, and operating times. Therefore, laparoscopy was largely abandoned for this procedure entirely [35–37]. However, the advanced capabilities of the newer generations of the da Vinci robot make completing ALIF laparoscopically both possible and possibly more efficient. Case series have shown successful dissection, exposure, and interbody placement without any vessel or ureteral complications [33].

Accuracy

Multiple randomized controlled trials (RCTs) and retrospective series have assessed the accuracy of RA vs FH as well as RA vs image-guided pedicle screw techniques. All data show significantly higher rates of accuracy for RA versus FH. Most studies involve the various iterations of the Mazor robotic systems, as Mazor was the first to obtain FDA approval.

Many authors use the Gertzbein-Robbins classification system [38] to determine the accuracy of pedicle screws. This system grades pedicle screws based on the screw tract in relation to the cortical margins of the pedicle, with increasing error based on increase distance breached past the medial or lateral cortex (Table 16.1).

The concept of clinically acceptable pedicle screws (GR A/B), which lie in the safe zone [38], is important to understand when comparing accuracy rates. The risk for neurologic injury is much smaller within the first 2-mm breach past the medical pedicle cortex due to inherent epidural fat, veins, and ligamentum flavum. Many head-on comparisons that note superior or equivalent accuracy rates for FH vs RA techniques are often referring to *acceptable* pedicle screw placement rather than *perfect* pedicle screw placement. When comparing just GR A PS accuracy, most studies actually show significantly higher accuracy for RA group and, similarly, better improved accuracy for major breach (GR C, D, E) where image guidance, FH, or RA groups can be more reliable than pure FH techniques.

Table 16.1 Gertzbein-Robbins classification of pedicle screw accuracy based on presence of implant breach past the pedicle cortical margin and distance of breach beyond the cortical margin in millimeters. *GR, Gertzbein-Robbins*

GR grade	Breach distance (mm)
A	0
B	<2
C	<4
D	<6
E	<8

The ROSA system was also studied by a single-surgeon small retrospective series of 20 patients. In that series, the authors found superior accuracy of 97.3% with the RA technique versus 92% with the FH technique [39].

Although no prospective controlled trials have been conducted comparing ExcelsiusGPS™ to other commercial robotic systems or image-guided techniques, early case reports and cohort series suggest high accuracy, efficacy, and safety [40–43]. Huntsman et al. [44] and Godzik et al. [45] have reported accuracy rates (based on the Gertzbein-Robbins scale) ranging from 96.6% to 99%. Jiang et al. [40] also reported minimal screw deviation with the ExcelsiusGPS™ compared with a pre-planned trajectory in a small lumbar fusion case series.

A 2017 systematic review of RA spinal instrumentation by Joseph et al. identified 22 studies assessing accuracy of spinal robotic systems, including 4 RCTs [27]. They found that RA instrumentation was highly accurate and safe with clinically acceptable instrumentation (GR A or B) in 85% to 100% cases. Most studies investigating robot-guided pedicle screw placement versus FH placement demonstrated an accuracy benefit with robotic assistance.

Only one early RCT from 2012 found diminished accuracy of the SpineAssist® (Mazor Robotics) system compared with FH placement for 1- and 2-level lumbar fusions [46]. 30 FH patients were compared to 30 RA patients, and the authors found increased screw accuracy for the FH vs RA groups (93% vs. 85%, respectively). In this study, 10 RA screws required revision, whereas only 1 FA screw required the same. Although this was a single-center study, the study population was split among 3 experienced spine surgeons who were familiar with both techniques. The smaller size of the RA cohort (which is further subdivided among 3 surgeons) and the study results noting longer surgical time for screw placement for the RA group, suggest that the surgeons in this group were early in the learning curve and utilizing first-generation technology for using RA.

An even more recent systematic review and meta-analysis of over 50,000 pedicle screws compared CT navigation-guided (CTNav), fluoroscopy-assisted (FA), RA, and FH techniques [47]. Out of 78 studies encompassing 7858 patients and 51,161 screws, 3614 breaches were noted. In a subgroup analysis, breaches were subdivided into minor and major breaches defined by a 4-mm cutoff (i.e., GR grade B/C vs D/E). The authors reported overall pooled accuracy rates of 95.5% for the CTNav; 93.1% for the FH alone; 91.5% with FA, and 90.5% with RA. 48% of the breaches were noted in the thoracic spine, with a breach rate of 12% for FH, 10% for FA, 5% for CTNav, and <1% for RA, suggesting that the anatomy of the narrower thoracic pedicles with relatively flatter pedicle entry points favors navigated technologies. Also telling is the rate of lateral breach among screw placement, which is closely related to lumbar facet anatomic factors (hypertrophy) and entry point preparation (i.e., open procedures, which are required for FH, vs percutaneous, which is more common in CTNav and RA cases). Lateral breach rates were highest for early RA cases at 10.8% and were lowest at 3% for FH, where direct visual inspection can significantly reduce risk during pedicle cannulation. Interestingly, in subgroup univariate analysis, the rate of major breach for FH was significantly higher ($p = 0.04$) than CTNav and RA groups, while CTNav was the only group to have significantly lower minor breach rates compared to the other 3 techniques. This suggests that navigated and robotic cohorts did better overall in terms of reducing neurologic risk from major pedicle violations. Although the CTNav group remained the lowest for minor pedicle violations, it is possible that the learning curve and technique aspects of the robotic cohort created more error that could lead to higher minor breaches.

Another meta-analysis of 6 RCTs [48] using primarily the Mazor system, including a combined 158 RA patients vs 148 FH, perfect screw placement (GR A) in the RA group was found to be superior to FH (RR 1.03, $p = 0.04$) while clinically acceptable screws (GR A+B) did not differ ($P = 0.29$). This conclusion is very similar to the large single-surgeon series published by Mao et al. [49]. Interestingly, they noted that proximal facet joint violation, a major cause of proximal junctional kyphosis, was significantly lower in the RA group compared to FH (RR = 0.07, $P = 0.01$). The RA group did have slightly longer operation times, with a mean difference of 21 min ($P = 0.009$).

Han et al. carried out an RCT at a single center, using the TiRobot system [50]. They found significantly higher accuracy for RA vs FH in thoracolumbar cases. 234 patients were randomized 1:1 to RA vs FH. The authors noted similar surgical time and hospital length of stay. Cumulative radiation exposure was significantly higher for the FH group (71 microSievert) than for the RA group (22 microSievert). Mean screw deviation was only 1.5 mm in the RA group, with 95.3% of the screws measured with GR grade A accuracy compared with 86.1% in the FH group. The TiRobot is a multi-indication orthopedic surgical robot that can be used in spinal, pelvic, and limb surgeries performed via an open or a minimally invasive approach [51–53]. The TiRobot is the first orthopedic surgical robot created entirely in China, and it received China's Food and Drug Administration approval in 2016 but is not currently approved for use in the US. Thoracolumbar surgeries resulted in a higher percentage of both radiographically and clinically acceptable outcomes in the robot-assisted cohort compared to a matched FA cohort [29].

The updated meta-analysis of 10 RCTs and cohort studies in 2018 by Fan et al. concluded statistically significant superiority in accuracy using robotic-assisted techniques compared with conventional methods [54]. After the recent advent of the first real-time image-guided spinal robotic system (ExcelsiusGPS™), accuracy rates have increased to range from 96.6% to 99% [44, 45].

In terms of direct comparisons for existing image-guidance systems against robotic assistance in pedicle screw placement, Mao et al. examined a consecutive series of 46 single-surgeon Mazor X cases vs 39 O-arm navigation cases for a mixture of indications, ranging from adult degenerative deformity to trauma [49]. The accuracy of the screw placement was examined both in terms of significant screw misplacement versus clinically acceptable trajectories and was further divided into categories based on the Gertzbein-Robbins classification system for screw accuracy. The robotic outcomes were found to have significantly improved accuracy of pedicle screw placement compared to the O-arm image guidance with respect to GR grade A screws ("perfect," no cortical breach) at rates of 86% vs 66%. The authors also found superior, although not statistically significant, accuracy in the Mazor X cases with respect to clinically acceptable screws (GR A or B) 97.5% vs 95%.

Radiation Safety

Minimally invasive surgery is in part characterized by the lack of standard visual landmarks that are afforded by a larger exposure. Nonetheless, MIS is on the rise—but to overcome the limited visualization, it has increasingly relied on image guidance and navigation. The growing use of intraoperative fluoroscopy naturally leads to concerns regarding the radiation exposure risk to both the surgeon and the patient on the operating room table. More recent technologies, such as intraoperative CT-based guidance (e.g., O-arm [Medtronic], AIRO [Brainlab]), three-dimensional fluoroscopy (e.g., Orbic 3D, [Siemens]), and automatic image registration-navigation using preoperatively acquired CT (e.g., BrainLab) have been shown to reduce radiation exposure to OR staff based on small cohorts [55, 56].

The National Council on Radiation Protection and Measurements and the International Commission on Radiological Protection have published "maximal limits" for exposure for those that work with radiation. These proposed safe limits take into account both yearly cumulative dose (i.e., "deterministic" effects) and a lifetime cumulative dose (i.e., "stochastic" effects). Currently, guidelines recommend no more than 20 millisievert (mSv) per year averaged over 5 years, or 50 mSv/year in any 1 year. For nonradiation workers, the recommended limit of exposure to radiation is 1 mSv/year.

An early retrospective series by Kantelhardt et al. [12] looked at the differences in exposure among a consecutive series of 112 patients, with 35 percutaneous procedures, 57 conventional open procedures, and 20 RA procedures. 94.5% of RA and 91.4% of conventionally placed screws were found to be accurate without significant differences between percutaneous robotic and open robotic-guided subgroups. Average X-ray exposure per screw was 34 s in robotic-guided compared to 77 s in conventional cases. Subgroup analysis indicates that percutaneously operated patients required fewer opioids, had a shorter length of stay, and lower rate of adverse events in the perioperative period, suggesting that the use of robotic guidance significantly increased accuracy of screw positioning while reducing X-ray exposure.

Radiation exposure is also dependent on the robotic technology, workflow, and amount of fluoroscopy required for the RA procedure. Lonjon et al. reported outcomes from an early series of 10 patients using the ROSA robotic system placing 40 pedicle screws vs 10 FA procedure placing 50 pedicle screws [39]. The average exposure was 821 cGy cm^2 over 1.2 min for RA procedures vs 406 cGy cm^2 over 0.40 min for FA procedures. The limitations in the technology of the robotics system, particularly with respect to initial registration of the patient's anatomy to enable the image guidance, and the experience and efficiency of the surgeon naturally also increase the radiation exposure especially for low-volume surgical series.

A 2018 meta-analysis of various RCTs found that radiation time (mean difference of -12.38; $P < 0.001$) and radiation dosage (standard mean difference of -0.64; $P < 0.001$) were significantly decreased in the RA group compared with the FH group [48].

A 2019 meta-analysis of radiation exposure studies across the literature in thoracolumbar fusion procedures [57] found that patient radiation exposure per screw placed for each modality was highest for intraoperative CT-based navigation (1.20 ± 0.91 mSv), similar for conventional fluoroscopy without navigation (0.26 ± 0.38 mSv) and conventional fluoroscopy with preoperative CT-based navigation (0.027 ± 0.010 mSv), and lowest for robot-assisted instrumentation (0.04 ± 0.30 mSv). Although all image-guidance modalities are associated with surgeon radiation exposures well below current safety limits, RA procedures were superior in reducing radiation risk to both the OR staff members and the patient.

An RCT by Hyun et al. [58] compared radiation exposure of 1- or 2-level lumbar cases for RA MIS vs FA open procedures in 2 arms of 30 patients each. Both arms had equivalent clinical outcomes as measured by visual analog scale and Oswestry Disability Index, while the screw accuracy rate was 100% in the RA group and breached in 2/30 (7%) of FA cases. More importantly, the RA arm showed 62.5% reduction in per-screw radiation exposure compared to the FA group as measured by thermoluminescent dosimeters.

In children, for whom the long-term effects of radiation exposure are even more detrimental, RA surgery can be helpful. Sensakovic et al. evaluated a new low-dose radiation CT protocol for patients undergoing pediatric idiopathic scoliosis deformity correction performed using the Mazor robot [59]. In this protocol, patients either underwent traditional preoperative CT or low-dose CT. The authors reported that images were adequate for robotic screw placement although accuracy of screw placement was not graded postoperatively.

Estimated Blood Loss

Direct comparisons of RA against FH or FA cases generally show significantly less estimated blood loss associated with RA procedures [49, 50, 60]. This is likely secondary to the bias of RA cases toward more minimally invasive paramedian exposures rather than midline open exposures. Conventional FH techniques rely on a more extensive, and destructive, soft tissue exposure to adequately expose anatomic landmarks needed to safely place pedicle screws. Image-guided and RA techniques do not require such wide exposures, and in many ways suffer from midline exposures, which necessitate rigid retractors that can block the precise placement of the instruments. In bigger patients with bulky paraspinous musculature or increased subcutaneous adipose tissue, forceful tissue retraction can also distort the regional anatomy, which then imperceptibly shifts with respect to the reference frame, causing failure of the image guidance.

Learning Curve

Robotic systems also have inherent learning curves. Surgeons need to work to understand the available features of the system and to gain mastery over those systems, which includes learning how to incorporate them efficiently into the operating room workflow.

Likewise, surgeons should also be cognizant of the inherent limitations of each respective technology, whether the issue is related to intermittent failure of intraoperative image-guidance features in newer robotic systems, or the anatomic variations of the patient such as hypertrophied facet joints that predispose to a lateral deviation of the cannulation process and subsequent screw placement. The accuracy and safety features of robotic systems depend not only on the normal functioning of the technology, but also on the surgeon's ability to anticipate, obviate, and occasionally promptly diagnose any intraoperative issues to prevent a mistake from snowballing due to non-recognition. Common robotic errors, whether from registration issues (e.g., wrong level co-registration), or frame-shift issues, will remain for entirety of the case, so they can easily propagate in severity and cause neurologic issues when a surgeon is not paying adequate attention and does not identify the issue early. These technical, mechanical, or surgical errors can lead to significant morbidity for the patient and length to the overall operating time.

Several single-center case series have looked at the learning curve primarily using either operative time or screw accuracy as a metric of familiarity and efficiency with the robotic system. The literature suggests that the learning curve for robotic systems lies in the range of 20–50 cases [61, 62], with 1 group recommending a minimum of 25 cases to gain proficiency [61]. The largest series to date, by Schatlo et al. [61], summarized 258 cases by 13 surgeons using the legacy Mazor SpineAssist system. The authors mainly analyzed the screw accuracy rates with cases grouped 5 at a time in chronological order and misplacement defined by ≥3 mm breach outside the pedicle. They noted a clear difference in screw misplacement before and after the first 20 cases in the series. Interestingly enough, the misplacement rate was low in the first 5 cases (2.4%), suggesting high surgeon's caution, and gradually increased to a peak of 7.1% for cases 16–20 before declining steadily afterward to 2–3% after the first 50 cases.

A series from Melbourne [62] analyzed 80 consecutive RA spinal fusion cases using the older Mazor Renaissance System. This series benefitted from a more homogenous pathology (86% degenerative spondylosis; 73% single level performed) and technique using involving only percutaneous screw placement. The authors divided the cases chronologically into 4 quartiles and noted no difference in GR A screws ($P = 0.11$) or clinically acceptable screw placement rate ($P = 0.31$) over time. More importantly, they also noted no difference in mean time per screw across the quartiles ($P = 0.61$), concluding that the learning curve must be quite short and less than the first 20 cases of the initial quartile.

A key issue with the learning curve for different systems lies with the design of the software systems and mechanical systems, which are key in planning and intraoperative control of the robotic system, respectively. Earlier robotic assisted such as the Mazor SpineAssist and first-generation Mazor X robot had inherent issues with secure fixation of the robotic arm to the patient and guidewires to align the screws during placement. These issues are less threatening in smaller degenerative cases; however, they can lead to bigger challenges for longer spinal deformity cases. A single-surgeon series of surgeons using the older Mazor X spine system analyzed 39 consecutive cases of spinal oncology, trauma, and deformity cases that involved longer constructs (mean fused levels 5.4). Though the addition of corpectomies and osteotomies certainly complicates the picture, this series did demonstrate strong evidence of a more gradual learning curve, with the mean operation time per level decreasing 50% over the initial 30–35 cases. Due to the smaller sample size and high case complexity, there were no significant differences in the operation times between the O-arm and RA cohorts in this comparison. It is possible that the learning curve progression will advance faster with successive newer systems as the software design is iteratively improved and image-guidance features become more reliable, already eliminating the need for any guidewires in many newer robotic systems.

The most recent data from Jiang et al. [60] found that improvements in workflow are achieved relatively rapidly in the Globus ExcelsiusGPS system in a small case-control series. Assessing 56 cases (28 RA and 28 FH) 1- and 2-level lumbar fusion procedures, their series reported the duration of RA cases improving to the speed of FH operations by the twentieth procedure. The RA cohort also experienced significantly less blood loss (300 cc difference, $p < 0.001$) and shorter length of stay (1d difference, $p = 0.01$). The authors concluded that if operative efficiency can be taken as an effective proxy of mastery, then it is likely that >30 cases must be performed before the learning curve is meaningfully reduced.

Limitations of Current Technology

Limitations of these robotic spine surgery systems are largely related to the high initial capital expenditure requirement to acquire the robot and the longer operative times related to the learning curve for adoption of the technology and techniques.

Use of these complex machines necessitates additional training for both the surgeon and staff in the operating room. Additionally, robotic equipment has a high initial cost, often exceeding $1,000,000 [14]. Because of these factors, further studies are required to justify their extra labor and expense [17]. In addition, technological limitations of the effector arm, force feedback, and end effector design currently limit the indication mainly to pedicle screw placement and soft tissue retraction.

In addition, several studies have evaluated reasons for failure of the robot during spine instrumentation. Reasons for aborting the robotic procedure included failure of registration software and failure to obtain adequate fluoroscopic images. In several studies, soft tissue pressure on the guiding arm led to inaccurate placement [46, 63]. Other reasons for failure included the inability to adequately obtain surgically the necessary angles determined by the registration software. Other studies describe difficulties with keeping the drill guide in position on the slope of the facet, causing a lateral and inferior deviation [46, 64]. Macke et al. found that patients who had preoperative CTs performed in a prone position had a screw misplacement rate of 2.4%, compared with a misplacement rate of 7.6% in patients whose preoperative CTs were performed in the standard supine position [65].

Most studies conclude that robotic systems work in synergy with both traditional open and MIS techniques, improving the accuracy, safety, and postoperative surgical site pain of fusion cases. However, some heterogeneous studies question that paradigm. Lieber et al. [66] performed a retrospective analysis of data in the Nationwide Inpatient Sample database, comparing 257 patients who underwent robot-assisted lumbar fusion with 257 matched controls who underwent conventional lumbar fusion. After controlling for various patient factors, they did not find a significant difference in minor or major complications between the two groups. However, they report increased hospital costs and length of stay in the RA group, compared with the conventional lumbar fusion group. Due to inherent limitations of database queries, the authors were only able to look at certain major and minor complications coded in the Nationwide Inpatient Sample database. They were unable to assess important spine-specific metrics, such as operation duration, estimated blood loss, pedicle screw accuracy, return to the operating suite, radiographic results, and patient-reported functional outcomes. They also did not have access to long-term follow-up data, so they were unable to assess adjacent segment disease, pseudarthrosis rates, proximal junctional failure, and other factors, which limit their ability to truly assess differences between robot-assisted and conventional lumbar fusion cases. It is also important to keep in mind that these data were obtained from 2010 to 2014. At the time, there was only one FDA-approved, commercially available robot in the US for spinal surgery (Renaissance™, Medtronic). As a result, this study does not reflect recent innovations and techniques available with spinal surgery robots currently on the market.

Conclusion

Initial clinical studies regarding RA spinal surgery suggest that it may be more accurate, more efficient, and safer for pedicle screw instrumentation and other spinal procedures compared to traditional fluoroscopic-assisted freehand approaches. Current evidence suggests that robotic-assisted pedicle screw placement offers decreased radiation exposure to the surgical team, and that the combination of robotics and MIS techniques reduces the use of intraoperative fluoroscopy and length of hospital stay. Though robotic-assisted spine surgery is still in its infancy, the potential for augmenting surgeon performance and improving patient outcomes is significant. Unfortunately, one of the main issues limiting the widespread adoption of robots in spinal surgery worldwide is its associated costs—there remains a lack of studies on the cost-effectiveness of these procedures [67]. There are probably specific clinical scenarios, such as tumor, infection, and deformity cases, where robotic systems have a more profound advantage for MIS; however, further investigation is needed to fully explore the benefits in application of robotic guidance for MIS procedures. Robotics have made their way into the armamentarium of today's spinal surgeon. Given the ongoing adoption of this technology, it will undoubtedly become a common tool in the treatment of spinal disorders.

References

1. Theodore N, Ahmed A, Karim B. The history of robotics in spine surgery. Spine (Phila PA 1976). 2018;43(7):S23. https://doi.org/10.1097/BRS.0000000000002553.
2. Childers CP, Maggard-Gibbons M. Estimation of the acquisition and operating costs for robotic surgery. JAMA. 2018;320(8):835–6. https://doi.org/10.1001/jama.2018.9219.
3. Roser F, Tatagiba M, Maier G. Spinal robotics: current applications and future perspectives. Neurosurgery. 2013;72(Suppl 1):12–8. https://doi.org/10.1227/NEU.0b013e318270d02c.
4. Narain AS, Hijji FY, Duhancioglu G, Haws BE, Khechen B, Manning BT, et al. Patient perceptions of minimally invasive versus open spine surgery. Clin Spine Surg. 2018;31(3):E184–92. https://doi.org/10.1097/BSD.0000000000000618.
5. Djurasovic M, Gum JL, Crawford CH, Owens K, Brown M, Steele P, et al. Cost-effectiveness of minimally invasive midline lumbar interbody fusion versus traditional open transforaminal lumbar interbody fusion. J Neurosurg Spine. 2019:1–5. https://doi.org/10.3171/2019.6.SPINE1965.
6. Mobbs RJ, Li J, Sivabalan P, Raley D, Rao PJ. Outcomes after decompressive laminectomy for lumbar spinal stenosis: comparison between minimally invasive unilateral laminectomy for bilateral decompression and open laminectomy: clinical article. J Neurosurg Spine. 2014;21(2):179–86. https://doi.org/10.3171/2014.4.SPINE13420.
7. D'Souza M, Gendreau J, Feng A, Kim LH, Ho AL, Veeravagu A. Robotic-assisted spine surgery: history, efficacy, cost, and future trends. Robot Surg. 2019;6:9–23. https://doi.org/10.2147/RSRR.S190720.
8. Schurr PH, Merrington WR. The Horsley-Clarke stereotaxic apparatus. Br J Surg. 1978;65(1):33–6. https://doi.org/10.1002/bjs.1800650110.
9. Okada S, Tanaba Y, Kimura K, Yamauchi H, Sato S. Thoracoscopic surgery using voice controlled robot for spontaneous pneumothorax. Kyobu Geka. 1998;51(7):561–3.
10. Kim MJ, Ha Y, Yang MS, Yoon DH, Kim KN, Kim H, et al. Robot-assisted anterior lumbar interbody fusion (ALIF) using retroperitoneal approach. Acta Neurochir. 2010;152(4):675–9. https://doi.org/10.1007/s00701-009-0568-y.
11. Yang MS, Kim KN, Yoon DH, Pennant W, Ha Y. Robot-assisted resection of paraspinal schwannoma. J Korean Med Sci. 2011;26(1):150–3. https://doi.org/10.3346/jkms.2011.26.1.150.
12. Kantelhardt SR, Martinez R, Baerwinkel S, Burger R, Giese A, Rohde V. Perioperative course and accuracy of screw positioning in conventional, open robotic-guided and percutaneous robotic-guided, pedicle screw placement. Eur Spine J. 2011;20(6):860–8. https://doi.org/10.1007/s00586-011-1729-2.
13. Schroerlucke SR, Wang MY, Cannestra AF, Good CR, Lim J, Hsu VW, et al. Complication rate in robotic-guided vs fluoro-guided minimally invasive spinal fusion surgery: report from MIS Refresh Prospective Comparative Study. Spine J. 2017;17(10):S254–5. https://doi.org/10.1016/j.spinee.2017.08.177.
14. Lanfranco AR, Castellanos AE, Desai JP, Meyers WC. Robotic surgery: a current perspective. Ann Surg. 2004;239(1):14–21. https://doi.org/10.1097/01.sla.0000103020.19595.7d.

15. Kim VB, Chapman WH, Albrecht RJ, Bailey BM, Young JA, Nifong LW, et al. Early experience with telemanipulative robot-assisted laparoscopic cholecystectomy using da Vinci. Surg Laparosc Endosc Percutan Tech. 2002;12(1):33–40. https://doi.org/10.1097/00129689-200202000-00006.
16. Devito DP, Kaplan L, Dietl R, Pfeiffer M, Horne D, Silberstein B, et al. Clinical acceptance and accuracy assessment of spinal implants guided with SpineAssist surgical robot: retrospective study. Spine (Phila Pa 1976). 2010;35(24):2109–15. https://doi.org/10.1097/BRS.0b013e3181d323ab.
17. Shweikeh F, Amadio JP, Arnell M, Barnard ZR, Kim TT, Johnson JP, et al. Robotics and the spine: a review of current and ongoing applications. Neurosurg Focus. 2014;36(3):E10. https://doi.org/10.3171/2014.1.FOCUS13526.
18. Overley SC, Cho SK, Mehta AI, Arnold PM. Navigation and robotics in spinal surgery: where are we now? Neurosurgery. 2017;80(3S):S86–99. https://doi.org/10.1093/neuros/nyw077.
19. Kazemi N, Crew LK, Tredway TL. The future of spine surgery: new horizons in the treatment of spinal disorders. Surg Neurol Int. 2013;4(Suppl 1):S15–21. https://doi.org/10.4103/2152-7806.109186.
20. Kim HJ, Jung WI, Chang BS, Lee CK, Kang KT, Yeom JS. A prospective, randomized, controlled trial of robot-assisted vs freehand pedicle screw fixation in spine surgery. Int J Med Robot. 2017;13(3) https://doi.org/10.1002/rcs.1779.
21. Ravi B, Zahrai A, Rampersaud R. Clinical accuracy of computer-assisted two-dimensional fluoroscopy for the percutaneous placement of lumbosacral pedicle screws. Spine (Phila Pa 1976). 2011;36(1):84–91. https://doi.org/10.1097/BRS.0b013e3181cbfd09.
22. Hamilton DK, Smith JS, Sansur CA, Glassman SD, Ames CP, Berven SH, et al. Rates of new neurological deficit associated with spine surgery based on 108,419 procedures: a report of the scoliosis research society morbidity and mortality committee. Spine (Phila Pa 1976). 2011;36(15):1218–28. https://doi.org/10.1097/BRS.0b013e3181ec5fd9.
23. Wang MY, Goto T, Tessitore E, Veeravagu A. Introduction. Robotics in neurosurgery. Neurosurg Focus. 2017;42(5):E1. https://doi.org/10.3171/2017.2.FOCUS1783.
24. Bertelsen A, Melo J, Sánchez E, Borro D. A review of surgical robots for spinal interventions. Int J Med Robot. 2013;9(4):407–22. https://doi.org/10.1002/rcs.1469.
25. Tjardes T, Shafizadeh S, Rixen D, Paffrath T, Bouillon B, Steinhausen ES, et al. Image-guided spine surgery: state of the art and future directions. Eur Spine J. 2010;19(1):25–45. https://doi.org/10.1007/s00586-009-1091-9.
26. Kim HJ, Lee SH, Chang BS, Lee CK, Lim TO, Hoo LP, et al. Monitoring the quality of robot-assisted pedicle screw fixation in the lumbar spine by using a cumulative summation test. Spine (Phila Pa 1976). 2015;40(2):87–94. https://doi.org/10.1097/BRS.0000000000000680.
27. Joseph JR, Smith BW, Liu X, Park P. Current applications of robotics in spine surgery: a systematic review of the literature. Neurosurg Focus. 2017;42(5):E2. https://doi.org/10.3171/2017.2.FOCUS16544.
28. Hu X, Ohnmeiss DD, Lieberman IH. Robotic-assisted pedicle screw placement: lessons learned from the first 102 patients. Eur Spine J. 2013;22(3):661–6. https://doi.org/10.1007/s00586-012-2499-1.
29. Jiang B, Azad TD, Cottrill E, Zygourakis CC, Zhu AM, Crawford N, et al. New spinal robotic technologies. Front Med. 2019;13(6):723–9. https://doi.org/10.1007/s11684-019-0716-6.
30. Crawford N, Johnson N, Theodore N. Ensuring navigation integrity using robotics in spine surgery. J Robot Surg. 2020;14(1):177–83. https://doi.org/10.1007/s11701-019-00963-w.
31. Moskowitz RM, Young JL, Box GN, Paré LS, Clayman RV. Retroperitoneal transdiaphragmatic robotic-assisted laparoscopic resection of a left thoracolumbar neurofibroma. JSLS. 2009;13(1):64–8.
32. Yang MS, Yoon DH, Kim KN, Kim H, Yang JW, Yi S, et al. Robot-assisted anterior lumbar interbody fusion in a swine model in vivo test of the da Vinci surgical-assisted spinal surgery system. Spine (Phila Pa 1976). 2011;36(2):E139–43. https://doi.org/10.1097/BRS.0b013e3181d40ba3.

33. Lee JY, Bhowmick DA, Eun DD, Welch WC. Minimally invasive, robot-assisted, anterior lumbar interbody fusion: a technical note. J Neurol Surg A Cent Eur Neurosurg. 2013;74(4):258–61. https://doi.org/10.1055/s-0032-1330121.
34. Perez-Cruet MJ, Welsh RJ, Hussain NS, Begun EM, Lin J, Park P. Use of the da Vinci minimally invasive robotic system for resection of a complicated paraspinal schwannoma with thoracic extension: case report. Neurosurgery. 2012;71(1 Suppl Operative):209–14. https://doi.org/10.1227/NEU.0b013e31826112d8.
35. Liu JC, Ondra SL, Angelos P, Ganju A, Landers ML. Is laparoscopic anterior lumbar interbody fusion a useful minimally invasive procedure? Neurosurgery. 2002;51(5 Suppl):S155–8.
36. Chung SK, Lee SH, Lim SR, Kim DY, Jang JS, Nam KS, et al. Comparative study of laparoscopic L5-S1 fusion versus open mini-ALIF, with a minimum 2-year follow-up. Eur Spine J. 2003;12(6):613–7. https://doi.org/10.1007/s00586-003-0526-y.
37. Kaiser MG, Haid RW Jr, Subach BR, Miller JS, Smith CD, Rodts GE Jr. Comparison of the mini-open versus laparoscopic approach for anterior lumbar interbody fusion: a retrospective review. Neurosurgery. 2002;51(1):97–103.; discussion 103-5. https://doi.org/10.1097/00006123-200207000-00015.
38. Gertzbein SD, Robbins SE. Accuracy of pedicular screw placement in vivo. Spine (Phila Pa 1976). 1990;15(1):11–4. https://doi.org/10.1097/00007632-199001000-00004.
39. Lonjon N, Chan-Seng E, Costalat V, Bonnafoux B, Vassal M, Boetto J. Robot-assisted spine surgery: feasibility study through a prospective case-matched analysis. Eur Spine J. 2016;25(3):947–55. https://doi.org/10.1007/s00586-015-3758-8.
40. Jiang B, Ahmed AK, Zygourakis CC, Kalb S, Zhu AM, Godzik J, et al. Pedicle screw accuracy assessment in ExcelsiusGPS® robotic spine surgery: evaluation of deviation from pre-planned trajectory. Chin Neurosurg J. 2018;4:23. https://doi.org/10.1186/s41016-018-0131-x.
41. Godzik J, Walker CT, Theodore N, Uribe JS, Chang SW, Snyder LA. Minimally invasive transforaminal interbody fusion with robotically assisted bilateral pedicle screw fixation: 2-dimensional operative video. Oper Neurosurg (Hagerstown). 2019;16(3):E86–7. https://doi.org/10.1093/ons/opy288.
42. Walker CT, Godzik J, Xu DS, Theodore N, Uribe JS, Chang SW. Minimally invasive single-position lateral interbody fusion with robotic bilateral percutaneous pedicle screw fixation: 2-dimensional operative video. Oper Neurosurg (Hagerstown). 2019;16(4):E121. https://doi.org/10.1093/ons/opy240.
43. Zygourakis CC, Ahmed AK, Kalb S, Zhu AM, Bydon A, Crawford NR, et al. Technique: open lumbar decompression and fusion with the ExcelsiusGPS robot. Neurosurg Focus. 2018;45(VideoSuppl1):V6. https://doi.org/10.3171/2018.7.FocusVid.18123.
44. Huntsman KT, Ahrendtsen LA, Riggleman JR, Ledonio CG. Robotic-assisted navigated minimally invasive pedicle screw placement in the first 100 cases at a single institution. J Robot Surg. 2020;14(1):199–203. https://doi.org/10.1007/s11701-019-00959-6.
45. Godzik J, Walker CT, Hartman C, de Andrada B, Morgan CD, Mastorakos G, et al. A quantitative assessment of the accuracy and reliability of robotically guided percutaneous pedicle screw placement: technique and application accuracy. Oper Neurosurg (Hagerstown). 2019;17(4):389–95. https://doi.org/10.1093/ons/opy413.
46. Ringel F, Stüer C, Reinke A, Preuss A, Behr M, Auer F, et al. Accuracy of robot-assisted placement of lumbar and sacral pedicle screws: a prospective randomized comparison to conventional freehand screw implantation. Spine (Phila Pa 1976). 2012;37(8):E496–501. https://doi.org/10.1097/BRS.0b013e31824b7767.
47. Perdomo-Pantoja A, Ishida W, Zygourakis C, Holmes C, Iyer RR, Cottrill E, et al. Accuracy of current techniques for placement of pedicle screws in the spine: a comprehensive systematic review and meta-analysis of 51,161 screws. World Neurosurg. 2019;126:664–678.e3. https://doi.org/10.1016/j.wneu.2019.02.217.
48. Gao S, Lv Z, Fang H. Robot-assisted and conventional freehand pedicle screw placement: a systematic review and meta-analysis of randomized controlled trials. Eur Spine J. 2018;27(4):921–30. https://doi.org/10.1007/s00586-017-5333-y.

49. Mao G, Gigliotti MJ, Myers D, Yu A, Whiting D. Single-surgeon direct comparison of O-arm neuronavigation versus Mazor X robotic-guided posterior spinal instrumentation. World Neurosurg. 2020;137:e278–85. https://doi.org/10.1016/j.wneu.2020.01.175.
50. Han X, Tian W, Liu Y, Liu B, He D, Sun Y, et al. Safety and accuracy of robot-assisted versus fluoroscopy-assisted pedicle screw insertion in thoracolumbar spinal surgery: a prospective randomized controlled trial. J Neurosurg Spine. 2019:1–8. https://doi.org/10.3171/2018.10.SPINE18487.
51. Tian W. Robot-assisted posterior C1-2 transarticular screw fixation for atlantoaxial instability: a case report. Spine (Phila Pa 1976). 2016;41(Suppl 19):B2–5. https://doi.org/10.1097/BRS.0000000000001674.
52. Tian W, Wang H, Liu YJ. Robot-assisted anterior odontoid screw fixation: a case report. Orthop Surg. 2016;8(3):400–4. https://doi.org/10.1111/os.12266.
53. Wang JQ, Wang Y, Feng Y, Han W, Su YG, Liu WY, et al. Percutaneous sacroiliac screw placement: a prospective randomized comparison of robot-assisted navigation procedures with a conventional technique. Chin Med J. 2017;130(21):2527–34. https://doi.org/10.4103/0366-6999.217080.
54. Fan Y, Du JP, Liu JJ, Zhang JN, Qiao HH, Liu SC, et al. Accuracy of pedicle screw placement comparing robot-assisted technology and the free-hand with fluoroscopy-guided method in spine surgery: an updated meta-analysis. Medicine (Baltimore). 2018;97(22):e10970. https://doi.org/10.1097/MD.0000000000010970.
55. Mendelsohn D, Strelzow J, Dea N, Ford NL, Batke J, Pennington A, et al. Patient and surgeon radiation exposure during spinal instrumentation using intraoperative computed tomography-based navigation. Spine J. 2016;16(3):343–54. https://doi.org/10.1016/j.spinee.2015.11.020.
56. Noriega DC, Hernández-Ramajo R, Rodríguez-Monsalve Milano F, Sanchez-Lite I, Toribio B, Ardura F, Torres R, Corredera R, Kruger A. Risk-benefit analysis of navigation techniques for vertebral transpedicular instrumentation: a prospective study. Spine J. 2017;17(1):70–5. https://doi.org/10.1016/j.spinee.2016.08.004.
57. Pennington Z, Cottrill E, Westbroek EM, Goodwin ML, Lubelski D, Ahmed AK, et al. Evaluation of surgeon and patient radiation exposure by imaging technology in patients undergoing thoracolumbar fusion: systematic review of the literature. Spine J. 2019;19(8):1397–411. https://doi.org/10.1016/j.spinee.2019.04.003.
58. Hyun SJ, Kim KJ, Jahng TA, Kim HJ. Minimally invasive robotic versus open fluoroscopic-guided spinal instrumented fusions: a randomized controlled trial. Spine (Phila Pa 1976). 2017;42(6):353–8. https://doi.org/10.1097/BRS.0000000000001778.
59. Sensakovic WF, O'Dell MC, Agha A, Woo R, Varich L. CT radiation dose reduction in robot-assisted pediatric spinal surgery. Spine (Phila Pa 1976). 2017;42(7):E417–24. https://doi.org/10.1097/BRS.0000000000001846.
60. Jiang B, Pennington Z, Azad T, Liu A, Ahmed AK, Zygourakis CC, et al. Robot-assisted versus freehand instrumentation in short-segment lumbar fusion: experience with real-time image-guided spinal robot. World Neurosurg. 2020;136:e635–45. https://doi.org/10.1016/j.wneu.2020.01.119.
61. Schatlo B, Martinez R, Alaid A, von Eckardstein K, Akhavan-Sigari R, Hahn A, Stockhammer F, Rohde V. Unskilled unawareness and the learning curve in robotic spine surgery. Acta Neurochir. 2015;157(10):1819–23.; discussion 1823. https://doi.org/10.1007/s00701-015-2535-0.
62. Kam JKT, Gan C, Dimou S, Awad M, Kavar B, Nair G, et al. Learning curve for robot-assisted percutaneous pedicle screw placement in thoracolumbar surgery. Asian Spine J. 2019;13(6):920–7. https://doi.org/10.31616/asj.2019.0033.
63. Barzilay Y, Liebergall M, Fridlander A, Knoller N. Miniature robotic guidance for spine surgery--introduction of a novel system and analysis of challenges encountered during the clinical development phase at two spine centres. Int J Med Robot. 2006;2(2):146–53. https://doi.org/10.1002/rcs.90.

64. Kuo KL, Su YF, Wu CH, Tsai CY, Chang CH, Lin CL, et al. Assessing the intraoperative accuracy of pedicle screw placement by using a bone-mounted miniature robot system through secondary registration. PLoS One. 2016;11(4):e0153235. https://doi.org/10.1371/journal.pone.0153235.
65. Macke JJ, Woo R, Varich L. Accuracy of robot-assisted pedicle screw placement for adolescent idiopathic scoliosis in the pediatric population. J Robot Surg. 2016;10(2):145–50. https://doi.org/10.1007/s11701-016-0587-7.
66. Lieber AM, Kirchner GJ, Kerbel YE, Khalsa AS. Robotic-assisted pedicle screw placement fails to reduce overall postoperative complications in fusion surgery. Spine J. 2019;19(2):212–7. https://doi.org/10.1016/j.spinee.2018.07.004.
67. Fiani B, Quadri SA, Farooqui M, Cathel A, Berman B, Noel J, et al. Impact of robot-assisted spine surgery on health care quality and neurosurgical economics: a systemic review. Neurosurg Rev. 2020;43(1):17–25. https://doi.org/10.1007/s10143-018-0971-z.

Part III
Rehabilitation and Assistive Robots

Chapter 17
Rehabilitation and Assistive Robotics: Shared Principles and Common Applications

Camilla Pierella and Silvestro Micera

Introduction

Predictions of the United Nations present the 2050 as the year when for the first time the world population of adults age 60 or older will surpass the world population of children [1]. Aging is the biggest factor in several neuromuscular conditions, like orthopedic and neurological. With the big advances in the medical and surgical care, there is and will be increasing survival rates and rehabilitation referrals [2] so increasing number of people requiring assistance and rehabilitation. This is a major challenge in terms of social and economic adaptation for society and that poses a significant pressure to create solutions and technologies to help in this direction. Therefore, technology can help in a broad scenario and in many places, inpatient assistance and rehabilitation both in the hospital and in a home-based setting, in outpatient clinics, and in visiting services.

These age-related neuromuscular disabilities are caused by various factors such as normal degeneration, stroke, and musculoskeletal conditions, resulting in sensorimotor dysfunction [3, 4], impaired mobility [5], and long-lasting motor

C. Pierella (✉)
Department of Neurosciences, Rehabilitation, Ophthalmology, Genetics, and Maternal and Children's Sciences (DINOGMI), University of Genoa, Genoa, Italy

Department of Informatics, Bioengineering, Robotics and Systems Engineering (DIBRIS), University of Genoa, Genoa, Italy
e-mail: camilla.pierella@edu.unige.it

S. Micera
Center for Neuroprosthetics and Institute of Bioengineering, School of Engineering, Ecole Polytechnique Federale de Lausanne, Lausanne, Switzerland

The Biorobotics Institute and Department of Excellence in Robotics and AI, Scuola Superiore Sant'Anna, Pisa, Italy
e-mail: silvestro.micera@epfl.ch

J. A. González Martínez, F. Cardinale (eds.), *Robotics in Neurosurgery*,
https://doi.org/10.1007/978-3-031-08380-8_17

disabilities [6–8], directly affecting their quality of life [9]. In addition to the deleterious effect on the quality of life, these disabilities can reduce life expectancy, increase the risk of injuries (particularly fall-related injuries), and result in further cognitive and sensorimotor deterioration.

According to the World Health Organization, 15 million people suffer stroke worldwide each year [10]. In particular, more than 1.1 million people are affected every year in Europe [11] by a stroke and about 800,000 in the United States [12]. Even though acute stroke care and intensive rehabilitation are improving, two-thirds of chronic stroke survivors have to cope with persisting neurologic deficits, and only 20% of them are able to go back to their normal professional and private life [13]. The most common impairments in the acute and chronic stages are cognitive conditions and motor deficits contralateral to the affected brain hemisphere [14], usually called "affected side." A profound neuromuscular reorganization occurs after stroke [8, 15, 16]. The affected limb is typically characterized by spasticity [17], stereotyped movement patterns, mainly caused by abnormal muscle co-activation and an enlarged activity of the antagonist muscles [16, 18], which result in a reduced range of motion against gravity, and, thus, to a limited workspace in three-dimensional reaching movements [19, 20] and in walking functions.

A lot of attention has been posed by researchers of different fields like robotics, engineering, neuroscience, medicine on the development of technological solutions for stroke which can be also used with patients with other pathologies such as Spinal Cord Injury (SCI) and Multiple Sclerosis (MS), that are among the world's most diffuse neurological disorders and affect the nervous system at various levels.

Spinal cord injury results in a damage of neural signal transmission at and below the level of injury, leading to loss of motor and/or sensory functions [21]. This condition is not only physically but also psychologically challenging for SCI people because one of the main and most impacting consequences is the loss of functional independence in Activities of Daily Living (ADLs), making recovery a priority for SCI individuals [22, 23]. To this aim, physical rehabilitation continues to remain a mainstay in the treatment of SCI because, so far, no curative treatments exist and only limited spontaneous recovery attributed to the natural and intrinsic neural plasticity of the remaining intact fibers happens after the lesion occurrence [21–23]. Furthermore, the loss of somatic and autonomic control results in secondary complications such as cardiovascular, respiratory, cutaneous, musculoskeletal, and psychological [2]. Therefore, interventions to promote physical activity after SCI are among the top goals of recovery and improvement in quality of life.

Multiple sclerosis is a chronic progressive disease that affects the entire Central Nervous System (CNS) characterized by inflammation, demyelination, and degenerative changes at the brain and spine levels and it is the first cause of non-traumatic disability in young adult population [24, 25]. The estimated prevalence of MS is 50–300 per 100,000 individuals, with approximately 2.3 million affected individuals worldwide [25]. MS predominantly occurs in early adult life, with increased awareness of presentation in childhood, and it strongly impacts mobility, function, and quality of life [25, 26]. The inflammatory state that characterizes the CNS of people with MS leads to deficits of motor, sensory, and cognitive functions that can relapse and remit for several years until the disease switches to a secondary progressive phase characterized by irreversible disability. The cause of MS is still unknown and its pathophysiology is poorly understood; pharmacological therapies are currently able to slow down the inflammatory-related disability progression, but cannot neither cure the disease nor restore functionality [24, 25].

In such variegated framework, for all these pathologies rehabilitation remains a key element to maximize the recovery process discouraging negative behavior and promoting the re-learning of appropriate motor synergies, strategies, and coordination patterns. People suffering of these pathologies have complex clinical, rehabilitative, but also psychological, relational, and social needs. For this reason, they require a multidisciplinary approach, as well as an individualized and specialized path. Indeed, an effective rehabilitative intervention represents the solution to prevent secondary complications due to the immobilization or to bad movements control, to reduce the disabilities, and to resume their ADLs also thanks to assistive tools avoiding social isolation and depression. Robotics can provide appropriate solutions and support to standard clinical rehabilitative approaches [27, 28] and at the same time can provide the right tools to assist these people while going back to their normal life [29, 30].

Indeed, assistive robotic aims at developing solutions (mechatronic devices, systems, and technologies) to assist and interact with individuals with reduced motor or cognitive abilities in order to increase their autonomy in the personal environment, while rehabilitation robotic proposes similar solutions for assisted therapy and objective functional assessment of these patients usually in a clinical context (Fig. 17.1). On the one hand, assistive robotic solutions are designed to be used on a lifelong perspective in activities of daily living and promote independent living and autonomy of disabled and elderly individuals. On the other hand, rehabilitation robotic intends to be complementary of existing therapeutic approaches in order to improve patient's functional recovery, to optimize and maximize clinical effectiveness of therapy. The constraints associated with assistive and rehabilitation robotics are therefore different, especially in terms of acceptability. Even though the differences are important between the two fields, from a technical and scientific point of view there are important similarities.

In the last decades, many research groups developed innovative robotic systems for assistance and neurorehabilitative treatments [31–34], under the intrinsic features of innovation technologies that can serve disable people providing efficient tools to improve activities of daily living and the scientific evidence that task-oriented, high-intensity movements can improve muscle strength and movement coordination in patients with impairments due to neurological lesions [35–42]. Indeed, some of them became commercial products [43–46] and are part of the rehabilitative programs of many hospitals and clinics around the world [47–51].

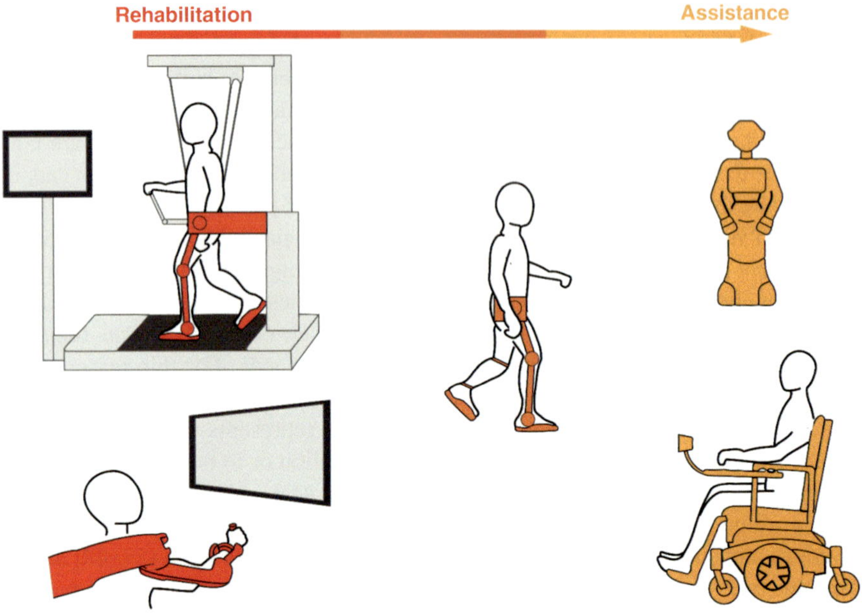

Fig. 17.1 From only rehabilitative (red) to only assistive (yellow) robots. Illustrative examples of rehabilitative robots (in red, left panel) that can be used only in the lab setting, robots that can have a dual function (in orange, central panel)—rehabilitative and assistive—and robots that have a mainly assistive function (in yellow, right panel)

Robots for Rehabilitation

Individuals engaged in rehabilitation to improve or restore their abilities often have diminished strength, endurance, or ability and that can limit the intensity and number of repetitions (the rehabilitation dosage) needed to achieve the desired training effects. As a result, rehabilitation robots combined with virtual reality are often used by therapists to facilitate musculoskeletal and cardiorespiratory fitness as well as other neurological, physiological, and psychological measures. The use of robots in therapeutic interventions has become increasingly widespread since they overcome some limits of traditional treatments, offering among other things intense, controllable, repetitive, reproducible, and quantifiable motor training [39, 83–86]. All of these have been shown to be critical factors for facilitating nervous system reorganization and potentially beneficial changes in the neuromuscular system [87–89]. Moreover, robotic systems can provide load bearing, suppress undesired motions, extend a person's range of motion, incorporate programmed load/motion disturbances. As described in several works from various research groups worldwide, i.e., in [38, 39, 41, 49, 90, 91], robotic technologies effectively help clinicians and physical therapists during the neurorehabilitation process in augmenting or recovering a person's capabilities speeding up the recovery process. However, such outcomes are challenging due to the complexities of the inherent physical human–machine interaction. For all the above-mentioned reasons, there are two main challenges when developing a robot for rehabilitation: (i) developing the appropriate mechanical product using front-edge technologies, (ii) designing effective training modalities supported by appropriate low-level control strategies.

Presently available rehabilitation robotic devices can be divided broadly into two categories: end-effector robots and exoskeletons. End-effector robots, which are the pioneer devices used in rehabilitation, are interfaced with the subjects only at their end-point, i.e., the hand of the subjects is the only body part that is mechanically attached at the end-effector of the robot. These robots are able to exsert forces only at the end-point and cannot measure the position of the entire kinematic chain, which can be estimated indirectly, but it still remains unconstrained. With this configuration, the human limb is completely free to move and react to external disturbances or to movements applied by the robot. The movement of the end-effector, depending on the robot, can be constrained on a plane or can move in the 3D space. Some examples of end-effector robots are for the upper limb MIT-Manus [50], Bi-Manu-Track [52], Braccio di Ferro [92], and for the lower limb the G-EO [67] and the Gait Trainer [69]. More information are in Table 17.1. In contrast, exoskeleton has a structure like the human limb and is attached to the surface of the limb at multiple locations. The axis of the joints of the exoskeleton matches that of the human limb. The physical interface at multiple locations on the device facilitates, differently from the end-effector robots, the determination of position and velocity of each Degree of Freedom (DoF) of the limb and also permits the control of the torque applied to each of them allowing to precisely determine position, velocity, and torque at each articular joint of the limb [93] and the independent or synergistic motion of shoulder, elbow, and wrist joints during the execution of functional movements [94, 95]. These advantages come with a cost that is the higher complexity for the control of the DoFs of the exoskeleton. With the exoskeleton robot, any part of upper or lower limb can be targeted for training and unlike an end-effector robot, an exoskeleton robot has a large range of motion. Examples of upper limb exoskeleton devices are Armeo Power [59], AlexRS [49], Mahi-EXO II [63], Gloreha [51]. While examples of lower limb exoskeletons are Lokomat [76], Rewalk [81], and Ekso [96]. More information are in Table 17.1. Nevertheless, despite the versatility of end-effector robot and exoskeletons, the outcome of robotic-based rehabilitation still do not significantly differ from the one of conventional therapy [91, 97], and patients improvements are not always transferred to the ADLs [85, 98]. The effectiveness of robot-assisted rehabilitation and therapy largely depends on its ability to assist patients' movement in different modes according to patients' recovery stages. The appropriate training mode should be determined by clinicians and physiotherapist's experience and subject's disability level, and the robot should be used as additional tool to boost this process.

Usually, most of the robots used in rehabilitation implement (i) a passive training modality (passive patient), where the robot imposes the trajectories, (ii) an active training modality (active patient), where the robot is mostly transparent to the user and follow his/her movements, i.e., it responses to the subject's intention to move, and (iii) an assisted training modality, where the robot partially helps participant to

Table 17.1 Some of the most common robot (exoskeleton and end-effector robot) used for rehabilitation and assistance. MS: multiple sclerosis, SCI: spinal cord injury

Body district	Type of device	Type of robot	Goal	Pathology
Upper limb	MIT-Manus	End-effector robot	Arm (and hand) rehabilitation	Stroke [50]
	Bi-Manu-track	End-effector robot	Arm rehabilitation	Stroke [52]
	Braccio di Ferro	End-effector robot	Arm rehabilitation	Stroke [53], MS [54]
	Wristbot	End-effector robot	Wrist rehabilitation	Stroke [55]
	Amadeo	End-effector robot	Hand fingers rehabilitation	MS [56], Stroke [57] and SCI [58]
	Armeo Spring/Power	Exoskeleton	Arm rehabilitation	MS [47], Stroke [59] and SCI [58]
	KinArm	Exoskeleton	Arm rehabilitation	MS [60], Stroke [61]
	Alex RS	Exoskeleton	Arm rehabilitation	Stroke [49, 62]
	Mahi-EXO II	Exoskeleton	Arm rehabilitation	Stroke and SCI [63]
	Wilmington robotic exoskeleton	Exoskeleton	Arm assistance	MS, stroke and SCI [45, 64]
	Armon	Exoskeleton	Arm assistance	
	Gloreha	Exoskeleton	Hand fingers rehabilitation	Stroke [51]
	JACO Arm	Robotic arm	Assistance	MS and SCI [43]
	Soft sixth-finger	Robotic finger	Assistance	Stroke [65]
Lower limb	G-Eo	End-effector robot	Gait rehabilitation	MS [66], SCI [67], Stroke [68]
	Gain Trainer	End-effector robot	Gait rehabilitation	MS [69], Stroke [70]
	CARR	End-effector robot	Ankle rehabilitation	Stroke and SCI [71]
	Hunova	End-effector robot	Ankle or pelvis rehabilitation	SCI [72], Stroke [73]
	Lokomat	Exoskeleton	Gait rehabilitation	MS [74], SCI [75], Stroke [76, 77]
	Ekso-GT	Exoskeleton	Gait rehabilitation/assistance	Stroke [78], SCI [79]
	Rewalk	Exoskeleton	Gait rehabilitation/assistance	MS [80], SCI [81]
	Caterwill	Powered wheelchair	Mobility assistance	SCI [44]
	SCEWO BRO	Powered wheelchair	Mobility assistance	SCI [82]

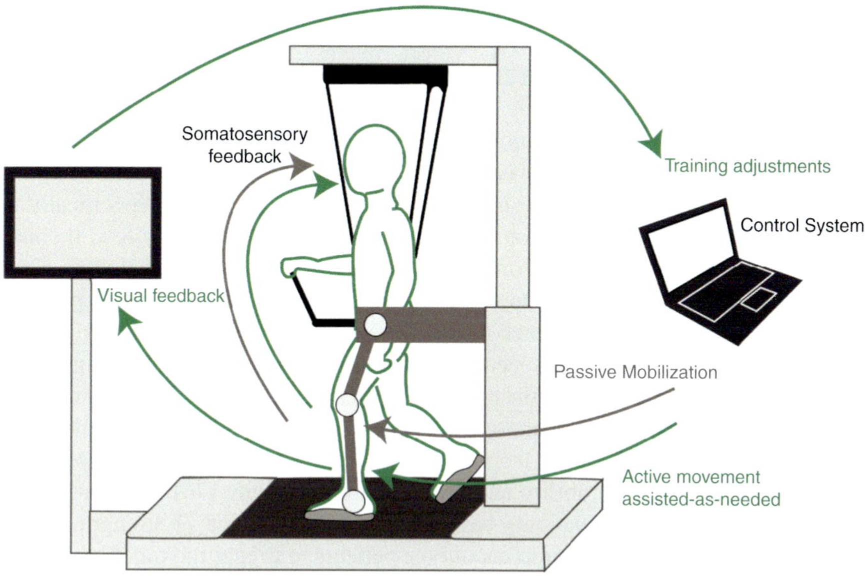

Fig. 17.2 Passive (gray) and assisted-as-needed (green) training modalities. In the passive training modality, the control system of the robot imposes the movement, the limb is moved by the robot and the subject is not actively involved in the exercise. He/she only receive somatosensory sensations. On the contrary, the assisted-as-needed training modality actively involves the subject that is assisted by the robot only when is needed. During this training the subject receives also visual feedback on a screen and based on the subject's performance the control system adjusts the training parameters and the level of assistance

move his/her impaired limbs according to the desired postures during grasping, reaching, or walking, reflecting the strategy adopted by conventional therapy [99, 100]. A schematic example of these modalities is illustrated in Fig. 17.2.

Specifically, among the assisted training modalities, the (iii-a) assistance-as-needed modality is widely employed because it reduces the patient risk of relying only on the robot to accomplish the rehabilitative task. Indeed, over-assistance could decrease the level of participation and, as a consequence, also the chance to induce neuroplastic changes [101]. This is called the "slacking" effect, and can be formally defined as a reduction of voluntary movement control when the patient undergoes repetitive passive mobilization of the limbs [102]. In addition to the assistance-as-needed modality, to avoid the slacking effect, the (iii-b) challenge-based modalities are used to make tasks more difficult or stimulating. Among them, there are controllers that provide resistance to the participant's limb movements during exercise [103, 104] or others called corrective strategies that limits the incorrect movement of the subjects, similarly to the approach of constraint induced by therapists. An example of this strategy is the creation of virtual haptic channels for the end-effector or the joints of the exoskeleton (tunneling) allow users to move only in delimited tunnels. Once they go out from the correct path, adopting compensatory movements, they are forced to go back into the channel [105, 106]. Moreover, error augmentation strategies that amplify movement errors have been proposed and proved successful since kinematic errors generated during movement are a fundamental neural signal that drives motor adaptation [107, 108].

Depending on the type and severity of the motor dysfunction and related impairment, one type of device could be more effective than the other [89]. Specifically, if the residual sensorimotor functionalities of the patient are extremely low, it could be more appropriate to apply forces to each joint by using exoskeletons [24]. Moreover, end-effector devices could be more effective to deliver complex patterns of forces (e.g., based on assistance-as-needed strategies) able to exploit the redundancy of the human body, thus speeding up sensorimotor recovery [25]. Same thing for the training modality. Thus, the patients might need to receive passive and active exercises in different recovery phases. For example, in early stage of rehabilitation, passive modality can be used to help patients to track the predefined trajectories for improving the movement ability and reduce muscle atrophy [76]. After an initial training period, once the patients have gained certain degree of strength, active modality should be carried out to encourage patients to trigger the robot assistance by their own active efforts. In this situation, active assist modality means that the robot provides assistance at subjects which have voluntary to move but perform inadequate movements, while active resist modality means that the subjects perform the exercise against a resistive force provided by the robot when muscle strengthening exercises are required [89]. In late rehabilitation stage, the robot is used to guarantee, for example, patients balance in the gait training and record data for further analysis.

Indeed, robotic devices in combination with sensors that can measure muscular (EMG) and/or brain (EEG) activity can help us assessing the neurobiological status of the patients. Combining aspects from other disciplines like neuroscience and motor control, we could quantify the motor impairment following an injury to the nervous system, the impact of the rehabilitative interventions using the data recorded through the exercise program [49] and also eventually adjust the training based on features extracted from these measures [62]. This is an asset that, if properly used, can make robotic rehabilitation reach further advancement in treating and also understanding pathologies like stroke, SCI, or MS [27, 28]. Indeed, understanding how the brain controls movements and which are the applied mechanisms to learn new skills or re-learn the lost ones is fundamental to plan an effective robot-based therapy, aimed at the promotion of sensorimotor recovery. In this framework, the design of the most appropriate and effective control strategy plays a crucial role [99] and can be achieved by exploiting and properly applying the latest findings in human neuroscience. For example, recent studies explored how stroke hemisphere localization plays a role in the different interaction with dynamic environments [109, 110]. Other studies tried to characterize muscular and brain changes while stroke subjects [49], SCI subjects [79], or people with MS [60] were trained with exoskeletons.

Robots for Assistance

As mentioned in the previous section, robotic systems have transformed the delivery of rehabilitation therapies assisting the gradual recovery of patients with sensorimotor disabilities. The other related, yet different, category of robotic systems developed to help patients with neuromuscular deficits is the assistive robotic field with its technologies. The primary difference is that assistive technologies are designed to immediately augment the sensorimotor capacity of those patients and help them in performing activities of daily living. They are designed to augment individual's functional abilities beyond neuro-restoration potential, and assist him/her in performing ADL, independently or with very little assistance from others (patients initially will require a therapist's guidance to help accustom them to the wearing technique and usability of the assistive robotic device). These devices are usually portable and can be worn in the home environment. The main outcomes of the use of assistive systems are enhanced independence, empowered mobility, and increased manipulability for individuals with degraded sensorimotor competence. In addition to helping to carry out the ADL, the use of an assistive robotic device can result in motor recovery when consistently used over a long period [33, 111]. Common use cases of assistive robots to improve the motor performance of patients living with neuromuscular deficits are: (i) orthosis and exoskeletons for patients with spinal cord injuries, stroke, and arm mobility [45, 46] or gait deficits [81, 111], (ii) smart motorized wheelchairs for patients with severe lack of mobility [44, 82], (iii) extra robotic arms and/or fingers [43, 65] for patients with the lack of manipulability (such as those aging with severe cerebral palsy or tetraplegic people).

In addition to the above-mentioned examples, which mainly focus on augmenting the users' motor abilities and independence, a second category of assistive robots and technologies are designed to augment the sensory perception of the patients and to boost up the perceptual awareness of users. These technologies ultimately help with activities of daily living. Sensory perception enhancing systems may be in the format of wearable suits and may provide auditory, vibrotactile, or visual cues for the patients. One example is wearable vibrotactile suit for helping individuals with degraded vision and sensory awareness, so they can navigate safely in daily environments while protecting them when encountering unexpected contacts, which may result in falls [112]. Another example is technology that provides cues to the user regarding their posture during walking to maintain a safer balance [113] that can result in danger and challenges during daily navigation (such as crossing a street, moving in an apartment, walking to the bathroom, etc.), resulting in limited mobility and independence. With the use of sensory augmentation technologies, all these subjects have shown to have significantly enhanced mobility and have recovered a high degree of movement fluency.

An ultimate category that falls within the family of assistive robots are called Social Robots. They are the last evolution of collaborative robots, specialized in social interactions with humans [114], and have been used for a variety of applications like social interaction [115], education [116], elderly care [117], helping people with autism [118], and depression [119]. Social robots may be actuated or have speech capabilities and can measure the user's mood, stress, and vital signs via various embedded sensors. Smart social robots have shown good potential in engaging the users in interactive social exercises. Social robotic systems have been shown to successfully benefit kids living with autism [118], and elderly living with mild cognitive impairments, Alzheimer's disease, and dementia [29]. This technology can be a major benefit, especially during this complicated period when COVID-19 is pandemic, when elderly people are isolated due to the concerns over disease spread. Long-term isolation, not only for patients with physical impairments but especially for patients who are already having cognitive disorders may have very serious consequences, and any technology which can engage these persons in interactive social exercises, while reducing the risk of human–human contact, can be significantly beneficial. They can have a dual role, in the field of both assistance and rehabilitation.

Perspectives

In the recent past, there have been several developments in and around the fields of assistive robotics and rehabilitation engineering. Advances in material sciences are allowing lighter, more customizable robotic and wearable structures with tightly integrated sensing and actuation. Furthermore, there is an increasing focus on combining robotics with non-invasive and invasive brain–machine interfaces or neuroprosthetics [27, 28], with the aim of increasing motor recovery and of promoting independence during ADL. It appears clear that assistive and rehabilitation robotics approaches can potentially provide better clinical outcomes after neurorehabilitation and facilitate the reintegration of people with neuromuscular injuries in the society, however the exploitation of their potential is hampered by several important issues. For example, future studies should focus on the investigation of more suitable control algorithms personalized based on each user's needs and characteristics; and on the design of new mechatronic structures to favor the adoption of these robotic devices, such as improving wearability, encumbrance, weight, and calibration procedure. However, this is not an easy task, especially for exoskeletons that have to deal with a high mechanical complexity [111, 120]: they should be lightweight, portable, compliant, and, at the same time, they must safely support the patient even when severe impairments, such as a complete SCI subject. Another important aspect which is still under investigation from many research groups is the transferring of functional improvements obtained through robotic rehabilitation to ADL [111, 121]. This is one of the main challenges to be faced to really improve quality of life of people with neuromuscular disorders. The integration of hybrid robotic systems within more realistic and life-like environments could help in this direction. Another crucial aspect that could definitely help to maximally exploit the potential that robots have in the rehabilitation and assistive fields is a better and deeper understanding of the mechanisms underlying robot-based neurorehabilitation. To this aim, the use of animal and computational models can be extremely useful to understand the role played by different brain areas during and after the neurological injury and how the rehabilitative process might favor their reorganization [27, 28, 122]. The use of computational models can also be extremely useful for a better prediction of the outcomes, treatment efficacy, and, thus, personalization of the neuromodulation approach [123]. In addition, artificial intelligence and machine learning techniques can support the above-mentioned computation models in understanding neural plasticity processes and motor recovery pathways putting together many multimodal data, i.e., EEG, neuroimaging, EMG, clinical scales ..., and defining significant biomarkers useful for the identification of the best therapeutic and robotic interventions for each individual patient.

Finally, the current trend of health care decentralization also applies to rehabilitation. If the patient can train at home with the remote supervision of a physiotherapist and, eventually, the help of a caregiver, he/she can train more and for a longer period of time, with the well-known benefits of intensive and prolonged training. Hybrid robotic systems can have a crucial role in this context, but important steps further are needed. One option is using small wireless and low-cost sensors and a user-friendly software that is able to transform a rehabilitative session in a game session at home, like in [124]. In this way, the users can receive two types of sensory feedback based on user's performance: from the physical therapist connected online checking the exercise, and from the sensor worn by the patient. Another recent option is the introduction of exosuits, clothing-like devices made of fabric or elastomers working in parallel with human muscles, may help in this direction [30, 125]. Exosuits are lightweight and wearable by definition, they improve comfort and safety since they do not require a perfect alignment with human joints and, therefore, they work perfectly for domestic use. Exosuits and other wearable mechatronic technologies can also display information to the user through biofeedback to support, assist, or augment the capabilities of the user. Smart wearables can also provide haptic-, vibro-, and electro-feedback stimulation to users.

All these advances will bring benefits to the development of newest robots, designed by strong collaboration between engineers, therapists, and clinicians that not only support sensorimotor rehabilitation but can also serve as assistive devices to compensate for persistent sensorimotor deficits.

References

1. "World Population Prospects." 2019.
2. Heinemann AW. State of the science on postacute rehabilitation: setting a research agenda and developing an evidence base for practice and public policy. An introduction. Assistive Technol. 2008;20(1):55–60. https://doi.org/10.1080/10400435.2008.10131932.
3. Degardin A, et al. Deficit of sensorimotor integration in normal aging. Neurosci Lett. Jul. 2011;498(3):208–12. https://doi.org/10.1016/j.neulet.2011.05.010.
4. Krakauer JW. Arm function after stroke: from physiology to recovery. Semin Neurol. 2005;25(4):384–95. https://doi.org/10.1055/s-2005-923533.

5. Wesselhoff S, Hanke TA, Evans CC. Community mobility after stroke: a systematic review. Topics Stroke Rehabil. 2018. Taylor and Francis Ltd.;25(3):224–38. https://doi.org/10.1080/10749357.2017.1419617.
6. Sosnoff JJ, Gappmaier E, Frame A, Motl RW. Influence of spasticity on mobility and balance in persons with multiple sclerosis. J Neurol Phys Ther. 2011;35(3):129–32. https://doi.org/10.1097/NPT.0b013e31822a8c40.
7. Pila O, Duret C, Gracies JM, Francisco GE, Bayle N, Hutin E. Evolution of upper limb kinematics four years after subacute robot-assisted rehabilitation in stroke patients. Int J Neurosci. 2018;128(11):1030–9. https://doi.org/10.1080/00207454.2018.1461626.
8. Cirstea MC, Mitnitski AB, Feldman AG, Levin MF. Interjoint coordination dynamics during reaching in stroke. Exp Brain Res. 2003;151(3):289–300. https://doi.org/10.1007/s00221-003-1438-0.
9. Muren MA, Hütler M, Hooper J. Functional capacity and health-related quality of life in individuals post stroke. Top Stroke Rehabil. 2008;15(1):51–8. https://doi.org/10.1310/tsr1501-51.
10. WHO. World health statistics. World Health Organization; 2008.
11. Wafa HA, Wolfe CDA, Emmett E, Roth GA, Johnson CO, Wang Y. Burden of stroke in Europe: thirty-year projections of incidence, prevalence, deaths, and disability-adjusted life years. Stroke. Aug. 2020;51(8):2418–27. https://doi.org/10.1161/STROKEAHA.120.029606.
12. Virani SS, et al. Heart disease and stroke statistics—2020 update: A report from the American Heart Association. Circulation. 2020. Lippincott Williams and Wilkins.;141(9):E139–596. https://doi.org/10.1161/CIR.0000000000000757.
13. Di Carlo A. Human and economic burden of stroke. Age Ageing. 2009;38(1):4–5.
14. Lee KB, et al. Six-month functional recovery of stroke patients: a multi-time-point study. Int J Rehabil Res. 2015;38(2):173–80. https://doi.org/10.1097/MRR.0000000000000108.
15. Levin MF. Interjoint coordination during pointing movements is disrupted in spastic hemiparesis. Brain. 1996;119(1):281–93.
16. Huitema RB, Hof AL, Mulder T, Brouwer WH, Dekker R, Postema K. Functional recovery of gait and joint kinematics after right hemispheric stroke. Arch Phys Med Rehabil. 2004;85(12):1982–8. https://doi.org/10.1016/j.apmr.2004.04.036.
17. Sommerfeld DK, Gripenstedt U, Welmer A-K. Spasticity after stroke. Am J Phys Med Rehabil. 2012;91(9):814–20. https://doi.org/10.1097/PHM.0b013e31825f13a3.
18. Coscia M, Monaco V, Martelloni C, Rossi B, Chisari C, Micera S. Muscle synergies and spinal maps are sensitive to the asymmetry induced by a unilateral stroke. J Neuroeng Rehabil. 2015;12(1):39. https://doi.org/10.1186/s12984-015-0031-7.
19. Sukal TM, Ellis MD, Dewald JPA. Shoulder abduction-induced reductions in reaching work area following hemiparetic stroke: neuroscientific implications. Exp Brain Res. 2007;183(2):215–23.
20. Ellis MD, Sukal T, DeMott T, Dewald JPA. Augmenting clinical evaluation of hemiparetic arm movement with a laboratory-based quantitative measurement of kinematics as a function of limb loading. Neurorehabil Neural Repair. 2008;22(4):321–9.
21. Jazayeri SB, Beygi S, Shokraneh F, Hagen EM, Rahimi-Movaghar V. Incidence of traumatic spinal cord injury worldwide: a systematic review. Eur Spine J. 2015;24(5):905–18.
22. Curt A, Van Hedel HJA, Klaus D, Dietz V. Recovery from a spinal cord injury: significance of compensation, neural plasticity, and repair. J Neurotrauma. 2008;25(6):677–85. https://doi.org/10.1089/neu.2007.0468.
23. Lynch J, Cahalan R. The impact of spinal cord injury on the quality of life of primary family caregivers: a literature review. Spinal Cord. 2017. Nature Publishing Group.;55(11):964–78. https://doi.org/10.1038/sc.2017.56.
24. Browne P, et al. Atlas of multiple sclerosis 2013: a growing global problem with widespread inequity. Neurology. 2014. Lippincott Williams and Wilkins.;83(11):1022–4. https://doi.org/10.1212/WNL.0000000000000768.

25. Thompson AJ, Baranzini SE, Geurts J, Hemmer B, Ciccarelli O. Multiple sclerosis. Lancet. 391(10130):1622, 2018. Lancet Publishing Group.–36. https://doi.org/10.1016/S0140-6736(18)30481-1.
26. Confavreux C, Vukusic S. Natural history of multiple sclerosis: a unifying concept. Brain. 2006;129(3):606–16. https://doi.org/10.1093/brain/awl007.
27. Coscia M, et al. Neurotechnology-aided interventions for upper limb motor rehabilitation in severe chronic stroke. Brain. 2019;142(8). Oxford University Press:2182–97. https://doi.org/10.1093/brain/awz181.
28. Micera S, Caleo M, Chisari C, Hummel FC, Pedrocchi A. Advanced Neurotechnologies for the restoration of motor function. Neuron. 2020;105:604–20. https://doi.org/10.1016/j.neuron.2020.01.039.
29. Góngora Alonso S, Hamrioui S, de la Torre Díez I, Motta Cruz E, López-Coronado M, Franco M. Social robots for people with aging and dementia: a systematic review of literature. Telemed e-Health. 2019;25(7):533–40. https://doi.org/10.1089/tmj.2018.0051.
30. Majidi H, Vatan F, Nefti-Meziani S, Davis S, Saffari Z, El-Hussieny H. A review: a comprehensive review of soft and rigid wearable rehabilitation and assistive devices with a focus on the shoulder joint. J Intell Robot Syst. 2021;102(9) https://doi.org/10.1007/s10846-021-01353-x.
31. Iandolo R, et al. Perspectives and challenges in robotic neurorehabilitation. Appl Sci. 2019;9(15):3138. https://doi.org/10.3390/app9153183.
32. Beckerle P, et al. A human-robot interaction perspective on assistive and rehabilitation robotics. Front Neurorobotics. 2017;11(MAY). Frontiers Media S.A.:1. https://doi.org/10.3389/fnbot.2017.00024.
33. Khalid S, Alnajjar F, Gochoo M, Shimoda S. Robotic assistive and rehabilitation devices leading to motor recovery in upper limb: a systematic review. Disabil Rehabil Assist Technol. 2021:1–15. https://doi.org/10.1080/17483107.2021.1906960.
34. Atashzar SF, Carriere J, Tavakoli M. Review: how can intelligent robots and smart mechatronic modules facilitate remote assessment, assistance, and rehabilitation for isolated adults with neuro-musculoskeletal conditions? Front Robot AI. 2021;8:48. https://doi.org/10.3389/frobt.2021.610529.
35. Reinkensmeyer DJ, Emken JL, Cramer SC. Robotics, motor learning, and neurologic recovery. Annu Rev Biomed Eng. 2004;6:497–525. https://doi.org/10.1146/annurev.bioeng.6.040803.140223.
36. Reinkensmeyer DJ, Boninger ML. Technologies and combination therapies for enhancing movement training for people with a disability. J Neuroeng Rehabil. 2012;9(1):17. https://doi.org/10.1186/1743-0003-9-17.
37. Riener R, Nef T, Colombo G. Robot-aided neurorehabilitation of the upper extremities. Med Biol Eng Comput. 2005;43(1):2–10, [Online]. Available: https://www.ncbi.nlm.nih.gov/pubmed/15742713.
38. Riener R, Lunenburger L, Colombo G. Human-centered robotics applied to gait training and assessment. J Rehabil Res Dev. 2006;43(5):679–94, [Online]. Available: https://www.ncbi.nlm.nih.gov/pubmed/17123208.
39. Veerbeek JM, Langbroek-Amersfoort AC, van Wegen EEHH, Meskers CGMM, Kwakkel G. Effects of robot-assisted therapy for the upper limb after stroke: a systematic review and meta-analysis. Neurorehabil Neural Repair. 2017;31(2):107–21. https://doi.org/10.1177/1545968316666957.
40. Lamers I, et al. Upper limb rehabilitation in people with multiple sclerosis: a systematic review. Neurorehabil Neural Repair. 2016;30(8):773–93. https://doi.org/10.1177/1545968315624785.
41. Krebs HI, Volpe BT. Robotics: a rehabilitation modality. Curr Phys Med Rehabil Rep. 2015;3(4):147–243. https://doi.org/10.1007/s40141-015-0101-6.
42. Calabrò RS, et al. Robotic gait rehabilitation and substitution devices in neurological disorders: where are we now? Neurol Sci. 2016;37(4). Springer-Verlag Italia s.r.l.:503–14. https://doi.org/10.1007/s10072-016-2474-4.

43. Maheu V, Archambault PS, Frappier J, Routhier F. Evaluation of the JACO robotic arm: Clinico-economic study for powered wheelchair users with upper-extremity disabilities; 2011. https://doi.org/10.1109/ICORR.2011.5975397.
44. Caterwil. Caterwill electric stair-climbing wheelchair. https://caterwil.com/product-category/power-wheelchairs/stair-climbing-wheelchairs-gts/.
45. Haumont T, et al. Wilmington robotic exoskeleton: A novel device to maintain arm improvement in muscular disease. J Pediatr Orthop. 2011;31(5) https://doi.org/10.1097/BPO.0b013e31821f50b5.
46. Armon. Zero gravity gadget. http://www.armonproducts.com/.
47. Gijbels D, Lamers I, Kerkhofs L, Alders G, Knippenberg E, Feys P. The Armeo Spring as training tool to improve upper limb functionality in multiple sclerosis: a pilot study. J Neuroeng Rehabil. 2011;8(1):5. https://doi.org/10.1186/1743-0003-8-5.
48. Esquenazi A, Lee S, Wikoff A, Packel A, Toczylowski T, Feeley J. A comparison of locomotor therapy interventions: partial-body weight−supported treadmill, Lokomat, and G-EO training in people with traumatic brain injury. PM R. Sep. 2017;9(9):839–46. https://doi.org/10.1016/j.pmrj.2016.12.010.
49. Pierella C, et al. A multimodal approach to capture post-stroke temporal dynamics of recovery. J Neural Eng. 2020;17(4):45,002. https://doi.org/10.1088/1741-2552/ab9ada.
50. Krebs HI, et al. Rehabilitation robotics: pilot trial of a spatial extension for MIT-Manus. J Neuroeng Rehabil. 2004;1(1):1–15. https://doi.org/10.1186/1743-0003-1-5.
51. Milia P, et al. Rehabilitation with robotic glove (Gloreha) in poststroke patients. Digit Med. 2019;5(2):62. https://doi.org/10.4103/digm.digm_3_19.
52. Hesse S, Schulte-Tigges G, Konrad M, Bardeleben A, Werner C. Robot-assisted arm trainer for the passive and active practice of bilateral forearm and wrist movements in hemiparetic subjects. Arch Phys Med Rehabil. 2003;84(6):915–20. https://doi.org/10.1016/S0003-9993(02)04954-7.
53. Casadio M, Morasso P, Sanguineti V, Giannoni P. Minimally assistive robot training for proprioception enhancement. Exp Brain Res. Apr. 2009;194(2):219–31. https://doi.org/10.1007/s00221-008-1680-6.
54. Vergaro E, et al. Adaptive robot training for the treatment of incoordination in multiple sclerosis. J Neuroeng Rehabil. 2010;7(1):37. https://doi.org/10.1186/1743-0003-7-37.
55. Squeri V, Masia L, Giannoni P, Sandini G, Morasso P. Wrist rehabilitation in chronic stroke patients by means of adaptive, progressive robot-aided therapy. IEEE Trans Neural Syst Rehabil Eng. 2014;22(2):312–25. https://doi.org/10.1109/TNSRE.2013.2250521.
56. Gandolfi M, et al. High-intensity robot-assisted hand training in individuals with multiple sclerosis: A randomized, controlled, single-blinded trial. In: Biosystems and biorobotics, vol. 21. Springer International Publishing; 2019. p. 528–32.
57. Sale P, Lombardi V, Franceschini M. Hand robotics rehabilitation: feasibility and preliminary results of a robotic treatment in patients with hemiparesis. Stroke Res Treat. 2012, 2012; https://doi.org/10.1155/2012/820931.
58. Jung JH, et al. Effects of combined upper limb robotic therapy in patients with tetraplegic spinal cord injury. Ann Rehabil Med. 2019;43(4):445–57. https://doi.org/10.5535/arm.2019.43.4.445.
59. Calabrò RS, et al. Who may benefit from Armeo power treatment? A neurophysiological approach to predict neurorehabilitation outcomes. PM R. Oct. 2016;8(10):971–8. https://doi.org/10.1016/j.pmrj.2016.02.004.
60. Simmatis LER, Jin AY, Taylor SW, Bisson EJ, Scott SH, Baharnoori M. The feasibility of assessing cognitive and motor function in multiple sclerosis patients using robotics. Mult Scler J Exp Transl Clin. 2020;6(4) https://doi.org/10.1177/2055217320964940.
61. Keeling AB, Piitz M, Semrau JA, Hill MD, Scott SH, Dukelow SP. Robot enhanced stroke therapy optimizes rehabilitation (RESTORE): a pilot study. J Neuroeng Rehabil. 2021;18(1):10. https://doi.org/10.1186/s12984-021-00804-8.

62. Pierella C et al.. Personalizing exoskeleton-based upper limb rehabilitation using a statistical model: a pilot study, vol. 21; 2019.
63. French JA, Rose CG, O'Malley MK, System characterization of MAHI Exo-II: a robotic exoskeleton for upper extremity rehabilitation. In: ASME 2014 dynamic systems and control conference, DSCC 2014; 2014, vol. 3. doi: https://doi.org/10.1115/DSCC2014-6267.
64. Gunn M, Shank TM, Eppes M, Hossain J, Rahman T. User evaluation of a dynamic arm orthosis for people with neuromuscular disorders. IEEE Trans Neural Syst Rehabil Eng. 2016;24(12):1277–83. https://doi.org/10.1109/TNSRE.2015.2492860.
65. Hussain I, Salvietti G, Spagnoletti G, Prattichizzo D. The soft-SixthFinger. IEEE Robot Autom Lett. 2021;1(2):1000–6. https://doi.org/10.1109/LRA.2016.2530793.
66. Munari D, et al. Effects of robot-assisted gait training combined with virtual reality on motor and cognitive functions in patients with multiple sclerosis: a pilot, single-blind, randomized controlled trial. Restor Neurol Neurosci. 2020;38(2):151–4. https://doi.org/10.3233/RNN-190974.
67. De Luca A, et al. Functional evaluation of robot end-point assisted gait re-education in chronic stroke survivors. IEEE Int Conf Rehabil Robot; 2013. https://doi.org/10.1109/ICORR.2013.6650513.
68. Hesse S, Waldner A, Tomelleri C. Innovative gait robot for the repetitive practice of floor walking and stair climbing up and down in stroke patients. J Neuroeng Rehabil. 2010;7(1):30. https://doi.org/10.1186/1743-0003-7-30.
69. Gandolfi M, et al. Robot-assisted vs. sensory integration training in treating gait and balance dysfunctions in patients with multiple sclerosis: a randomized controlled trial. Front Hum Neurosci. 2014;8(MAY):318. https://doi.org/10.3389/fnhum.2014.00318.
70. Iosa M, et al. Driving electromechanically assisted gait trainer for people with stroke. J Rehabil Res Dev. 2011;48(2):135–46. https://doi.org/10.1682/JRRD.2010.04.0069.
71. Zhang M, et al. A preliminary study on robot-assisted ankle rehabilitation for the treatment of drop foot. J Intell Robot Syst Theory Appl. 2018;91(2):207–15. https://doi.org/10.1007/s10846-017-0652-0.
72. Marchesi G et al., A robot-based assessment of trunk control in Spinal Cord Injured athletes. In Proceedings of the IEEE RAS and EMBS international conference on biomedical robotics and biomechatronics; 2020, vol. 2020-November, pp. 497–502. doi: https://doi.org/10.1109/BioRob49111.2020.9224337.
73. De Luca A, et al. Dynamic stability and trunk control improvements following robotic balance and core stability training in chronic stroke survivors: a pilot study. Front Neurol. 2020;11:494. https://doi.org/10.3389/fneur.2020.00494.
74. Calabrò RS, et al. Robotic gait training in multiple sclerosis rehabilitation: can virtual reality make the difference? Findings from a randomized controlled trial. J Neurol Sci. 2017;377:25–30. https://doi.org/10.1016/j.jns.2017.03.047.
75. Nam KY, Kim HJ, Kwon BS, Park JW, Lee HJ, Yoo A. Robot-assisted gait training (Lokomat) improves walking function and activity in people with spinal cord injury: a systematic review. J Neuroeng Rehabil. 2017;14(1):1–13. https://doi.org/10.1186/s12984-017-0232-3.
76. Jezernik S, Colombo G, Keller T, Frueh H, Morari M. Robotic orthosis Lokomat: a rehabilitation and research tool. Neuromodulation Technol Neural Interface. 2003;6(2):108–15. https://doi.org/10.1046/j.1525-1403.2003.03017.x.
77. van Kammen K, Boonstra AM, van der Woude LHV, Visscher C, Reinders-Messelink HA, den Otter R. Lokomat guided gait in hemiparetic stroke patients: the effects of training parameters on muscle activity and temporal symmetry. Disabil Rehabil. 2020;42(21):2977–85. https://doi.org/10.1080/09638288.2019.1579259.
78. Calabrò RS, et al. Shaping neuroplasticity by using powered exoskeletons in patients with stroke: a randomized clinical trial. J Neuroeng Rehabil. 2018;15(1):35. https://doi.org/10.1186/s12984-018-0377-8.

79. De Luca A, et al. Exoskeleton for gait rehabilitation: Effects of assistance, mechanical structure, and walking aids on muscle activations. Appl Sci. 2019;9(14):2868. https://doi.org/10.3390/app9142868.
80. Kozlowski AJ, Fabian M, Lad D, Delgado AD. Feasibility and safety of a powered exoskeleton for assisted walking for persons with multiple sclerosis: a single-group preliminary study. Arch Phys Med Rehabil. 2017;98(7):1300–7. https://doi.org/10.1016/j.apmr.2017.02.010.
81. Esquenazi A, Talaty M, Packel A, Saulino M. The ReWalk powered exoskeleton to restore ambulatory function to individuals with thoracic-level motor-complete spinal cord injury. Am J Phys Med Rehabil. 2012;91(11):911–21. https://doi.org/10.1097/PHM.0b013e318269d9a3.
82. Scewo wheelchair. Powere Wheelchair BRO. https://www.scewo.ch/en/bro/.
83. Kwakkel G, Kollen BJ, Krebs HI. Effects of robot-assisted therapy on upper limb recovery after stroke: a systematic review. Neurorehabil Neural Repair. 2008;22(2):111–21. https://doi.org/10.1177/1545968307305457.
84. Veerbeek JM, et al. What is the evidence for physical therapy poststroke? A systematic review and meta-analysis. PLoS One. 2014;9(2):e87987. https://doi.org/10.1371/journal.pone.0087987.
85. Brewer BR, McDowell SK, Worthen-Chaudhari LC. Poststroke upper extremity rehabilitation: a review of robotic systems and clinical results. Top Stroke Rehabil. 2007;14(6):22–44. https://doi.org/10.1310/tsr1406-22.
86. Hesse S, Schmidt H, Werner C, Bardeleben A. Upper and lower extremity robotic devices for rehabilitation and for studying motor control. Curr Opin Neurol. 2003;16(6):705–10. https://doi.org/10.1097/01.wco.0000102630.16692.38.
87. Edgerton VR, et al. Retraining the injured spinal cord. J Physiol. 2001;533(1). Wiley-Blackwell:15–22. https://doi.org/10.1111/j.1469-7793.2001.0015b.x.
88. Edgerton VR, Roy RR. Paralysis recovery in humans and model systems. Curr Opin Neurobiol. 2002;12(6). Elsevier Ltd:658–67. https://doi.org/10.1016/S0959-4388(02)00379-3.
89. Gassert R, Dietz V. Rehabilitation robots for the treatment of sensorimotor deficits: A neurophysiological perspective. J NeuroEng Rehabil. 2018;15(1). BioMed Central Ltd.:1–15. https://doi.org/10.1186/s12984-018-0383-x.
90. Colombo R, Sanguineti V. Rehabilitation robotics. 1st ed. Academic Press; 2018.
91. Klamroth-Marganska V, et al. Three-dimensional, task-specific robot therapy of the arm after stroke: a multicentre, parallel-group randomised trial. Lancet Neurol. 2014;13(2):159–66. https://doi.org/10.1016/S1474-4422(13)70305-3.
92. Casadio M, Sanguineti V, Morasso PG, Arrichiello V. Braccio di Ferro: a new haptic workstation for neuromotor rehabilitation. Technol Health Care. 2006;14(3):123–42. [Online]. Available: http://www.ncbi.nlm.nih.gov/pubmed/16971753.
93. Lo HS, Xie SQ. Exoskeleton robots for upper-limb rehabilitation: state of the art and future prospects. Med Eng Phys. 2012;34(3):261–8. https://doi.org/10.1016/j.medengphy.2011.10.004.
94. Milot M-H, et al. A crossover pilot study evaluating the functional outcomes of two different types of robotic movement training in chronic stroke survivors using the arm exoskeleton BONES. J Neuroeng Rehabil. 2013;10(1):112.
95. Proietti T, Guigon E, Roby-Brami A, Jarrassé N. Modifying upper-limb inter-joint coordination in healthy subjects by training with a robotic exoskeleton. J Neuroeng Rehabil. 2017;14(1):1–19. https://doi.org/10.1186/s12984-017-0254-x.
96. Bach Baunsgaard C, et al. Gait training after spinal cord injury: safety, feasibility and gait function following 8 weeks of training with the exoskeletons from Ekso bionics article. Spinal Cord. Feb. 2018;56(2):106–16. https://doi.org/10.1038/s41393-017-0013-7.
97. Frisoli A, et al. Positive effects of robotic exoskeleton training of upper limb reaching movements after stroke. J Neuroeng Rehabil. 2012;9(1):36.
98. Hornby TG, Campbell DD, Kahn JH, Demott T, Moore JL, Roth HR. Enhanced gait-related improvements after therapist- versus robotic-assisted locomotor training in subjects with chronic stroke: a randomized controlled study. Stroke. 2008;39(6):1786–92. https://doi.org/10.1161/STROKEAHA.107.504779.

99. Marchal-Crespo L, Reinkensmeyer DJ. Review of control strategies for robotic movement training after neurologic injury. J NeuroEng Rehabil. 2009;6(1). BioMed Central:20. https://doi.org/10.1186/1743-0003-6-20.
100. Meng W, Liu Q, Zhou Z, Ai Q, Sheng B, Xie SS. Recent development of mechanisms and control strategies for robot-assisted lower limb rehabilitation. Mechatronics. 2015;31:132–45. https://doi.org/10.1016/j.mechatronics.2015.04.005.
101. Wolbrecht ET, Chan V, Le V, Cramer SC, Reinkensmeyer DJ, Bobrow JE, Real-time computer modeling of weakness following stroke optimizes robotic assistance for movement therapy. In Proceedings of the 3rd International IEEE EMBS Conference on Neural Engineering, pp. 152–158; 2007. doi: 10.1109/CNE.2007.369635.
102. Casadio M, Sanguineti V. Learning, retention, and slacking: a model of the dynamics of recovery in robot therapy. IEEE Trans Neural Syst Rehabil Eng. May 2012;20(3):286–96. https://doi.org/10.1109/TNSRE.2012.2190827.
103. Lambercy O, Dovat L, Gassert R, Burdet E, Teo CL, Milner T. A haptic knob for rehabilitation of hand function. IEEE Trans Neural Syst Rehabil Eng. Sep. 2007;15(3):356–66. https://doi.org/10.1109/TNSRE.2007.903913.
104. Stienen AHA et al. Dampace: Dynamic force-coordination trainer for the upper extremities. In 2007 IEEE 10th international conference on rehabilitation robotics, ICORR'07, pp. 820–826; 2007. doi: https://doi.org/10.1109/ICORR.2007.4428519.
105. Proietti T, Crocher V, Roby-Brami A, Jarrassé N, et al. Upper-limb robotic exoskeletons for neurorehabilitation: a review on control strategies. IEEE Rev Biomed Eng. 2016;9:4–14.
106. Guidali M, Duschau-Wicke A, Broggi S, Klamroth-Marganska V, Nef T, Riener R. A robotic system to train activities of daily living in a virtual environment. Med Biol Eng Comput. 2011;49(10):1213–23. https://doi.org/10.1007/s11517-011-0809-0.
107. Liu LY, Li Y, Lamontagne A. The effects of error-augmentation versus error-reduction paradigms in robotic therapy to enhance upper extremity performance and recovery post-stroke: a systematic review. J NeuroEng Rehabil. 2018;15(1). BioMed Central Ltd.:65. https://doi.org/10.1186/s12984-018-0408-5.
108. Patton JL, Stoykov ME, Kovic M, Mussa-Ivaldi FA. Evaluation of robotic training forces that either enhance or reduce error in chronic hemiparetic stroke survivors. Exp Brain Res. 2006;168(3):368–83. https://doi.org/10.1007/s00221-005-0097-8.
109. Pellegrino L, et al. Effects of hemispheric stroke localization on the reorganization of arm movements within different mechanical environments. Life. 2021;11(5):383. https://doi.org/10.3390/life11050383.
110. Maenza C, Good DC, Winstein CJ, Wagstaff DA, Sainburg RL. Functional deficits in the less-impaired arm of stroke survivors depend on hemisphere of damage and extent of paretic arm impairment. Neurorehabil Neural Repair. 2020;34(1):39–50. https://doi.org/10.1177/1545968319875951.
111. Fritz H, Patzer D, Galen SS. Robotic exoskeletons for reengaging in everyday activities: promises, pitfalls, and opportunities. Disabil Rehabil. 2019;41(5):560–3. https://doi.org/10.1080/09638288.2017.1398786.
112. Bharadwaj A, Shaw SB, Goldreich D. Comparing tactile to auditory guidance for blind individuals. Front Hum Neurosci. 2019;13:443. https://doi.org/10.3389/fnhum.2019.00443.
113. Viseux F, Lemaire A, Barbier F, Charpentier P, Leteneur S, Villeneuve P. How can the stimulation of plantar cutaneous receptors improve postural control? Review and clinical commentary. Neurophysiologie Clinique. 2019;49(3). Elsevier Masson SAS.:263–8. https://doi.org/10.1016/j.neucli.2018.12.006.
114. Campa R. The rise of social robots: a review of the recent literature. J Evol Technol. 2016;26:106–13.
115. Recchiuto CT, Sgorbissa A. A feasibility study of culture-aware cloud services for conversational robots. IEEE Robot Autom Lett. 2020;5(4):6559–66. https://doi.org/10.1109/LRA.2020.3015461.

116. Belpaeme T, Kennedy J, Ramachandran A, Scassellati B, Tanaka F. Social robots for education: a review. Sci Robotics. 2018;3(21). American Association for the Advancement of Science.:5954. https://doi.org/10.1126/scirobotics.aat5954.
117. Broekens J, Heerink M, Rosendal H. Assistive social robots in elderly care: a review. Gerontechnology. 2009;8:94–103.
118. Pennisi P, et al. Autism and social robotics: a systematic review. Autism Res. 2016;9(2):165–83. https://doi.org/10.1002/aur.1527.
119. Chen SC, Jones C, Moyle W. Social robots for depression in older adults: a systematic review. J Nurs Scholarsh. 2018;50(6):612–22. https://doi.org/10.1111/jnu.12423.
120. Hobbs B, Artemiadis P. A review of robot-assisted lower-limb stroke therapy: unexplored paths and future directions in gait rehabilitation. Front Neurorobotics. 2020;14. Frontiers Media S.A.:19. https://doi.org/10.3389/fnbot.2020.00019.
121. Resquín F, et al. Hybrid robotic systems for upper limb rehabilitation after stroke: a review. Med Eng Phys. 2016;38(11):1279–88. https://doi.org/10.1016/j.medengphy.2016.09.001.
122. Capogrosso M, et al. A computational model for epidural electrical stimulation of spinal sensorimotor circuits. J Neurosci. 2013;33(49):19,326–40. https://doi.org/10.1523/JNEUROSCI.1688-13.2013.
123. Antonietti A, Casellato C, D'Angelo E, Pedrocchi A. Model-driven analysis of eyeblink classical conditioning reveals the underlying structure of cerebellar plasticity and neuronal activity. IEEE Trans Neural Networks Learn Syst. 2017;28(11):2748–62. https://doi.org/10.1109/TNNLS.2016.2598190.
124. Pierella C, et al. Learning new movements after paralysis: Results from a home-based study. Sci Rep. 2017;7(1):4779. https://doi.org/10.1038/s41598-017-04930-z.
125. Sutandi AC, Rahman SF. Robotic exosuit to improve walking and gait rehabilitation for stroke survivors: a review. AIP Conf Proc. 2021;2344(1):050014. https://doi.org/10.1063/5.0047186.

Chapter 18
A Brief Summary of the Article: "An Exoskeleton Controlled by an Epidural Wireless Brain-Machine Interface in a Tetraplegic Patient: A Proof-of-Concept Demonstration"

Francesco Cardinale

In 2019, Benabid and coworkers published a seminal article entitled "An exoskeleton controlled by an epidural wireless brain-machine interface in a tetraplegic patient: a proof-of-concept demonstration" [1]. The authors reported proof-of-concept findings from one of five patients planned in an ongoing trial registered with ClinicalTrials.gov, NCT02550522. This is likely the highest level of integration between different technologies ever published in the field of assistive robotics for neurological disorders.

The **patient** was a 28-year-old man suffering from tetraplegia caused by a C4-C5 spinal cord injury with a residual little motor control of the upper limbs. He was able just to drive a wheelchair controlled by a left-arm support-joystick. The patient applied to take part of the trial online.

The **system** included:

- WIMAGINE, an implantable recording machine for bilateral epidural implantation over the sensory-motor cortex able to radio-emit recorded data;
- EMY, a four-limb robotic neuroprosthetic exoskeleton;
- Adaptive decoding algorithms and software.

Operative and postoperative **methods** can be schematically summarized as follows.

- Surgical steps, from planning to postoperative imaging:

F. Cardinale (✉)
"Claudio Munari" Center for Epilepsy Surgery, Azienda Socio-Sanitaria Territoriale Grande Ospedale Metropolitano Niguarda, Milano, Italy

Dipartimento di Medicina e Chirurgia, Università degli Studi di Parma, Parma, Italy
e-mail: francesco.cardinale@ospedaleniguarda.it

J. A. González Martínez, F. Cardinale (eds.), *Robotics in Neurosurgery*,
https://doi.org/10.1007/978-3-031-08380-8_18

  - The sensory-motor cortex was located by means of repeat functional Magnetic Resonance (fMR) and Magnetoencephalography (MEG) datasets acquired during virtual or real execution of upper and lower limbs movements;
  - Coregistered fMR and MEG datasets provided main information for the pre-operative neuronavigation planning;
  - WINIMAGE was bilaterally implanted over the sensory-motor cortex;
  - The correct positioning was verified acquiring post-implant Computed Tomography (CT) and registering it to preoperative MR.

- Postoperative methods:

  - Calibration, training, assessments of performance and progress were performed by means of brain–computer interface tasks.

    In the first phase of every experiment, a decoder was created or updated (calibration).
    In the second phase, the performance of the decoder was estimated until it was satisfactory.

  - A number of tasks were executed by the patient in different modalities.

    Continuous spatial movements:

    - Simple video games:

      - A Pong-like video game task, in which the patient mentally controlled a paddle to intercept a falling ball (1D unidirectional movements);
      - A reach-and-touch-target video game (2D movements);

    - Controlling a virtual avatar:

      - A reach-and-touch-target task (3D one-handed movements);
      - Multi-limb activation of the avatar (2D and 3D two-handed movements);

    - Wearing the exoskeleton:

      - A reach-and-touch-target task (3D one-handed movements);
      - Multi-limb activation of the exoskeleton (2D and 3D two-handed tasks);
      - Bimanual tasks with pronation and supination of both hands (8D tasks).

    Triggered on-off events:

    - Video game to initiate a:

      - Manikin walking;
      - Avatar walking;
      - Worn suspended exoskeleton.

- The adaptive decoding algorithm was calibrated and updated regularly.

The **results** were satisfactory. In fact, during a two-year long period, the patient was able to cortically control a program to simulate walking or to make upper-limb movements with both hands, using a virtual avatar at home or the real exoskeleton in the laboratory. The rate of success during several reach-and-touch tasks and wrist rotations made with EMY was 70.9% (Standard Deviation 11.6).

The adaptive decoder remained efficient up to 7 weeks without the need of recalibration.

The epidural array of electrodes, despite its semi-invasiveness, showed similar efficiency compared to microelectrodes directly implanted in the cortex that had been implemented in previous studies.

Compared to the baseline, the neurological performance did not improve. No complications occurred.

In **conclusion**, this is the first paper reporting the combination of epidural recording, wireless power, and emission and online decoding of many electrocorticographic channels in a unique, totally embedded system. As the authors reported in their discussion, "the successful control of eight degrees of freedom (the patient had permanent access to all dimensions), suspended walking capability during the 24 months after surgical implantation, and continued control after several weeks without recalibration are the highest performances reported so far."

This brief summary is certainly not exhaustive, of course. The reader is strongly invited to enjoy the original paper by Benabid and coworkers, a true milestone in the fields of neurosurgical robotics and brain–computer interface.

Reference

1. Benabid AL, Costecalde T, Eliseyev A, et al. An exoskeleton controlled by an epidural wireless brain-machine interface in a tetraplegic patient: a proof-of-concept demonstration. Lancet Neurol. 2019;18:1112–22.

Part IV
Special Topics

Chapter 19
Robotics in Neurosurgical Training

Michael Y. Bai, Hussam Abou-Al-Shaar, Zachary C. Gersey, Daryl P. Fields, and Nitin Agarwal

Introduction

A surgical robot is a powered computer controlled manipulator with artificial sensing that can be reprogrammed to move and position tools to carry out a range of surgical tasks [1].The Czech novelist and playwright, Karel Čapek, first coined the word robot to describe automated machines in his science-fiction play, "R.U.R—Rossumovi Univerzální Roboti" in 1921, originating from the Czech word robota for forced labor [2]. The first industrial applications of robotics can be traced back to the partnership forged between George Devol and Joseph Engelberger. In 1959, General Motors installed the fruits of their labor, the Unimate #001 (which Devol termed a "Programmed Article Transfer Device") at its die casting production line in New Jersey, ushering in a new era of manufacturing. It was not until 25 years later when robotic technology was first used in the operating theater. An industrial robotic arm, the PUMA 200 (Programmable Universal Machine for Assembly), was used to perform a stereotactic brain biopsy with 0.05 mm accuracy. This system was the prototype for the dawn of robotic-assisted neurosurgery.

Since then, technological advances continue to the present day with several integrated systems allowing improved precision, high accuracy, and decreased complications, and thereby increasing the capabilities of the surgeon in minimally invasive surgical procedures. As a result, the use of diverse robotic devices has rapidly expanded into the medical and surgical arena to completely revolutionize the provision of care. Robots are perceived to relieve some amount of labor from surgeons, but robotic surgery still requires a considerable amount of skill and training to

M. Y. Bai · H. Abou-Al-Shaar · Z. C. Gersey · D. P. Fields · N. Agarwal (✉)
Department of Neurological Surgery and Epilepsy Center, University of Pittsburgh Medical Center, Pittsburgh, PA, USA
e-mail: aboualshaarh@upmc.edu; gerseyzc@upmc.edu; fieldsdp@upmc.edu; agarwaln@upmc.edu

J. A. González Martínez, F. Cardinale (eds.), *Robotics in Neurosurgery*,
https://doi.org/10.1007/978-3-031-08380-8_19

perform on the part of the operator. Today, robotics mainly support the desire for minimally invasive, stereotactic surgery with robots being physical extensions of computer systems that interact with surgeons to provide improved accuracy in surgical site location, reduced invasiveness, increased precision of surgical tool motion, and overall better surgical outcomes. Since the first use of surgical robots in 1985, the field has exploded and represents a new paradigm shift in medicine and surgery. While the use of robotics in neurosurgery is still in its early stages, its use has become widespread in laparoscopy, gynecology, vascular surgery, cardiothoracic surgery, urology, and respiratory interventions [3].

Neurorobotics is accelerating at a rapid pace. Technological and economic advances will allow robots to become smaller, stronger, faster, and more precise than ever before. Their ability to perform complex tasks with great accuracy and reliability is what makes robots ideal for neurosurgery. Robots can also enhance the visual and manual dexterity of surgeons and allow them to see and reach areas of the brain that were previously inaccessible. It can also allow for unconventional approaches to access areas of the brain that would previously have been considered "too risky" or "inoperable" and therefore reduce harm to patients, increase the chances of surgical success, and improve postoperative recovery and quality of life. In many academic centers, robotic surgery became part of the training for residents and fellows (Fig. 19.1), which had been incorporated into the academic curriculum.

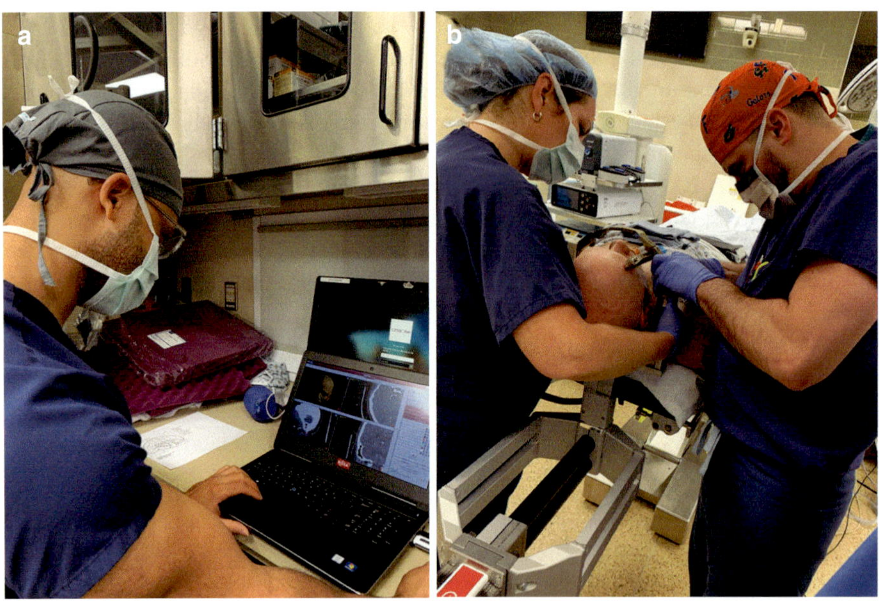

Fig. 19.1 Intraoperative image depicting active resident participation in robotic-assisted surgery for a patient with medically refractory epilepsy undergoing SEEG. The robot is utilized during various parts of the procedure including preoperative planning (**a**), registration (**b**), SEEG drilling (**c**), and SEEG lead implantation (**d**)

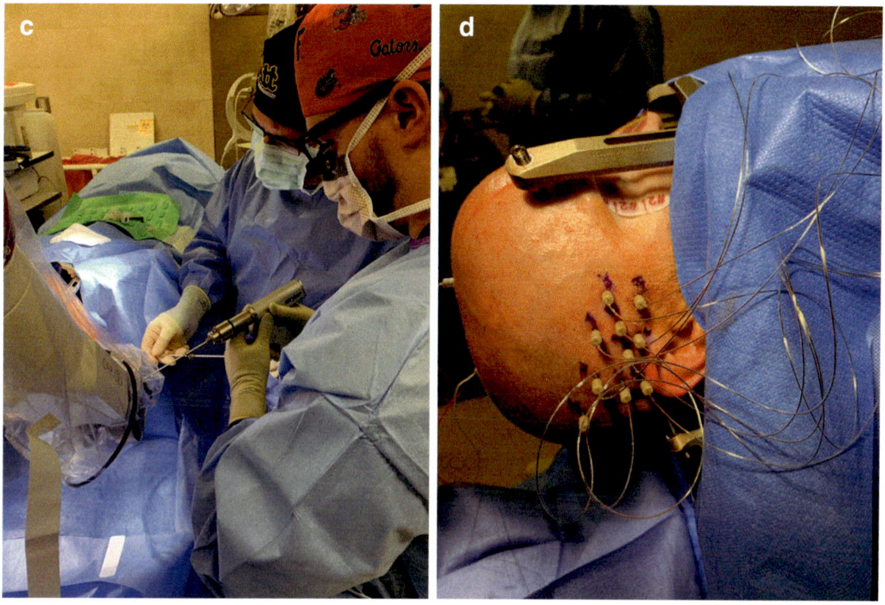

Fig. 19.1 (continued)

We anticipate that robotic surgery competency will become a necessary step for a complete neurosurgical training as imaging guiding surgery, as an example. This chapter provides an overview of robotics utilization in neurosurgical procedures and training of residents and fellows, spanning from their origin, current perspective, and future implications.

Historical Perspective

The first robotic surgery systems were designed for brain tumor biopsies [4]. In April 1985, Dr. Yik San Kwoh used the Unimation PUMA (Programmable Universal Machine for Assembly) 200 robot, which was a machine designed for industrial use, to position a needle precisely using computed tomography (CT) guidance in a 52-year-old male when performing a stereotactic biopsy of a deep intracerebral lesion [4]. The ability of the robot to calculate its movements based on the stereotactic frame resulted in delivery of faster and more accurate results than any other method available at the time. Kwoh et al. demonstrated that robots assistance could be safely employed along with the use of a stereotactic frame during neurosurgical procedures [5]. This development was soon followed by the use of the same robot (PUMA 200) as an assistant to retract delicate neural structures during the surgical resection of low-grade thalamic tumors in children [6]. However, the PUMA 200 robot was limited in neurosurgical applications and was eventually surpassed in capabilities by the MINERVA (University of Lausanne, Switzerland) robot in 1995, which allowed the use of real-time CT to guide stereotactic biopsy probes [5].

The concept of robotics progressed further, and technological advancements led to a multitude of diverse robotic devices such as the ROSA, which gained FDA approval in 2012 [7] (Robotic Stereotactic Assistance—Medtech, Montpellier, France) NeuroArm (2007 launch, technology acquired in 2010 by IMRIS, Minnetonka, MN) [8], NeuroBlate (2013 release, Monteris Medical. Plymouth MN) [9], Pathfinder (consortium) [10], Renaissance (technology acquired by Medtronic 2018, Minneapolis, MN), and Neuromate (Renishaw plc, Wotton-under-Edge, UK) [11].

Robotic Types

The differences in the function and application of a robot as well as the type of robot–surgeon interaction is key to describing different types of surgical robots [12]. The three basic categories of surgical robots are:

- Dependent: the surgeon controls every movement of the robot such as with the da Vinci Surgical System.
- Autonomous: the robot can perform pre-programmed actions with close supervision of the surgeon.
- Shared control: both the surgeon and robot control actions concurrently.

Dependent Systems

Dependent systems are the most popular type of robots as the surgeon retains full control over the actions of the robot. Also known as master-slave systems, these robots enhance the capabilities of the human surgeon by allowing the surgeon greater comfort, precision, visualization, and ability to operate remotely while simultaneously reducing the size of the surgical field, operative time, and complications [12].

Autonomous Systems

The robots assist the surgeon to carry out precise tasks. They are pre-programmed to perform a specific motion or move tools to set locations. The success of this type of system is dependent on the technology itself, and complications can arise if the system has not been programmed correctly. As a result, a great deal of trust is associated when using these systems [12].

Robots like the Minerva (University of Lausanne, Lausanne, Switzerland) [5] and Pathfinder (consortium) [10] perform stereotactic tasks with or without a frame and have progressed from guiding biopsy needles and depth electrodes in the brain to planning and inserting pedicle screws in the spine. Supervised robots like the SpineAssist [13] and Renaissance [14] (both systems acquired by Medtronics, Minneapolis, MN) systems are now widely utilized in spinal instrumentation, and more recently have been approved for use in intracranial procedures [7, 15].

Shared Control Systems

Shared control systems are a combination of autonomous and dependent systems and involve the surgeon and the robot jointly controlling the instruments used to manipulate and dissect neural structures [12]. In this way, the precise actions of the robot can be combined with the manipulative skills and manual dexterity of the neurosurgeon. The instrument is held by the surgeon and the robot, allowing for finer dissection and elimination of tremor and muscle fatigue.

Utilization of Robotics in Neurosurgery

Robots have various applications in neurosurgery, including functional, spine, tumor, endovascular, and epilepsy surgery. Functional neurosurgery, in particular, witnessed a great deal of robotics integration and advancements throughout the years. The use of frameless robots in deep brain stimulation (DBS) and stereo electroencephalography (SEEG) is of particular interest [16, 17]. Examples of these in the field of deep brain stimulation include the work of Candela et al. [18] who used the Neuromate stereotactic robot (Renishaw plc, Wotton-under-Edge, UK) to assess the accuracy and safety of this device when used for electrode placement bilaterally in the globus pallidus internus (GPi) for deep brain stimulation in six pediatric patients suffering from hyperkinetic movement disorders. Primary outcome measurements were a comparison of actual electrode position placement determined by CT imaging compared with the preoperative planned coordinates, and through comparison of validated scales of dystonia and myoclonus acquired 1 month preoperatively and 6 months postoperatively. They concluded that the robot was both an accurate and safe tool for use in the placement of GPi electrodes. Neudorfer et al. [19] conducted a retrospective study comparing the accuracy, precision, reliability, duration of surgery, intraoperative imaging quality, safety, and maintenance between robot-assisted (ROSA Brain, MedTech, Montpellier, France) and conventional DBS surgical procedures. Their analysis of the outcomes of 80 patients led to the conclusion that robot-assisted DBS procedures were superior in terms of accuracy, precision, and operation time when compared to conventional DBS surgeries. Shorter procedure times were also observed to be a benefit of robot-assisted DBS surgeries by Vansickle et al. [20] in their study on 128 Parkinson's disease patients. Using the Renaissance robot (Medtronics, Minneapolis, MN), they aimed to demonstrate the effectiveness of DBS surgeries with asleep patients and fusion of preoperative magnetic resonance imaging (MRI) scans with intraoperative CT scans. Not only did they observe shorter operation times to the benefit of the patient, but also electrode placement was found to be accurate.

Another field in robot-assisted neurosurgery that has blossomed is in SEEG, in particular for epilepsy patients. In an earlier study [21] that evaluated SEEG safety and accuracy, using conventional and the ROSA robotic system (MedTech, Montpellier, France) for electrode placement, the authors found that use of the robotic device was equally successful at mapping the epileptogenic zone as use of conventional procedures. This result was also confirmed in two separate studies also employing the ROSA device with adult [22] and pediatric [23] patients. Almost simultaneous to these reports, a review of neurosurgical treatments of pediatric epilepsy also underscored the value of robotic assistance in SEEG as well as in laser interstitial thermal therapy [24]. Gonzalez-Martinez's group has since moved forward to investigate the validity of using the ROSA robot-assistive device for placement of electrodes for the Responsive Neurostimulator System (RNS, NeuroPace Inc., Mountainview, California) compared to frame-based or frameless stereotactic systems [25]. Their conclusion was again similar, pointing to the usefulness of robotic-assistive devices in neurosurgery: that robotic-assisted stereotaxis can be used to provide an accurate and safe method for implantation of RNS electrodes. Debenedictis et al. [26] have documented their extensive experience of the use of the ROSA robot-assisted device in 128 pediatric neurosurgical procedures (SEEG, neuroendoscopy, stereotactic biopsy, pallidotomy, shunt placement, deep brain stimulation procedures, and stereotactic cyst aspiration). Their results touted the versatility of the ROSA device for many different neurosurgical applications while maintaining safety and minimizing operative times. The future of robot-assisted neurosurgeries is bright and will be highlighted by further applications and technological advances including those in curvilinear needle guiding and brain imaging technologies [27].

Robotics also have applications in pain-related surgeries and treatments of psychiatric diseases such as depression and obsessive-compulsive disorder. MRI-guided robots are used in biopsies and telesurgery, as well as endoscopic endonasal trans-sphenoidal surgery for pituitary tumors and skull base lesions. Recently, the use of robotics in spinal surgery has gained an interest among neurosurgeons [28].

Another area in which robotics plays a role is in the development of the exoscope for surgical site visualization. Several different systems are available, each with their own advantages and limitations and choice will depend upon the type of surgery involved. However, they are all associated with much improved ergonomics in the operating theater when it comes to surgical site visualization and are also valuable for training and educational purposes [29–31]. Description of these systems is beyond the scope of this chapter.

Benefits and Limitations of Robotics in Neurosurgery

The benefits of robotic integration in neurosurgical procedures are numerous, which include increased dexterity for surgeons, minimally invasive access without loss of surgical ability, motion scaling (conversion of large movements to short movements of hands during surgery), and easier manipulation of small delicate structures. Neurosurgical robots have an advantage of integration with image guidance systems yielding increased precision, consistency, and accuracy minimizing the risk of iatrogenic injury to critical neurovascular structures. For example, in the placement of electrodes for DBS, robots allow for the precise alignment of multiple trajectories and ensure accurate placement of the leads in the desired location [32, 33]. An important aspect of neurosurgical robots is that they help to improve patient's comfort, shorten surgical procedure time, and reduce surgeon's fatigue during microscopic surgery [7, 34].

Robotic systems, however, are not without their own set of inherent limitations, which are predominantly related to elements of robotic systems (the technology) and aspects of training of surgeons regarding their application and use. Other concerns include the cost/benefit ratio, which could offset observed benefits and integration difficulties due to the bulky size of robotic systems. As with other forms of technology where the drive is for smaller and better, this should become less of a problem in the near future. Latency in movement, lack of tactile feedback, and risks of mechanical failure and malfunction are other apprehensions of robotics use in surgery [1, 12, 33, 35].

Augmented Reality

Augmented reality (AR) or virtual reality (VR) refers to the ability to overlay artificial images or other useful information onto the operative visual field [12]. This would enable surgeons to incorporate patient specific preoperative images obtained from CT, MRI, or X-ray into their live view of the patient and therefore enhance their awareness of important unperceived structures within the patient's anatomy and plan surgical procedures.

Technologies such as the Google Glasses (Google Inc., Mountain View, CA), HoloLens (Microsoft Inc., Redmond, WA) allow 3D reconstruction of useful images in front of the surgical field [36, 37]. They can display information such as tumor location, pedicle screw trajectories, and nearby important neurovascular structures.

AR can be combined with surgical robotics to achieve an integrated system comprising of a slave system performing the surgery, a master system controlling the slave system, an imaging system with live images of the operating field, and an AR display attaching markers to the images [38]. Such combined robotic and AR surgery has been reported in laparoscopic procedures, including nephrectomies and liver segmentectomies [39–41].

In the future, AR visualization may be taken from the robot's point of view, with surgeons controlling the system from outside of the sterile field. With advances in live, intraoperative imaging, this technology has the capability of completely revolutionizing neurosurgery with enhanced accuracy and reduced complications. In fact, in a recent review, it was determined that AR is constantly improving the effectiveness of training physicians and the overall outcomes of the treatment [42]. AR can be combined with other technologies that give surgeons greater control, such as intuitive, responsive controls with sensitive haptic feedback. This will allow surgeons to become fully immersed in AR while protecting the patient from the limitations of a human operator (such as fatigue, muscle tremor, and orientation).

Neurosurgical Training

The first surgical training program, established by William Stewart Halsted at Johns Hopkins, set the foundation for modern surgical residency programs [43]. His program comprised the basic sciences, research, and graduated responsibility of patients in the operating room, now supplemented by the observation of experts, practice on cadavers, and VR platforms. The latter has been developed and grown in a manner analogous to avionic flight simulators [44] for a variety of procedures, including simulations of ventriculostomies, pedicle screw placement, image-guided microsurgical procedures, planning of stereotactic radiosurgery, and remote surgical assistance of cadaveric surgery. Amongst the first of these VR platforms designed specifically for neurosurgery was described by Kockro et al. [45] They developed the VIVIAN (Virtual Intracranial Visualization and Navigation) system for the Dextroscope (Bracco, Milan, Italy), a virtual reality environment, which has since proven valuable in several neurosurgical training scenarios [46–48]. However, it lacked haptic feedback. Malone et al. [49] have reviewed some of the earlier developments in neurosurgical simulations. In 2012, Delorme et al. [50] outlined their efforts at designing a VR platform that incorporated haptic feedback (Neurotouch/NeuroVR, Saint-Laurent, Québec, Canada), which consisted of a stereovision system, bimanual haptic tool manipulators, and a powerful (at that time) computer and set up for beta testing at 7 teaching hospitals in Canada. A more complete training framework surrounding the Neurotouch was then established [51]. The framework consisted of five modules deemed representative of basic and advanced neurosurgical skill. These were ventriculostomy, endoscopic nasal navigation, tumor debulking, hemostasis, and microdissection. Further improvements of the Neurotouch system were later developed for the extraction of data which was used for further evaluation and metrics of trainee performance [52]. This simulator was later used to show through force pyramid analysis that certain tumor regions required greater psychomotor ability to resect. This knowledge could then be used as a focus for further resident training efforts [53, 54], with expertise in technique now being evaluated with the assistance of artificial intelligence and machine learning algorithms [55, 56]. The technology has now advanced to the point where it can evaluate and quantify neurosurgeon tremor [57].Other simulators continue to be developed to address the important issue of surgeon training, for example, a recent system that combines real brain tissue with 3D printing and augmented reality [58].Another example is a method of training fine-motor skills such as Microscopic Selection Task (MST) using virtual reality (VR) with objective quantification of performance and introduction of vibrotactile feedback (VTFB) to study its impact on training performance. The results were promising, as MST with VTFB led to faster completion of MST with higher precision and accuracy compared to that without VTFB [59].

Though these advances in virtual reality for surgical technique and evaluation are helpful training aids, the training of surgeons in robotics remains a challenging issue. It is time consuming, placing emphasis on proficiency, dexterity, robotics knowledge, and skills acquisition. It involves learning the basic kinematics of using machines and their control systems, which can involve AR and VR platforms and/or cadavers. Surgeons are trained to improve their technical, clinical, and cognitive abilities and skills to assist their adoption of these new technologies [41, 60–62]. Thus, with the application of robot-assisted surgery, there is an increased need for training, and while the traditional methods have been effective, more modern methods such as dual robotic consoles and AR and VR platforms show great promise, but not yet widely adopted [63].

Training programs should aim to integrate theory and training across simulated and cadaveric domains. The first step in robotics training of surgeons starts with theoretical training followed by simulation. Inanimate simulation exercises are characterized by good construct validity and have been employed in criterion-based training [64]. Simulation has gained acclaim over the last two decades [65–67], and a plethora of simulation platforms and software are available today from companies such as Mimic Technologies (Seattle WA), Simulab (Seattle WA), Insimo (Strasbourg, France), FundamentalVR (London UK), among others.

Examples of these training programs include VR surgery training that can utilize pre-designed scenarios to allow trainees to practice particular skills. Both AR and VR have been associated with greater improvement of skills and provide the advantage of remote robotically assisted surgeries [68]. They can also be designed around a patient's specific anatomy involving rare and challenging cases and to allow pre-operative preparation in a personalized approach to treatment [12, 69]. The advantage of VR training is that surgeons are able to receive tuned haptic feedback, which is often cited as an important feature of surgical robots [1, 12, 70]. Haptic feedback in robotic surgery is especially important, and is believed to reduce operative time and surgical errors. In a recent study, the importance of adding a superior haptic feedback device in telerobotic surgery for standardization of surgery and care was evaluated. The conclusion clearly showed that the choice of haptic hand controller was very significant in the outcomes [71]. Indeed, results indicate that haptic feedback in VR training is especially important during early phase acquisition of psychomotor skills [69]. Applications of VR include case planning, playback, and rehearsal, which will become especially beneficial for neurosurgical training. Incorporation of VR simulators in surgical curricula is of great interest for robot-assisted training. Many VR simulators exist, but the most prominent include the dV trainer (Mimic Technologies, Seattle WA; mimicsimulation.com), the robotic surgical simulator "RoSS" system (Simulated Surgical Systems, San Jose CA), RobotiX mentor (3D Systems, Littleton CO), and the da Vinci skills stimulator (Intuitive Surgical Inc., Sunnyvale CA) [72].

The da Vinci system (Intuitive Surgical, Inc., Sunnyvale, CA) is the most widely used surgical robot approved by the FDA for various operations. In just 9 years since its introduction to the market, the da Vinci system is now used in 80% of radical prostatectomies conducted in the US. The system also provides a platform for trainees to develop expertise in robotic skills. In addition, this system has shown good construct validity of an in vivo exercise testing which discriminates novice and expert surgeon competencies, hence supporting evidence of benefit associated with VR exercises [73]. The da Vinci Research Kit (dVRK) has been instrumental in development of novel software frameworks to prototype and test gradations of human–robot interactions and automation in surgical robots according to trainees' performance levels [74]. In fact, the framework developed by Enayati et al. [75] highlighted the potential of robotic assistance in visuomotor training though further research is needed to validate generalizability of their findings.

Although the da Vinci surgical system offers seven degrees of freedom in range of motion (equivalent to the human arm) and is considered to be the most widely used robotic system in the world [2], its adoption into neurosurgery has been hindered due to the limited tools available, the number of ports needed, and size of the machinery. The steady hand system is the only version reported to be in use in micro-neurosurgery [12].

Perhaps superior to the completely robotic and digital approaches described above, robotic systems training through cadaveric surgeries allows utility of proprioceptive feedback. Trainees can improve their technique by conducting experiments on human cadavers. For this reason, the coordination of cadaveric use to increase the availability of human training sites is recommended [35]. Though considerably more expensive, it is still considered the best way to practice because it gives a better representation of the surgical field [12]. Cadaveric training is, however, limited by single time use and leading some to conclude that inanimate training including VR exercises is most effective in standardized curricula [76].

Robot-Assisted Surgical Training

Advantages

Computer simulations paired with robotics such as in the previously mentioned RobotiX mentor (3D Systems, Littleton CO) and the da Vinci skills stimulator (Intuitive Surgical Inc., Sunnyvale CA; intuitive.com) systems produce high quality programs for trainee surgeons to equip them with dexterity, precision, and speed so that they can work efficiently whilst ensuring patients' safety [77]. Neurosurgical training makes use of surgical based simulations, which exhibit high performance and are cost efficient [78]. Robotic surgical systems also provide better 3D visualization of surgery, with increasing capability for sensory immersion [35, 79].

Limitations

Similar to robotic utilization in surgical procedures, there are several limitations for using robots in surgery training. Surgical robotic systems are expensive, with hefty prices involved in the maintenance of a robot and the use of instruments [78]. In robot-assisted surgery, the robots and instruments must be changed every 8–10 operations [78, 79]. Furthermore, the Da Vinci Surgical System is the most modern and most developed system for surgery, but requires large operating rooms [79]. 3D spatial navigation and visual spatial coordination have in the past been cited as two additional limitations in robotic neurosurgery [80], as for the machine to think in a complex 3D environment is computationally demanding and limited by sensor technology.

Prerequisites

Although robotically assisted surgeries have spiked worldwide in the last two decades, there is no standardized training or unified credentialing system in place. As the demand for this technology grows, it is imperative to devise a formal comprehensive robotic neurosurgical training program and validated assessment tool to achieve safe practices and best patient outcomes with the greater goal to prepare trainees for independent practice. Combined simulation-based training and didactic lessons support training through progressive skills acquisition [81].

As prerequisites, trainees should have knowledge about robot-assisted surgery, its parameters, and its functions. Information about surgical procedures should also be known. Surgical procedures involving robots include how to select patients for surgery, what to do in the event of complications, and the appropriate distance between the robotic system and patient [77]. Secondly, training for robotic neurosurgery should be performed as much as possible in the laboratory using robotic simulator systems; using operating theater robotic systems extensively for training is not cost effective [77, 82]. Thirdly, trainees should be familiar with VR training, which has a vital role in learning to use robots in robot-assisted neurosurgery [77]. Lastly, a trainee should be aware of how to use human and animal cadavers for robotics training. Animal simulation models can be used but due to ethical concerns their use is limited [83].

Mentoring, proctoring, and precepting are valuable throughout the training period and beyond. Institutions should provide necessary resources needed for supporting these experiences. Training should proceed from surgical observation and assistance to autonomous performance of surgical tasks. Therefore, active trainee involvement during procedures has to be addressed either through surgeon shifts during procedure or employing surgical robotic systems. In a survey of residents regarding their attitude and compliance towards robotic surgery training, the authors identified that the non-mandatory structured robotic training curriculum used at their institution was insufficient in helping them gain fundamental robotic skills. Specific problems identified were the amount of time they needed to invest in the program and lack of access to a simulator [84].

The scarcity of assessment tools and methods specifically employed in neurosurgical robotics training is strikingly evident. The Global Evaluative Assessment of Robotic Skills (GEARS) [85] is a validated tool to differentiate expertise in robotic surgery which can be integrated with metrics available in robotic surgery simulators. Other assessment tools in use include the Non-Technical Skills for Surgeons (NOTSS) [86] rating system designed for non-technical skills and the Observational Teamwork Assessment for Surgery (OTAS) [87] rating scale that assesses team performance. Guru et al. [88] have highlighted that assessment of cognitive abilities (i.e., processes involving information-gathering, visual scanning, and sustained attention) is a good marker of differentiation between beginners, competent, proficient, and expert surgeons. Nevertheless, it requires further research for external validation. It is clear that the design and development of a targeted, standardized, and integrated assessment tool remain an unmet need to reflect the capabilities of surgeons worldwide.

Future Directions

The scope for improvement in robotics in the field of neurosurgery is immense [33], however, communication latency remains one of the biggest hurdles to overcome in order to increase the scope of robotics in the field. Future advancements will be seen in sensors, computers, and manipulation components of surgical robots to improve the identification of tissues, nerves, blood vessels, and tumors. Advancing sensors for haptic feedback aim to address the primary complaints of surgeons. Another arena where technology is being advanced is manipulators and end-effectors [33]. Robots such as the da Vinci system are progressing to reduce their size and footprint within the operating room. This will make them more accessible, safer, and cheaper, increasing their adoption in years to come.

Shared control robots, rather than completely autonomous or dependent systems, will likely dominate the field as surgeons combine the sense of control with allowing robots to assist in pre-programmed ways [12]. The ability of some neurosurgical robots to assume autonomous tasks will continue into the future. Such abilities will include the use of artificial intelligence to automatically adjust cutting speed or applied force or will be able to sense delicate boundaries and warn surgeons before they proceed [5]. This will enhance our capability to operate in small spaces and reach previously "inoperable" lesions within the brain while simultaneously reducing the risk of harm to the patient.

In order to arrive to this state, surgeons need to be trained in a cost-effective manner on all aspects of robot-assisted surgery. Robotic simulators combined with AR/VR will continue to evolve to decrease the steep learning curve. At the same time, regulatory agencies will discuss standardization of credentials and residency programs to ensure all practicing robot-assisted surgeons are educated and trained equivalently.

Acknowledgements *Funding Statement:* This chapter received no specific grant from any funding agency in the public, commercial or not-for-profit sectors.

Competing Interests Statement: The authors declare no conflicts of interest regarding the production of this article.

References

1. Davies B. A review of robotics in surgery. Proc Inst Mech Eng H. 2000;214(1):129–40. https://doi.org/10.1243/0954411001535309.
2. Moore E. Robotic surgery. Encyclopædia Britannica, Inc.. Accessed 12th June, 2020. https://www.britannica.com/science/robotic-surgery
3. Leal Ghezzi T, Campos CO. 30 years of robotic surgery. World J Surg. 2016;40(10):2550–7. https://doi.org/10.1007/s00268-016-3543-9.
4. Kwoh YS, Hou J, Jonckheere EA, Hayati S. A robot with improved absolute positioning accuracy for CT guided stereotactic brain surgery. IEEE Trans Biomed Eng. 1988;35(2):153–60. https://doi.org/10.1109/10.1354.
5. Smith JA, Jivraj J, Wong R, Yang V. 30 years of neurosurgical robots: review and trends for manipulators and associated navigational systems. Ann Biomed Eng. 2016;44(4):836–46. https://doi.org/10.1007/s10439-015-1475-4.
6. Drake JM, Joy M, Goldenberg A, Kreindler D. Computer- and robot-assisted resection of thalamic astrocytomas in children. Neurosurgery. 1991;29(1):27–33. https://doi.org/10.1227/00006123-199107000-00005.
7. D'Souza M, Gendreau J, Feng A, Kim LH, Ho AL, Veeravagu A. Robotic-assisted spine surgery: history, efficacy, cost, and future trends. Robotic Surg Res Rev. 2019;6:9–23. https://doi.org/10.2147/RSRR.S190720.
8. Sutherland GR, Wolfsberger S, Lama S, Zarei-nia K. The evolution of neuroArm. Neurosurgery. 2013;72:A27–32. https://doi.org/10.1227/NEU.0b013e318270da19.
9. Sloan AE, Ahluwalia MS, Valerio-Pascua J, et al. Results of the NeuroBlate system first-in-humans phase I clinical trial for recurrent glioblastoma. J Neurosurg. 2013;118(6):1202–19. https://doi.org/10.3171/2013.1.JNS1291.
10. Deacon G, Harwood A, Holdback J, et al. The pathfinder image-guided surgical robot. Proc Inst Mech Eng H J Eng Med. 2010;224(5):691–713. https://doi.org/10.1243/09544119JEIM617.
11. Varma TR, Eldridge P. Use of the NeuroMate stereotactic robot in a frameless mode for functional neurosurgery. Int J Med Robot. 2006;2(2):107–13. https://doi.org/10.1002/rcs.88.
12. Doulgeris JJ, Gonzalez-Blohm SA, Filis AK, Shea TM, Aghayev K, Vrionis FD. Robotics in neurosurgery: evolution, current challenges, and compromises. Cancer Control. 2015;22(3):352–9. https://doi.org/10.1177/107327481502200314.
13. Devito DP, Kaplan L, Dietl R, et al. Clinical acceptance and accuracy assessment of spinal implants guided with SpineAssist surgical robot: retrospective study. Spine (Phila Pa 1976). 2010;35(24):2109–15. https://doi.org/10.1097/BRS.0b013e3181d323ab.

14. Theodore N, Ahmed AK. The history of robotics in spine surgery. Spine. 2018;43:S23. https://doi.org/10.1097/BRS.0000000000002553.
15. Bagga V, Bhattacharyya D. Robotics in neurosurgery. Ann Roy Coll Surg Engl. 2018;100(6_sup):23–6. https://doi.org/10.1308/rcsann.supp1.19.
16. Lefranc M, Le Gars D. Robotic implantation of deep brain stimulation leads, assisted by intra-operative, flat-panel CT. Acta Neurochir. 2012;154(11):2069–74. https://doi.org/10.1007/s00701-012-1445-7.
17. McBeth PB, Louw DF, Rizun PR, Sutherland GR. Robotics in neurosurgery. Am J Surg. 2004;188(4):68–75. https://doi.org/10.1016/j.amjsurg.2004.08.004.
18. Candela S, Vanegas MI, Darling A, et al. Frameless robot-assisted pallidal deep brain stimulation surgery in pediatric patients with movement disorders: precision and short-term clinical results. J Neurosurg Pediatr. 2018;22(4):416–25. https://doi.org/10.3171/2018.5.PEDS1814.
19. Neudorfer C, Hunsche S, Hellmich M, El Majdoub F, Maarouf M. Comparative study of robot-assisted versus conventional frame-based deep brain stimulation stereotactic neurosurgery. Stereotact Funct Neurosurg. 2018;96(5):327–34. https://doi.org/10.1159/000494736.
20. VanSickle D, Volk V, Freeman P, Henry J, Baldwin M, Fitzpatrick CK. Electrode placement accuracy in robot-assisted asleep deep brain stimulation. Ann Biomed Eng. 2019;47(5):1212–22. https://doi.org/10.1007/s10439-019-02230-3.
21. Serletis D, Bulacio J, Bingaman W, Najm I, González-Martínez J. The stereotactic approach for mapping epileptic networks: a prospective study of 200 patients. J Neurosurg. 2014;121(5):1239–46. https://doi.org/10.3171/2014.7.JNS132306.
22. González-Martínez J, Bulacio J, Thompson S, et al. Technique, results, and complications related to robot-assisted Stereoelectroencephalography. Neurosurgery. 2016;78(2):169–80. https://doi.org/10.1227/NEU.0000000000001034.
23. McGovern RA, Knight EP, Gupta A, et al. Robot-assisted stereoelectroencephalography in children. J Neurosurg Pediatr. 2018;23(3):288–96. https://doi.org/10.3171/2018.7.PEDS18305.
24. Roland JL, Smyth MD. Recent advances in the neurosurgical treatment of pediatric epilepsy: JNSPG 75th Anniversary Invited Review Article. J Neurosurg Pediatr. 2019;23(4):411–21. https://doi.org/10.3171/2018.12.PEDS18350.
25. McGovern RA, Alomar S, Bingaman WE, Gonzalez-Martinez J. Robot-assisted responsive neurostimulator system placement in medically intractable epilepsy: instrumentation and technique. Oper Neurosurg (Hagerstown). 2019;16(4):455–64. https://doi.org/10.1093/ons/opy112.
26. De Benedictis A, Trezza A, Carai A, et al. Robot-assisted procedures in pediatric neurosurgery. Neurosurg Focus. 2017;42(5):E7. https://doi.org/10.3171/2017.2.FOCUS16579.
27. Audette MA, Bordas SPA, Blatt JE. Robotically steered needles: a survey of neurosurgical applications and technical innovations. Robot Surg. 2020;7:1–23. https://doi.org/10.2147/RSRR.S224446.
28. Lonjon N, Chan-Seng E, Costalat V, Bonnafoux B, Vassal M, Boetto J. Robot-assisted spine surgery: feasibility study through a prospective case-matched analysis. Eur Spine J. 2016;25(3):947–55. https://doi.org/10.1007/s00586-015-3758-8.
29. Murai Y, Sato S, Yui K, et al. Preliminary clinical microneurosurgical experience with the 4K3-dimensional microvideoscope (ORBEYE) system for microneurological surgery: observation study. Oper Neurosurg (Hagerstown). 2019;16(6):707–16. https://doi.org/10.1093/ons/opy277.
30. Langer DJ, White TG, Schulder M, Boockvar JA, Labib M, Lawton MT. Advances in intra-operative optics: a brief review of current exoscope platforms. Oper Neurosurg (Hagerstown). 2020;19(1):84–93. https://doi.org/10.1093/ons/opz276.
31. Kanzaki S, Takahashi S, Toda M, Yoshida K, Ogawa K. Pros and cons of the exoscope for otologic surgery. Surg Innov. 2020:1553350620964151. https://doi.org/10.1177/1553350620964151.
32. Ahmed SI, Javed G, Mubeen B, et al. Robotics in neurosurgery: a literature review. JPMA J Pak Med Assoc. 2018;68(2):258–63.

33. Vazhayil V, Rao M, Beniwal M, Sadashiva N, Lakshmi N, Somanna S. An overview of robotics in functional neurosurgery. Indian J Neurosurg. 2019;08(01):006–10. https://doi.org/10.1055/s-0039-1687715.
34. Schroerlucke SR, Wang MY, Cannestra AF, et al. Complication rate in robotic-guided vs fluoro-guided minimally invasive spinal fusion surgery: report from MIS refresh prospective comparative study. Spine J. 2017;17(10):S254–5. https://doi.org/10.1016/j.spinee.2017.08.177.
35. Schreuder HWR, Verheijen RHM. Robotic surgery. BJOG Int J Obstet Gynaecol. 2009;116(2):198–213. https://doi.org/10.1111/j.1471-0528.2008.02038.x.
36. Wei NJ, Dougherty B, Myers A, Badawy SM. Using Google glass in surgical settings: systematic review. JMIR Mhealth Uhealth. 2018;6(3):e54. https://doi.org/10.2196/mhealth.9409.
37. Al Janabi HF, Aydin A, Palaneer S, et al. Effectiveness of the HoloLens mixed-reality headset in minimally invasive surgery: a simulation-based feasibility study. Surg Endosc. 2020;34(3):1143–9. https://doi.org/10.1007/s00464-019-06862-3.
38. Lee HK, Hwang WJ, Roh KS, Choi JY, Inventors. Augmented reality image display system and surgical robot system comprising the same; 2017.
39. Pessaux P, Diana M, Soler L, Piardi T, Mutter D, Marescaux J. Towards cybernetic surgery: robotic and augmented reality-assisted liver segmentectomy. Langenbeck's Arch Surg'. 2015;400(3):381–5. https://doi.org/10.1007/s00423-014-1256-9.
40. Su L-M, Vagvolgyi BP, Agarwal R, Reiley CE, Taylor RH, Hager GD. Augmented reality during robot-assisted laparoscopic partial nephrectomy: toward real-time 3D-CT to stereoscopic video registration. Urology. 2009;73(4):896–900. https://doi.org/10.1016/j.urology.2008.11.040.
41. Vávra P, Roman J, Zonča P, et al. Recent development of augmented reality in surgery: a review. J Healthc Eng. 2017;2017:4574172. https://doi.org/10.1155/2017/4574172.
42. Liu T, Tai Y, Zhao C, et al. Augmented reality in neurosurgical navigation: a survey. Int J Med Robot. 2020:e2160. https://doi.org/10.1002/rcs.2160.
43. Rankin JS. William Stewart Halsted: a lecture by Dr. Peter D. Olch. Ann Surg. 2006;243(3):418–25. https://doi.org/10.1097/01.sla.0000201546.94163.00.
44. Schmitt PJ, Agarwal N, Prestigiacomo CJ. From planes to brains: parallels between military development of virtual reality environments and virtual neurological surgery. World Neurosurg. 2012;78(3–4):214–9. https://doi.org/10.1016/j.wneu.2012.06.014.
45. Kockro RA, Serra L, Tseng-Tsai Y, et al. Planning and simulation of neurosurgery in a virtual reality environment. Neurosurgery. 2000;46(1):118–35; discussion 135-7.
46. Wong GK, Zhu CX, Ahuja AT, Poon WS. Stereoscopic virtual reality simulation for microsurgical excision of cerebral arteriovenous malformation: case illustrations. Surg Neurol. 2009;72(1):69–72; discussion 72-3. https://doi.org/10.1016/j.surneu.2008.01.049.
47. Agarwal N, Schmitt PJ, Sukul V, Prestigiacomo CJ. Surgical approaches to complex vascular lesions: the use of virtual reality and stereoscopic analysis as a tool for resident and student education. BMJ Case Rep. 2012;2012 https://doi.org/10.1136/bcr.02.2012.5859.
48. Marinho P, Thines L, Verscheure L, Mordon S, Lejeune JP, Vermandel M. Recent advances in cerebrovascular simulation and neuronavigation for the optimization of intracranial aneurysm clipping. Comput Aided Surg. 2012;17(2):47–55. https://doi.org/10.3109/10929088.2011.653403.
49. Malone HR, Syed ON, Downes MS, D'Ambrosio AL, Quest DO, Kaiser MG. Simulation in neurosurgery: a review of computer-based simulation environments and their surgical applications. Neurosurgery. 2010;67(4):1105–16. https://doi.org/10.1227/NEU.0b013e3181ee46d0.
50. Delorme S, Laroche D, DiRaddo R, Del Maestro RF. NeuroTouch: a physics-based virtual simulator for cranial microneurosurgery training. Neurosurgery. 2012;71(1 Suppl Operative):32–42. https://doi.org/10.1227/NEU.0b013e318249c744.
51. Choudhury N, Gélinas-Phaneuf N, Delorme S, Del Maestro R. Fundamentals of neurosurgery: virtual reality tasks for training and evaluation of technical skills. World Neurosurg. 2013;80(5):e9–19. https://doi.org/10.1016/j.wneu.2012.08.022.

52. Alotaibi FE, AlZhrani GA, Sabbagh AJ, Azarnoush H, Winkler-Schwartz A, Del Maestro RF. Neurosurgical assessment of metrics including judgment and dexterity using the virtual reality simulator NeuroTouch (NAJD metrics). Surg Innov. 2015;22(6):636–42. https://doi.org/10.1177/1553350615579729.
53. Sawaya R, Bugdadi A, Azarnoush H, et al. Virtual reality tumor resection: the force pyramid approach. Oper Neurosurg (Hagerstown). 2018.;14;(6):686–96. https://doi.org/10.1093/ons/opx189.
54. Sawaya R, Alsideiri G, Bugdadi A, et al. Development of a performance model for virtual reality tumor resections. J Neurosurg. 2018;131(1):192–200. https://doi.org/10.3171/2018.2.JNS172327.
55. Winkler-Schwartz A, Yilmaz R, Mirchi N, et al. Machine learning identification of surgical and operative factors associated with surgical expertise in virtual reality simulation. JAMA Netw Open. 2019;2(8):e198363. https://doi.org/10.1001/jamanetworkopen.2019.8363.
56. Winkler-Schwartz A, Bissonnette V, Mirchi N, et al. Artificial intelligence in medical education: best practices using machine learning to assess surgical expertise in virtual reality simulation. J Surg Educ. 2019;76(6):1681–90. https://doi.org/10.1016/j.jsurg.2019.05.015.
57. Siyar S, Azarnoush H, Rashidi S, Del Maestro RF. Tremor assessment during virtual reality brain tumor resection. J Surg Educ. 2020;77(3):643–51. https://doi.org/10.1016/j.jsurg.2019.11.011.
58. Grosch AS, Schröder T, Onken J, Picht T. Development and initial evaluation of a novel simulation model for comprehensive brain tumor surgery training. Acta Neurochir (Wien). 2020;162(8):1957–65. https://doi.org/10.1007/s00701-020-04359-w.
59. Vasudevan MK, Isaac JHR, Sadanand V, Muniyandi M. Novel virtual reality based training system for fine motor skills: towards developing a robotic surgery training system. Int J Med Robot. 2020;16(6):1–14. https://doi.org/10.1002/rcs.2173.
60. Tergas AI, Sheth SB, Green IC, Giuntoli RL, Winder AD, Fader AN. A pilot study of surgical training using a virtual robotic surgery simulator. JSLS: J Soc Laparoendoscopic Surg. 2013;17(2):219–26. https://doi.org/10.4293/108680813X13654754535872.
61. Williams MA, McVeigh J, Handa AI, Lee R. Augmented reality in surgical training: a systematic review. Postgrad Med J. 2020;96(1139):537–42. https://doi.org/10.1136/postgradmedj-2020-137600.
62. Gierwiało R, Witkowski M, Kosieradzki M, Lisik W, Groszkowski Ł, Sitnik R. Medical augmented-reality visualizer for surgical training and education in medicine. Appl Sci. 2019;9(13):2732. https://doi.org/10.3390/app9132732.
63. McDonnell JM, Ahern DP, Ó Doinn T, et al. Surgeon proficiency in robot-assisted spine surgery. Bone Joint J. 2020;102-B(5):568–72. https://doi.org/10.1302/0301-620X.102B5.BJJ-2019-1392.R2.
64. Jarc AM, Curet M. Face, content, and construct validity of four, inanimate training exercises using the da Vinci ® Si surgical system configured with single-site ™ instrumentation. Surg Endosc. 2015;29(8):2298–304. https://doi.org/10.1007/s00464-014-3947-2.
65. Agha RA, Fowler AJ. The role and validity of surgical simulation. Int Surg Feb 2015;100(2):350–357. doi:https://doi.org/10.9738/INTSURG-D-14-00004.1.
66. Abboudi H, Khan MS, Aboumarzouk O, et al. Current status of validation for robotic surgery simulators—a systematic review. BJU Int. 2013;111(2):194–205. https://doi.org/10.1111/j.1464-410X.2012.11270.x.
67. Ahmed K, Khan R, Mottrie A, et al. Development of a standardised training curriculum for robotic surgery: a consensus statement from an international multidisciplinary group of experts. BJU Int. 2015;116(1):93–101. https://doi.org/10.1111/bju.12974.
68. Madhavan K, Kolcun JPG, Chieng LO, Wang MY. Augmented-reality integrated robotics in neurosurgery: are we there yet? Neurosurg Focus. 2017;42(5):E3. https://doi.org/10.3171/2017.2.FOCUS177.
69. van der Meijden OAJ, Schijven MP. The value of haptic feedback in conventional and robot-assisted minimal invasive surgery and virtual reality training: a current review. Surg Endosc. 2009;23(6):1180–90. https://doi.org/10.1007/s00464-008-0298-x.

70. Wagner CR, Stylopoulos N, Howe RD. The role of force feedback in surgery: analysis of blunt dissection; 2002.
71. Baghdadi A, Hoshyarmanesh H, de Lotbiniere-Bassett MP, Choi SK, Lama S, Sutherland GR. Data analytics interrogates robotic surgical performance using a microsurgery-specific haptic device. Expert Rev Med Devices. 2020;17(7):721–30. https://doi.org/10.1080/17434440.2020.1782736.
72. Moglia A, Ferrari V, Morelli L, Ferrari M, Mosca F, Cuschieri A. A systematic review of virtual reality simulators for robot-assisted surgery. Eur Urol. 2016;69(6):1065–80. https://doi.org/10.1016/j.eururo.2015.09.021.
73. Ramos P, Montez J, Tripp A, Ng CK, Gill IS, Hung AJ. Face, content, construct and concurrent validity of dry laboratory exercises for robotic training using a global assessment tool. BJU Int. 2014;113(5):836–42. https://doi.org/10.1111/bju.12559.
74. Saracino A, Deguet A, Staderini F, et al. Haptic feedback in the da Vinci research kit (dVRK): a user study based on grasping, palpation, and incision tasks. Int J Med Robot Comp Assisted Surgery. 2019;15(4) https://doi.org/10.1002/rcs.1999.
75. Enayati N, Okamura AM, Mariani A, et al. Robotic assistance-as-needed for enhanced visuomotor learning in surgical robotics training: an experimental study. IEEE; 2018. p. 6631–6.
76. Aghazadeh MA, Mercado MA, Pan MM, Miles BJ, Goh AC. Performance of robotic simulated skills tasks is positively associated with clinical robotic surgical performance. BJU Int. 2016;118(3):475–81. https://doi.org/10.1111/bju.13511.
77. Schreuder HWR, Wolswijk R, Zweemer RP, Schijven MP, Verheijen RHM. Training and learning robotic surgery, time for a more structured approach: a systematic review. BJOG Int J Obstet Gynaecol. 2012;119(2):137–49. https://doi.org/10.1111/j.1471-0528.2011.03139.x.
78. Attalla K, Raza SJ, Rehman S, et al. Effectiveness of a dedicated robot-assisted surgery training program. Can J Urol. 2013;20(6):7084–90.
79. Corcione F, Esposito C, Cuccurullo D, et al. Advantages and limits of robot-assisted laparoscopic surgery: preliminary experience. Surg Endosc. 2005;19(1):117–9. https://doi.org/10.1007/s00464-004-9004-9.
80. Nathoo N, Çavuşoğlu MC, Vogelbaum MA, Barnett GH. In touch with robotics: neurosurgery for the future. Neurosurgery. 2005;56(3):421–33. https://doi.org/10.1227/01.NEU.0000153929.68024.CF.
81. Moit H, Dwyer A, De Sutter M, Heinzel S, Crawford D. A standardized robotic training curriculum in a general surgery program. JSLS J Soc Laparoendoscopic Surg. 2019;23(4):e2019.00045. https://doi.org/10.4293/JSLS.2019.00045.
82. Moles JJ, Connelly PE, Sarti EE, Baredes S. Establishing a training program for residents in robotic surgery. Laryngoscope. 2009;119(10):1927–31. https://doi.org/10.1002/lary.20508.
83. Hart R, Karthigasu K. The benefits of virtual reality simulator training for laparoscopic surgery. Curr Opin Obstet Gynecol. 2007;19(4):297–302. https://doi.org/10.1097/GCO.0b013e328216f5b7.
84. Tam V, Lutfi W, Novak S, et al. Resident attitudes and compliance towards robotic surgical training. Am J Surg. 2018;215(2):282–7. https://doi.org/10.1016/j.amjsurg.2017.08.051.
85. Sánchez R, Rodríguez O, Rosciano J, et al. Robotic surgery training: construct validity of global evaluative assessment of robotic skills (GEARS). J Robot Surg. 2016;10(3):227–31. https://doi.org/10.1007/s11701-016-0572-1.
86. Yule S, Flin R, Paterson-Brown S, Maran N, Rowley D. Development of a rating system for surgeons' non-technical skills. Med Educ. 2006;40(11):1098–104. https://doi.org/10.1111/j.1365-2929.2006.02610.x.
87. Undre S, Sevdalis N, Healey AN, Darzi A, Vincent CA. Observational teamwork assessment for surgery (OTAS): refinement and application in urological surgery. World J Surg. 2007;31(7):1373–81. https://doi.org/10.1007/s00268-007-9053-z.
88. Guru KA, Esfahani ET, Raza SJ, et al. Cognitive skills assessment during robot-assisted surgery: separating the wheat from the chaff. BJU Int. 2015;115(1):166–74. https://doi.org/10.1111/bju.12657.

Correction to: Image Guidance for Intracranial Surgery with Supervisory-Control Robots

Francesco Cardinale, Martina Revay, Piergiorgio d'Orio, Sergio Raspante, Lorenzo Maria Giuseppe Bianchi, Khalid Al Orabi, Luca Berta, and Giorgio Lo Russo

Correction to:
Chapter 4 in: J. A. González Martínez, F. Cardinale (eds.), *Robotics in Neurosurgery*, https://doi.org/10.1007/978-3-031-08380-8_4

The chapter was inadvertently published with the incorrect word "Stereotaxic Surgery" in Fig. 4.2. It has been updated as "Stereotactic Surgery" in this corrected version.

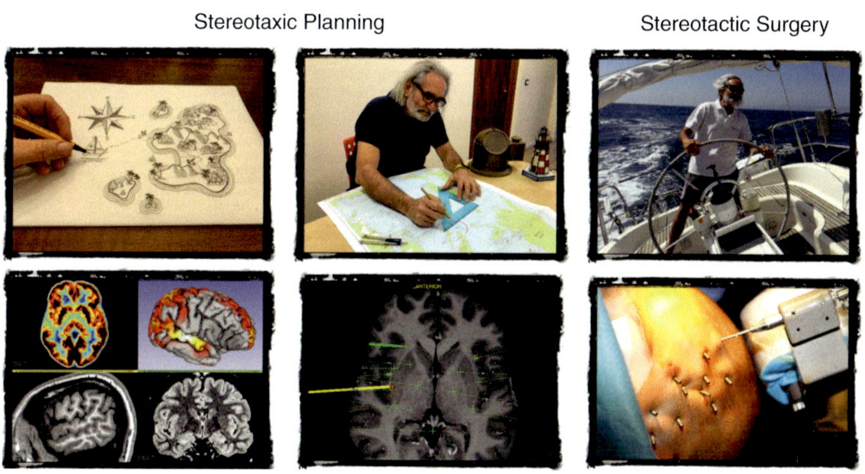

Fig. 4.2 Stereotaxic planning and stereotactic surgery
The stereotactic advancement of a probe to an intracranial target is performed after a stereotaxic planning has been done. Such planning includes the mapping of all information into the intracranial space, defined by a 3D coordinate system, and the use of the map to plan the trajectories

---

The updated original version of this chapter can be found at
https://doi.org/10.1007/978-3-031-08380-8_4

J. A. González Martínez, F. Cardinale (eds.), *Robotics in Neurosurgery*,
https://doi.org/10.1007/978-3-031-08380-8_20

Conclusions

Francesco Cardinale and Jorge Alvaro González Martínez

"The Skynet Funding Bill is passed. The system goes on-line August 4th, 1997. Human decisions are removed from strategic defense. Skynet begins to learn at a geometric rate. It becomes self-aware at 2:14 a.m. Eastern time, August 29th. In a panic, they try to pull the plug."[1]

With deep-touching voice, the Terminator tells when the Artificial Intelligence of Skynet, a computer network developed for strategic defense, became totally autonomous from human decisions. A vivid nightmare raises in the spectators viewing at military robots trying to terminate the human race. The loss of human decision power is the crucial point that transforms efficient robotic machines in a scary threat throughout all the Terminator saga.

In the real word, most people are still mistrustful of Driving Automation Systems for On-Road Motor Vehicles. High level of autonomy is not easily accepted, even if it is probable that such "robotic" motor vehicles will be able to drive better than humans in a relatively short time.

On the opposite, most patients like to know that their surgeon will operate with robotic assistance. This is probably due to the belief that surgical acts can be more

[1] Terminator's words, quoted from the movie *Terminator 2: Judgment Day*.

F. Cardinale
"Claudio Munari" Center for Epilepsy Surgery, Azienda Socio-Sanitaria Territoriale Grande Ospedale Metropolitano Niguarda, Milano, Italy

Department of Medicine and Surgery, Unit of Neuroscience, Università degli Studi di Parma, Parma, Italy
e-mail: francesco.cardinale@ospedaleniguarda.it

J. A. González Martínez
Department of Neurological Surgery and Epilepsy Center, University of Pittsburgh Medical Center, Pittsburgh, PA, USA
e-mail: gonzalezjo@upmc.edu

J. A. González Martínez, F. Cardinale (eds.), *Robotics in Neurosurgery*,
https://doi.org/10.1007/978-3-031-08380-8

accurate thanks to robotic assistance. This conviction is correct in most common neurological robot-assisted surgeries because appropriate image guidance and robot's mechanical features guarantee high accuracy in advancing a probe into the intracranial space. All along the several chapters of the present textbook we have read that supervisory-control robots allow to reach virtually any intracranial position with high accuracy and safety. However, the level of autonomy of the robots that are already available on the market is very limited. The question is: "Would the patients benefit from higher levels of robot autonomy?" Yes, probably. A simple example is the skiving of the twist drill on the skull surface while implanting SEEG electrodes, likely the most important source of errors in such surgeries. The bending of the thin perforator occurs because the cavity of the cylindric adaptor must be larger than the shaft of the drill to permit its rotation. Therefore, small planetary movements are unavoidable and they are not neglectable especially when the bony surface is curvilinear: the tip of the drill will skive and the stereotactic error will increase. This source of inaccuracy could be probably mitigated if the end effector was a short drill directly driven by an engine, instead of an adaptor that serves simply as a guide. The problem is that such a device would increase the level of autonomy of the robotic assistant. Actually, most supervisory control robots adopted in neurosurgery are passive, in that they do not operate directly the patient. On the opposite, if the above-mentioned solution would be implemented, the robot would drill the skull directly, without any human intervention. Whose responsibility is it if the drilling is too deep and the brain is therefore hurt? Robot's or surgeon's responsibility? Likely for this reason, manufacturers are reluctant to develop active robots with higher levels of autonomy. The paradox is that, due to a potential difficulty in assessing responsibilities, the risk of complications is larger than it could probably be. This circumstance illustrates the great challenge of matching medical advancements with legislation that allows more autonomy for robots.

Higher levels of autonomy should be welcome to increase patient's safety and treatment's efficacy, and the research in this direction should be strongly promoted. However, deep thinking is requested to regulate ethical and legal aspects for increasing levels of autonomy. Due to the rapid increase in robot usage in neurosurgery, some first papers have been recently published on the topic. We like to highlight the seminal editorial published by Yang et al. in 2017, entitled "Medical robotics—Regulatory, ethical, and legal considerations for increasing levels of autonomy" [1]. The authors proposed six levels of robot autonomy: (1) no autonomy, (2) robot assistance, (3) task autonomy, (4) conditional autonomy, (5) high autonomy, and (6) full autonomy. This reading can be fruitfully complemented by another paper recently published by Attanasio et al. providing several explanations and examples taken from the panorama of commercially available systems and main research projects [2]. These two papers will be certainly followed by many others because the equilibrium between the surgeon and the robot must be carefully analyzed, discussed and finely tuned. It is necessary to let patients, doctors and developers to understand how many further improvements can be obtained thanks to upcoming technologies. At the same time, it will be necessary to define limits and constraints. Robotics is not only mechanical dexterity and accuracy but it also includes high-level programmability. The intersection between medical decision and artificial-intelligence-driven robotic autonomy is a very delicate topic. As clearly suggested by Attanasio and co-workers, "at high autonomy levels, the robotic systems are supposed to make clinically-relevant decisions. This could introduce another regulatory dilemma: notified bodies like FDA lack the legal authority to regulate medicine, as this practice is usually left to medical societies. The latter, on the other hand, lack the technical competence to dominate complex and continuously evolving technologies such as robotics" [2]. However, we like to be optimistic and hope that this regulatory dilemma will be solved, whatever it takes. The progress must be well channeled into the groove of conscious balance between patient's protection and treatment improvements, avoiding to remain frozen by risks rather than stimulated by opportunities. Similar problems are tackled even in other fields of medicine such as genetics, but also in other areas of human life and progress. Artificial intelligence and machine learning analyses are enormous opportunities to improve many decisional processes, medical or not, but they must be governed with aware responsibility and diligence. New professional profiles will come out, expanding the horizon of co-operation between humans and machines, in the name of healthiness.

And finally, the Terminator saved the human race.

References

Yang GZ, Cambias J, Cleary K, et al. Medical robotics—regulatory, ethical, and legal considerations for increasing levels of autonomy. Sci Robot. 2017;2(4):1–3.

Attanasio A, Scaglioni B, De Momi E, Fiorini P, Valdastri P. Autonomy in surgical robotics. Annu Rev Control Robot Auton Syst. 2021;4(1):651–79.

Index

J. A. González Martínez, F. Cardinale (eds.), *Robotics in Neurosurgery*,
https://doi.org/10.1007/978-3-031-08380-8

MIX
Papier aus verantwortungsvollen Quellen
Paper from responsible sources
FSC® C105338

If you have any concerns about our products,
you can contact us on
ProductSafety@springernature.com

In case Publisher is established outside the EU,
the EU authorized representative is:
Springer Nature Customer Service Center GmbH
Europaplatz 3, 69115 Heidelberg, Germany

Printed by Libri Plureos GmbH
in Hamburg, Germany